# *Multiple Sclerosis*

# *Multiple Sclerosis*

## A GUIDE FOR THE NEWLY DIAGNOSED

*FIFTH EDITION*

**T. Jock Murray,** OC, ONS, MD, FRCPC, FAAN, MACP, FRCP, MCFP, FCAHS
Professor Emeritus, Dalhousie University
Dalhousie Multiple Sclerosis Research Unit
Halifax, Nova Scotia

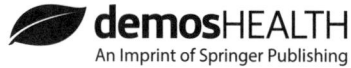
**demos**HEALTH
An Imprint of Springer Publishing

**Visit our website at www.demoshealth.com**

*ISBN:* 9780826165114
*e-book ISBN:* 9780826165121

*Acquisitions Editor:* Beth Barry
*Compositor:* diacriTech

**Library of Congress Cataloging-in-Publication Data**
Names: Murray, T. J., author.
Title: Multiple sclerosis : a guide for the newly diagnosed / T. Jock Murray,
   OC, ONS, MD, FRCPC, FAAN, MACP, FRCP, MCFP, FCAHS (honorary LLD, DSc,
   D.Litt, DFA, LLD) Professor Emeritus, Dalhousie University, Dalhousie
   Multiple Sclerosis Research Unit, Halifax, Nova Scotia.
Description: Fifth edition. | New York, NY : Demos Medical Publishing, [2017] |
   Includes bibliographical references and index.
Identifiers: LCCN 2017034850| ISBN 9780826165114 | ISBN 9780826165121 (e-book)
Subjects: LCSH: Multiple sclerosis—Popular works.
Classification: LCC RC377 .H65 2017 | DDC 616.8/34—dc23 LC record available at
   https://lccn.loc.gov/2017034850

Contact us to receive discount rates on bulk purchases.
We can also customize our books to meet your needs.
For more information please contact: sales@springerpub.com

Printed in the United States of America by McNaughton & Gunn.
17 18 19 20 21 / 5 4 3 2 1

***To my patients ...***

who taught me so many lessons. It has been a privilege to walk with you on the long road of life with MS. I continue to be inspired by your courage and strength. It was your generosity in teaching lessons to generations of physicians and to contributing to research that led to the advances that now benefit so many others.

# Contents

# *Preface*

It doesn't seem so long ago to me, but I first saw people with multiple sclerosis (MS) when I was a family doctor in a small community back in the early 1960s. I became part of their lives and struggles even though I had little to change the course of their disease. The patients taught me that what they really needed was someone who would be there when they needed help or information.

Later, as a neurologist, I was told by some patients that there was a lot of MS in their communities and I carried out studies to see if there were clusters of MS. Over those years the essential lessons I learned had nothing to do with the epidemiology of MS, but that so many MS patients in the communities felt abandoned. In the 1970s they were often told they had MS, there was no treatment, and the future would be for increasing disability and wheelchairs. In many instances, they were not given follow-up appointments because the neurologists had nothing to offer, and the family physicians said they didn't know much about MS.

It seemed to me then that what MS patients needed most was a place where they could seek help, ask questions, and relate to professionals who cared about them and were interested in them. I started an MS research center to provide care and education for MS patients and their families. It was also designed to carry out trials of new therapies and to initiate research programs that would tell us more about the patients and their ability to cope with the disease. We started with a computerized database, which recorded details about the assessment of every patient on every visit, unusual in the 1970s, but this has become a resource for research studies four decades later. It became especially useful to be able to assess the course of MS in decades before and after the new therapies for MS began to change the prognosis of MS.

Our MS Research Center offered a place of care and education provided by a multidisciplinary team, and in return the patients gave us their cooperation and support for our medical research.

It is now over a half century since I began to travel the long road of life with my MS patients. My gratitude is expressed by dedicating this volume to the patients who have taught me so much. With every new discovery, I feel a great sense of excitement about what is happening in care and research, and a tremendous sense of hope in the future for people with MS.

*Dr. T. Jock Murray*
*Dalhousie MS Research Unit*

# *Foreword*

Receiving a diagnosis of MS does not make a glad day. There is a blank space in those words when we first hear them because we know little about MS. Immediately the void fills with the few images we have – wheelchair, drooping head, slurred words. Sadly, what we fear is all we know. Every person, newly diagnosed with MS, needs a copy of Dr. Jock Murray's book *Multiple Sclerosis: A Guide for the Newly Diagnosed*. I have been in that place and revisited an old sense of foreboding in the face of my MS diagnosis.

Finding the right sort of knowledge was a challenge for me as Jock Murray's book did not exist at that time. An armload of library books alternately depressed, unsettled, or confused me. An older book gave a very bleak outlook, and so, was depressing; a more recent book was full of undecipherable medical language, thus confusing; another had lists of so many peculiar MS symptoms for "events" which could befall one, left me completely unsettled.

*Multiple Sclerosis: A Guide for the Newly Diagnosed* opens the door to knowledge, a wise antidote to fear. Here, facts about MS are presented in logical sequence. We gain a basic understanding of this disease that has mystified doctors for over a hundred years. We learn a new medical language and become comfortable with a discussion of neurological disease; of current treatment and management with sophisticated disease modifying drugs; of 21st century technology; of abundant support systems; and even of positive outcomes. The old pictures are erased from memory.

It is fascinating to read about advancements made as research moves forward. Dr. Murray continues to be a key player. Promising research is presented and by nature of its vital application in the hunt for understanding of and even cure for MS, one can feel excited about the future. No longer are the newly diagnosed told there is "no treatment and no cure." However committed researchers are to find a cure, we must appreciate the importance between curing and healing.

Importantly, *Multiple Sclerosis: A Guide for the Newly Diagnosed* makes clear the distinction between these two. The book has an encouraging, optimistic outlook which reflects Jock Murray's own character. That he knows so much about MS and is still positive is a testament to hope. This has a ripple effect on patients. Hope is real.

Having this book does make a glad day, like having Dr. Murray's wise counsel nearby when healing is what one needs. Upon being given a diagnosis of MS my overwhelming feeling was, "An obstacle has been placed in my way . . . . tomorrow will never be the same." While this is true, it is not exactly true.

Perhaps one day there will be a cure for MS. Right now we stand in need of healing. Thank you, Dr. Jock Murray, for that.

*Catherine Edward*

# *Acknowledgments*

I am indebted to the co-authors of previous editions of this book, Stephen Reingold, Nancy Holland, and Carol Saunders, and their wise advice from years of experience remains in this edition. I had excellent support from Beth Barry, Publisher at Demos Medical Publishing, who shepherded this project along. My friend Catherine Edward, who displayed her positive approach to living with MS in her book, *The Brow of Dawn: One Woman's Journey with MS*, kindly provided an introduction to this edition. Janet Murray, my in-house editor and supporter, assisted, as she does on all my efforts, with kind, gentle, and wise advice. She makes everything better.

# CHAPTER 1

# The History of Multiple Sclerosis

## Before MS Had a Name

We are now aware that multiple sclerosis, or MS, occurred in young adults for centuries but it was only in 1868 that a French neurologist, Jean Martin Charcot, outlined the characteristics of the disease and gave it a name. Prior to that, most people with a progressive neurological disease were all grouped together and identified with paraplegia or paralysis. From diaries and personal papers we have information about individuals who probably suffered from the disease before it had an official name.

## Early Cases of Multiple Sclerosis

The earliest case suggestive of MS was "the virgin Lidwina" (1380–1433), of Scheidam, Holland, who had a recurrent and progressive neurological condition over thirty years. She first noticed unsteadiness and falls when skating on the canals (she is the patron of the American Figure Skating Association). Her neurological symptoms increased and progressed for decades. She believed God wanted her to suffer for the sins of others, and because of her holiness and self-sacrifice she was made a saint by the Church. Her Saint Day is April 14th each year.

A young man, Augustus D'Este (1794–1848), a grandson of King George III, kept a diary for decades recording his recurrent and ultimately progressive neurological disease that we can now confidently say was MS. On the first page of his diary he wrote of an episode of blindness in one eye after attending a funeral, which he thought was due to his efforts to suppress tears, but was undoubtedly optic neuritis from MS. Over the next two decades he daily documented his progressive weakness and walking difficulty and the treatments by prominent physicians of the day, and provided insight on the treatments for neurological conditions in the early nineteenth century.

Margaret Gatty (1809–1873), a Victorian novelist and children's writer who wrote a respected guide to British seaweeds, had an episodic and progressive neurological disease that her physician thought was due to heavy gardening, using her muscles like a man. She was initially unaware that her case was published in the medical journal *The Lancet*, but pleased when she discovered this later. She wrote of her symptoms, especially in letters to her daughter.

### The Description by Charcot

When Charcot wrote his definitive description of MS he was aware that a dozen other physicians had described similar cases of young adults with a progressive neurological involvement with scattered grey patches, or lesions, in the central nervous system. In the mid-nineteenth century physicians were beginning to describe many "new" diseases and classifying types of illnesses further, taking lessons from the success of botanists and biologists who had classified the plant and animal kingdoms. Some disorders were already well known, such as apoplexy (stroke), epilepsy, and syphilis. Charcot and others in the nineteenth century were able to separate amyotrophic lateral sclerosis (Lou Gehrig's disease), Huntington's disease, Friedreich's ataxia, and other neurological condition from the general group of neurological disorders. An added incentive for physicians was to have the disease named for them, so we now remember Addison, Parkinson, Hodgkin, Huntington, Tourette, Alzheimer, and many others.

Charcot and his colleague, Edme Vulpian, at the Salpêtrière, the huge Paris hospital housing over 5,000 sick and poverty-stricken persons, were particularly effective in noting groups of patients who seemed to have similar neurological characteristics. Vulpian and Charcot presented some early cases of a condition they called *la sclérose en plaque disseminée* (disseminated patchy scarring) to a local medical society, which they published in a hospital journal, with Vulpian as first author. But it was three lectures by Charcot in 1868 that clarified the disease for the medical world and forever associated him with MS. He was not the first to recognize the disease, but his great contribution was describing the disease so clearly, and naming it, so that others around the world could now make the diagnosis. As he concluded his description of the clinical features, the pathology, the course, and prognosis, he came to the discussion of treatment and sadly concluded, "After what has preceded, need I detain you long over the question of treatment? The time has not yet come when such a subject can be seriously considered."

Once Charcot framed and named the disease, more and more information accumulated about the incidence, clinical patterns, family relationships, and pathology. But as often happens, the more that was known, the more questions arose about the genetics, geographical distribution, environmental relationships, and how to measure the disease and its symptoms.

## *Early Therapies of Neurological Diseases*

Early theories of disease centered around a belief in an imbalance in the four humors—black and yellow bile, phlegm, and blood—as the cause, so therapies attempted to effect some balance and remove harmful humors by vomiting, purging, bleeding, scarification, cupping, or other procedures.

There was a growing theory in the nineteenth century that nervous diseases could also be due to over- or understimulation of the nervous system, so complex remedies were concocted according to whether the condition was characterized as hot or cold, moist or dry, and by complex astrological measurements. Medicines administered contained such substances as musk, castor, asafoetida, valerian, garlic, oil of amber, skunk cabbage, coffee, and other "cerebral stimulants" such as henbane, deadly nightshade, and extract of hemp.

Stimulation could also be by chemicals, herbals, electricity, and various physical methods such as rough massage, horseback riding, cold water therapy, and irritating plasters. Paralysis required excitation and stimulation, so a person with a neurological disease would undergo stimulation by Galvanic or Faradic electrical charges, moxibustion, counter-irritation, wrapping in cold sheets, or hosing with torrents of icy water. Each physician might have preferred remedies, but the general list available was relatively unchanged over the century.

## Advances in the Twentieth Century

In the twentieth century, research focused on efforts to understand the pathological mechanisms underlying the disease. This initially did not result in any effective therapies, but it would be an error to think that there were no attempts at treatment. Various therapies were always offered to people with MS, in the hopes that they would provide some relief, even if they could not cure. During that time, the list of therapies applied to MS patients was long, longer than today. But looking at the list today we see that few would have provided any relief, and most would have been useless or even harmful. The therapeutic imperative was strong, however, as patients wanted some kind of therapy, and physicians of course wanted to try and help their patients.

Many of the new treatments developed for various diseases were applied to MS. When the magical x-ray made its appearance at the end of the nineteenth century, it was soon being directed to the spinal cords of MS patients as a form of radiation therapy, but without benefit. Those who believed MS was due to a toxin used many methods of "detoxification," an approach, despite its risks and lack of evidence of benefit, still has some current adherents. Others felt strongly that MS was due to infection and believed there would soon be a vaccine, but in the meantime gave any new anti-infection medicine to MS patients. To remove any possible source of infection, patients were subjected to removal of their teeth and tonsils, given sinus drainage, and prescribed any medication that was thought to treat infection. The list of remedies and procedures kept growing. Finally, a young and perceptive neurologist at the London Hospital, Dr. Russell Brain, reviewed the vast array of therapies administered to hopeful MS patients in 1930 and concluded: "No mode of therapy is successful enough to achieve, at the most, a greater improvement than might have occurred spontaneously." He felt none of the treatments were useful. But such skepticism did not stop the prescribing of these many therapies and in 1936 the neurologist Dr. Richard Brickner published a 29-page list evaluating 158 different therapies applied to MS patients. Perhaps it is not surprising that he concluded that the best approach was his own treatment.

A vascular theory for the cause of MS surfaced at various times, even before Charcot, and when anticoagulants were developed in 1940, they were given to MS patients in the hopes that a drug that prevents clotting and blocking of vessels might help. Unfortunately this was before the era of randomized clinical trials, which would have shown this to be a useless therapy that caused bleeding complications.

To clarify all the confusion, the newly formed National Multiple Sclerosis Society asked Dr. George Schumacher in 1950 to prepare a report on the state of MS therapy. He thought that the prognosis in MS was not as gloomy as most believed. He suggested a means of codifying the diagnostic criteria, which became known as the Schumacher Criteria, later superseded by the Poser and more recently, the McDonald Criteria (2010). Schumacher concluded that many treatments were useless, such as arsenic, fever therapy, vaccines and sera, autohemotherapy, lecithin, x-ray therapy, sympathectomy, belladonna, endocrine therapies, and penicillin. He thought more helpful would be good nutrition, avoidance of stress and pregnancy, and moderate physical therapy. He added that no patient benefited from anticoagulants, circulatory stimulants, vitamins, and other drugs applied to people with MS. In his final remarks, he was as negative about therapy as Russell Brain 20 years earlier:

Despite a recurring "wet blanket" being thrown over MS therapies, new claims would be made and new approaches tried. In the 1940s there were anticoagulants; in the 1950s histamine desensitization; in the 1960s, ACTH and cortisone (this helped in acute attacks but not when used long term); and in the 1970s, immunosuppressants such as the growing list of anti-cancer treatments. There was excitement over the claims that the Russians had a vaccine for MS, but it turned out to be a rabies vaccine and made MS patients worse. The list of claims for new therapies grew but without good evidence of benefit, and most faded from the scene as fast as they appeared.

Fad therapies came and went regularly over the last half of the twentieth century. These included vaccines, blood transfusions, serotherapy, plasma transfusions, anticoagulant therapy, antihistamines, snake venom, colonic irrigation, hyperbaric oxygen, magnetism, bee venom, and removal of dental amalgam. We now know that these were not helpful, and sometimes were harmful. Some of these periodically come back in vogue, advanced by enthusiasts, but without scientific evidence or any accepted trials to justify their use.

## The Modern Era

One of the most important steps forward occurred when Sylvia Lawry used her considerable personal energy and *chutzpah* to construct a National Multiple Sclerosis Society, which would catalyze an international movement in support of patients and research.

In the 1950s and 1960s, more scientists were exploring the immune reactions in MS. Epidemiological observations confirmed the unusual geographical distribution of the disease, with low incidence of the disease near the Equator, higher incidence in populations away from the Equator, and highest incidence in areas such as Scotland and Canada.

Efforts were being made to better classify the disease. Steroids appeared on the scene as the first convincing therapy for acute attacks of MS, supported by one of the first randomized clinical trials in MS in 1960. Early MS clinics were appearing in Montreal, Newcastle, and Atlanta. Diets became popular and the most popular was the diet developed by Dr. Roy Swank in Montreal. He was convinced lipids were responsible for MS and although the diet was complex, the essential goal was to lower fats in the diet. Many other diets followed, and although many were even more complex, they usually incorporated the lowering of animal fats. Diets such as elimination diets, low-gluten diet, MacDougall diet, Shatin diet, Evers diet, and so many others, have found little acceptance by most MS experts because of a lack of scientific evidence of benefit from randomized trials.

Although much was being learned, neurologists were generally negative about the treatments available. They also had a depressing view of the disease and its outcome and often avoided telling people they had MS, disguising the diagnosis with words that obscured the truth. Many neurologists who made the diagnosis did not continue to see the patients as they had little to offer.

## The Era of Clinical Trials

The idea that therapies should be objectively assessed by rules and designs that would minimize the influences of enthusiasm, bias, exaggeration, and placebo effects is surprisingly new. Over the centuries physicians depended on observation, experience, and patient responses to indicate if a remedy was helpful. But it was evident that these observations were often unreliable and we now know that medicines and procedures that seemed to be effective for many centuries were actually ineffective. So how do we know for sure that a therapy is effective? The gold standard is to subject the therapy to a randomized clinical trial.

The first well-designed randomized clinical trial was first used in the assessment of streptomycin for tuberculosis in 1948. This trial used the concept of similar groups of patients, randomly assigning one group of patients to the treatment group and another to a similar appearing placebo or comparison therapy, with the participants unaware of who is getting which treatment.

When cortisone came into clinical practice, there were exaggerated claims that it would cure rheumatoid disease, resulting in a premature Nobel Prize, and it seemed logical to use it in MS. A prominent neurologist, Dr. Henry Miller in Newcastle, England, who had started one of the earliest medical units dedicated to MS, did the earliest randomized clinical trial in MS, studying steroids. This indicated benefit of steroids on attacks of MS over placebo and was confirmed by a larger trial in the United States. Then the American Academy of Neurology presented guidelines on how trials should be conducted in MS to arrive at convincing conclusions about how much benefit and how much risk there was in any therapy. The methodology has been continually refined since then, and is used to support any approved therapy for MS.

Beware of any therapy that does not have supporting randomized clinical trials published in recognized, peer-reviewed, medical journals, and then confirmed by independent studies by other groups.

## The Modern Era of Therapy

The remarkable advances in laboratory sciences through the century and the development of magnetic resonance imaging (MRI), immunological studies, and modern genetic techniques added to our understanding of the intricacies and complexities of the disease. These advances led to the development of drugs that could be targeted toward very specific mechanisms of the disease.

In 1980 a number of meetings centered on the need for new approaches to MS therapy, better designs for trials, and collaborations that would foster clinical trials. Interferons were discovered in the 1950s, but it was decades later in the 1970s that their potential use in MS was recognized and clinical trials began. A series of trials resulted in the development of three interferon therapies (interferon beta-1b [Betaseron®], interferon beta-1a intramuscular [Avonex®], interferon beta-1a subcutaneous [Rebif®]) that reduced relapses of MS and also reduced the MRI evidence of inflammation in the brain. A different drug, copolymer-1, later called glatiramer acetate (Copaxone®), was shown to have a similar benefit. After a decade of clinical studies to demonstrate the place of these four drugs in the treatment of MS, other new agents have been approved for MS: mitoxantrone (Novantrone®) and natalizumab (Tysabri®), fingolimod (Gilenya®), interferon Ib (Extavia®), glatiramer acetate generic (Glatopa®), peginterferon (Plegridy®), daclizumab (Zinbryta®), teriflunomide (Aubagio®), dimethyl fumarate (Tecfidera), and alemtuzumab (Lemtrada®).

During the first two decades of new therapies for MS, all the new drugs with benefit targeted persons with relapsing–remitting MS, but these drugs did not have benefit in primary progressive MS. The only drug approved for the treatment of progressive MS is ocrelizumab (Ocrevus®), approved by the FDA for primary progressive MS in March 2017.

## *Changing Ideas*

Research has clarified many puzzling aspects of the disease. For instance, MS was thought to be an intermittent disease with inactivity between attacks. We now know from MRI studies that the activity of the disease goes on even when the person has no symptoms. It was always said to be a demyelinating disease, with damage to the myelin that covers the axons in the nerves, but we now know that damage to the axon in the center of the nerve is even more important in producing progressive disability. It was thought to be a white matter disease as the inflammatory patches of damage are evident in the white matter of the brain, but with new techniques we can see there is also grey matter damage, often early, and this correlates with cognitive symptoms and disability even more than the white matter changes. The disease was thought to begin when the first symptoms appeared, but we now have a lot of evidence that the disease starts many years before and there are often signs of old changes when symptoms are first noted by the patient. A lot more has been learned about how the immunological changes produce the inflammatory damage. Many of the advances of the last few decades are discussed in the following chapters of this book.

## *The Future*

More clinical trials for MS occur each year, and many new agents are on the horizon. As the search for therapies continues, there has also been progress in developing more therapies to treat the symptoms of MS as well. Research that shows more about the specific mechanisms in the immune system has allows researchers to develop specific therapies targeting specific steps in the immune system and even specific cells that are thought to be involved in MS.

Many alternative therapies are being studied and used by people living with MS. We hope there will be randomized clinical trials to see if any of these improve MS.

There is a long list of promising treatments under development and study so it is evident that the therapeutic era of MS is just beginning. To add to the sense of hope in MS research, we now see a great increase in the amount of research and funding dedicated to MS, and increased numbers of MS clinics, MS clinicians, researchers, and many other health professionals devoting their attention to people with MS, all striving for better outcomes and eventually a cure.

# CHAPTER 2

# *What Is Multiple Sclerosis and How Is It Diagnosed?*

The modern name *multiple sclerosis* refers to the multiple areas of "sclerosed" or hardened plaques of scar tissue throughout the central nervous system. Nerve fibers (axons) in the central nervous system are covered with a *myelin sheath,* which provides an insulating function similar to that of the insulation around electrical wires. This insulation is in segments that allow rapid conduction of electrical impulses. Plaques or patches of inflammation damage the myelin around the nerve and disrupt the transmission of messages to various parts of the body. For example, plaques that disrupt nerve fibers in the brain going to the legs could affect the ability to walk. Patients with MS often have a clinical history of episodes of neurological symptoms that are related to multiple patches of inflammation in the spinal cord, brain, and optic nerves.

Under the microscope, the lesions or plaques are seen as areas in which there is a preponderance of thickly myelinated fibers, the *white matter* of the brain, so called because it appears pale, due to the presence of myelin, compared to the *grey matter* in which there is little myelin. The area of plaque shows disruption of the myelin and some damage or loss of axons as well. There is an inflammatory reaction in these plaques, with some repair of fibers in older plaques and some scarring in very old plaques. More episodes of demyelination and more plaques may appear as years pass. Myelin can be repaired, allowing function to be restored, but conduction may be slower in these repaired fibers. Although repair can occur and may often be almost complete, the repeated myelin breakdown, incomplete repair, and accumulation of scarring lead to some progression of symptoms and signs of the disease after many years. Also when myelin repairs it is often thinner than before, and conducts more slowly.

Although a century ago MS was thought to be uncommon, we now know it is the most common serious neurological disease occurring in young adults. It occurs three times as often in women than men, and for reasons we don't understand, over the last century the disease seems to be increasing, but the increase is mostly in women.

MS follows a number of different patterns and courses, sometimes appearing more than once in the same family, more common in certain parts of the world, and more common in white people.

As the physicians and researchers seek answers and learn more about MS, they uncover more questions and more things to learn. But they are learning more, and there are more clinicians, researchers working to find the cause and cure of MS, and more research funding supporting the effort.

## *What Happens in Attacks of MS?*

Patches of inflammation occur in the central nervous system and some of these are in areas that produce various neurological symptoms. The episodes can be brief, a few days or more likely a few weeks or longer, and in the beginning the symptoms may completely clear. We can see by MRI scans that many inflammatory plaques do not produce symptoms. When there is a symptomatic attack of MS the person might experience numbness in a limb, or on the side of the body, blurred vision in one eye, or weakness in a leg, or perhaps a combination of symptoms. More surprisingly, some plaques may develop and heal without causing any symptoms.

At first there is an inflammatory response in the plaque, with cells involved that are often seen in immunologic reactions. This has led to the understanding that the episode of demyelination, or *attack*, is an immunologic reaction of the body to some target protein in the myelin sheath, which has not yet been identified (see Chapter 3). Why this happens is not certain. There are many other immunological diseases where the body's normal defense mechanism reacts to normal tissue as if it were "foreign" material, and then reacts against it.

When the episode of demyelination settles down, other cells clean away the debris and re-myelination, or repair of the myelin, begins. As a result, the symptoms improve or completely disappear, although some subtle changes may remain. When the symptoms disappear the patient may appear to be back to normal but special tests, such as evoked potential tests, can show that the repaired nerves may conduct more slowly.

Attacks of demyelination accompanied by symptoms of MS may occur over many years. This is another hallmark of the disease— plaques that occur not only in multiple areas of the central nervous system but also in multiple events over time. Neurologists refer to this characteristic of MS as "lesions in time and space."

## The Course of MS

The course of MS varies from person to person. We do not know why one person has a progressive course of symptoms and problems, while another has mild disease that produces little disability over many decades, or why different patterns can occur when MS is seen among family members.

The course of MS can be classified into four basic patterns:

***Relapsing-Remitting MS (RRMS).*** This form of MS is characterized by acute attacks, or relapses, followed either by full or partial recovery. The periods between relapses are characterized by a lack of new symptoms, although the underlying disease process may be continuing. About 85 percent of patients present with this pattern when they begin to have symptoms.

The term *benign MS* is sometimes used to refer to a small number of people with relapsing-remitting MS who have a mild form of the disease and who remain fully functional in all neurological systems fifteen years (some use ten years as the number of years) after disease onset. This is the most difficult form of MS to "label" because it requires many years to identify this pattern. Many people with this form of the disease have mostly sensory symptoms. Because it cannot be reliably predicted early, treatment decisions are not based on the possibility that this course may occur. Because someone who appears "benign" at ten or fifteen years may not be so benign in the next ten or fifteen years, some neurologists prefer not to use the term and it is not in the accepted classification of the disease (McDonald Classification, 2010).

***Secondary Progressive MS (SPMS)***. This pattern begins with a relapsing-remitting course, but after years may show progression over time. Prior to the recent treatments for MS, approximately 60 percent of those with a relapsing-remitting course entered a progressive phase within fifteen years. Patients may continue to have less frequent acute attacks or may stop having attacks altogether, but over the years show an increase in disability. Before deciding that a person has entered the secondary progressive phase of MS, neurologists usually wait to observe at least six months of progression, because an episode or worsening can be temporary. It is hoped and expected that the new therapies for MS will ultimately alter the long-term outcome of the disease, and delay the onset of secondary progression.

***Primary Progressive MS (PPMS)***. In this form of MS, the disease shows slow progression from the onset, without attacks, but sometimes has occasional plateaus and temporary minor improvements. This form of MS is more commonly seen in people who develop the disease after the age of forty, and more often in men. About 15 percent of people with MS are initially diagnosed with this course.

*Progressive-Relapsing MS (PRMS)*. This pattern of MS shows progression from onset, but later one or more attacks occur. This is an unusual pattern.

### Remissions in MS

Remissions can occur at any time in the course of MS and can last for months or for many years. Why remissions occur is not known, and we are not able to tell in whom they will occur or when. Remissions are more common in the early stages of the disease and in the relapsing-remitting type. Plateaus in the course, long periods when little change is seen in the affected person's symptoms, is quite common. Remissions become less frequent as the years go on. It is important to remember that the idea of remissions refers to symptoms—it does not mean that disease activity has necessarily stopped. There is a lot of information indicating that new lesions may still be developing in the nervous system, which will lead to later progression, even though the person may feel little or nothing is changing. Being in remission is not a reason to stop therapy—the therapy may be contributing to the reason for remission.

### The Diagnosis of MS

MS can be a difficult diagnosis to make. Although many patients who consult a neurologist can be diagnosed clinically on the first visit, and without any tests, other situations are more difficult, especially when a patient has recent vague complaints, shows no "findings" or abnormalities on examination, or has a symptom—such as numbness—that is common in many other conditions.

The diagnosis of MS is made by a physician, usually a neurologist, who takes a detailed history of the patient's symptoms and complaints, followed by a thorough physical and neurological examination. Although the disease is suspected and ultimately diagnosed by the clinician's diagnostic skills, two things can assist in the diagnostic process.

The first is a set of criteria for establishing the diagnosis, which were developed in 2001 by the International Panel on the Diagnosis of Multiple Sclerosis, supported by the National Multiple Sclerosis Society and the International Federation of Multiple Sclerosis Societies, and modified in 2005 and 2010 (Table 2.1). Although the terms may sound very general, the patient suspected of having MS is classified by the physician as having "possible" MS or "definite" MS. When a neurologist says that a person has MS, it means that he or she has had more than one episode or attack of symptoms occurring in multiple areas of the white matter of the central nervous system; in some instances, instead of attacks, there will have been progression over a long time, again characterized by changes typical of involvement of many areas of the white matter in the central nervous system.

When a person does not demonstrate all the criteria for MS, he or she may be classified as having possible MS after other conditions

**Table 2-1   Diagnostic Criteria**

Evidence of more than one area of central nervous system involvement (dissemination in "space") and central nervous system involvement at more than one time (dissemination in "time") are required for a diagnosis of MS

| CLINICAL PRESENTATION | ADDITIONAL DATA NEEDED |
|---|---|
| • Two or more attacks (relapses)<br>• Two or more objective clinical lesions | None; clinical evidence will suffice (additional evidence desirable but must be consistent with MS) |
| • Two or more attacks<br>• One objective clinical lesion | Dissemination in space, demonstrated by:<br>• MRI<br>• or a positive cerebrospinal fluid and twoor more MRI lesions consistent with MS<br>• or further clinical attack involving a different site |
| • One attack<br>• Two or more objective clinical lesions | Dissemination in time, demonstrated by:<br>• MRI<br>• or second clinical attack |

(continued)

**Table 2-1    *(continued)***

| CLINICAL PRESENTATION | ADDITIONAL DATA NEEDED |
|---|---|
| • One attack<br>• One objective clinical lesion (monosymptomatic presentation) | Dissemination in space demonstrated by:<br>• MRI<br>• or positive cerebrospinal fluid and two or more MRI lesions consistent with MS<br>**and**<br>Dissemination in time demonstrated by:<br>• MRI<br>• or second clinical attack |
| Insidious neurological progression suggestive of MS (primary progressive MS) | One year of disease progression (retrospectively or prospectively determined) and two of the following:<br>a. Positive brain MRI (nine T2 lesions or four or more T2 lesions with positive visual evoked potentials) |
| | b. Positive spinal cord MRI (two focal T2 lesions) |
| | c. Positive cerebrospinal fluid |

*Source:* Adapted from McDonald, et al. 2001. "Recommended Diagnostic Criteria for MS." *Annals of Neurology* 50: 121–27 and Polman, C., et al. 2005. "Revisions to the McDonald Diagnostic Criteria." *Annals of Neurology* 58: 840–46 and Polman, C., et al. 2010. "Diagnostic Criteria for Multiple Sclerosis: 2010 Revisions to the McDonald Criteria." *Annals of Neurology* 69: 292–302.

are ruled out, and in the likelihood that additional features of the disease may become evident in time. Common examples of patients who are initially classified as having possible MS are those who present with their first symptom (since they have had only one episode, they are identified with a "clinically isolated syndrome") or those who have had repeated episodes but always in one site (thus, not multiple symptoms in the areas involved).

The second helpful aid to the neurologist is a group of tests that may confirm the suspicion of MS. Remember, though, that the diagnosis is still a clinical decision, and there is no test that says definitively that MS is present. The test can only suggest changes that are compatible with the diagnosis, and the neurologist uses this to aid the clinical decision.

## Clinical Examination

The clinical examination has three major parts: history, examination, and tests.

### History

The history includes not only the story of your symptoms and complaints but also your general health during your lifetime, your operations and accidents, illnesses in your family, occupational information, and other details. This often is the most important part of the examination. The neurologist often makes the diagnosis during this part of the assessment, even before the neurological examination or diagnostic tests.

### Examination

To get a complete picture of your health and to better understand your symptoms, the neurologist performs a general physical examination that includes listening to your lungs and heart, taking your blood pressure, and examining your muscles and skin, as well as a neurological examination that includes examining your eyes, the cranial nerves to your head and face, your strength, sensation, and ability to detect vibration over various parts of the body, your reflexes, and your balance and walking. Sometimes a patient is surprised to have his or her feet and abdomen examined when the complaint is of numbness in a hand. However, this overall examination provides a picture of your nervous system and is able to identify other conditions that might explain the symptoms you are experiencing.

### Tests

A number of tests can help to confirm that MS may be present and also can identify other problems that mimic its symptoms. Some patients so clearly have MS when they are assessed that no tests are necessary, or only one test may be used to confirm the disease and rule out other problems that might be under suspicion. The following are only the most commonly used and valuable tests.

**Magnetic Resonance Imaging (MRI)** Decades ago, MRI would have seemed like science fiction—a test that produces a picture of your brain as you lie inside a huge electromagnet that momentarily spins the molecules in your body. Minutes later, the computer produces a remarkable picture of your nervous system that looks much like the illustrations in an anatomy textbook. More remarkable for those who care for people with MS, the MRI is particularly good at detecting the patchy areas of change in the white matter nervous system that occur with the disease. It has become the most accurate and helpful test for MS.

The MRI examination is done while you lie on a table that moves inside a tube-like space in a large machine that holds a magnet. You will need to lie very still while the magnet sends information to a computer that receives thousands of tiny bits of information and uses them to generate pictures. These images are like slices or views at many levels throughout the brain or the spinal cord, or wherever the scanner is set. Sometimes a dye or contrast material (gadolinium) is injected into a vein to obtain more detailed pictures.

No major discomfort is associated with the procedure, no x-rays are involved, and the scanners are becoming faster, so that the length of time you are in the scanner is getting much shorter. A few people have some feeling of claustrophobia and dislike the closed-in feeling of the narrow space and the noise the machine makes. Most people can tolerate it well, especially when they know how important it is and when they have received a clear explanation of the procedure and receive support and encouragement from the staff. However, the anxiety experienced by some people can be easily reduced by mild sedation, such as lorazepam (Ativan) or diazepam (Valium) taken prior to the MRI.

MRI is an amazing technologic advance that can help in the diagnosis of many diseases and also is helpful in research. However, there are some drawbacks to its completeness as a test for MS. Because it is so complex, the machinery, support systems, and personnel needed to operate them are very expensive. The cost of the test often is in the range of $800 to $1,500—higher if more complex procedures are necessary.

Another drawback is that the MRI is inconclusive in a few patients, especially if they are at an early stage in the disease and have had only a few or very mild symptoms. Furthermore, the test does not "show MS"; it shows changes that *could be* due to MS. We must remember that other conditions occasionally cause similar changes. That is why the clinical picture is most helpful and can indicate whether other problems should be considered or whether this is a typical story of MS symptoms, with typical findings of MS on examination, and with typical changes in keeping with MS on the MRI.

Finally, although the MRI can confirm the diagnosis, it does not tell us all the things you and we want to know, such as whether the disease is mild or advanced or whether it is getting worse (those are clinical features). Also, the standard MRI does not show changes that are less inflammatory, such as those in the grey matter and in areas that appear normal. Further developments in MRI techniques undoubtedly will allow us to answer many more of these questions.

**Cerebrospinal Fluid** The cerebrospinal fluid surrounds the brain and spinal cord and fills some cavities within the central nervous system. A fine needle can be inserted into the lower back (below the end of the spinal cord) to remove a sample of this clear fluid for examination of cells, protein, and electrolytes; this is a lumbar puncture, which is also called an LP or a spinal tap.

A number of tests can be done on the cerebrospinal fluid, but the most useful in MS is to examine the proteins for the presence of *oligoclonal bands*; the fluid is put on a gel and an electrical current is passed through it in the laboratory to separate its protein contents into these bands. Approximately nine of ten people who have a well-established pattern of MS have bands in the cerebrospinal fluid, but unfortunately this pattern is less common in early and very mild cases. The cerebrospinal fluid is usually examined if the MRI is not conclusive but the clinical picture is still suggestive of MS. It is also an important test if the pattern of involvement is primary progressive MS, to verify that the progressive disease is really MS.

Many people have heard that having a lumbar puncture is uncomfortable, but it usually does not cause much discomfort and can be done as an outpatient. Unfortunately, about one third of people get a headache when they sit up after the test, a problem that may last for days. Lying flat on the abdomen to facilitate closure of the puncture site and taking abundant oral fluids to replace cerebrospinal fluid lost through testing should minimize this side effect.

**Evoked Potential Studies** The principle of evoked potential studies is simple. Nerves that have experienced demyelination conduct impulses more slowly than normally, even if they have healed and re-myelinated. Evoked potential studies measure the rate and form of the impulse as it passes through specific nerves. The only evoked potential study that can strongly support the diagnosis of MS is the visual evoked potential study.

Visual evoked potential studies assess the conduction of messages through the optic nerves behind the eyes. To stimulate the visual system, a changing pattern of a checkerboard or some other pattern causes a stimulus that passes through the visual system at the back of the brain where vision is processed. Electrodes over the scalp measure the wave form and the speed of the impulse to determine whether one eye differs from the other or if there are other changes consistent with a diagnosis of MS.

The visual evoked potential study is most useful if there is evidence of neurological involvement in an area other than the visual system, and the neurologist is seeking involvement in another area; in this case, the optic nerve. If the person has a history of a definite optic neuritis, the test is of less value, as it is already known that the optic nerve is affected.

## Watchful Waiting

Uncertainty is difficult to cope with, and many people would like an answer to their problem even if it is unpleasant. Unfortunately, definitive answers are not always possible. In perhaps 10 to 15 percent of cases, the answer to the question "Is MS the cause of these symptoms?" remains uncertain even after all available examinations and tests have been done. By this time the neurologist will have eliminated other possibilities such as a tumor or a disc pressing on the spinal cord. The neurologist will know that MS could be causing the symptoms but that other conditions might also be responsible. This uncertainty can be upsetting, but the wise approach at this point is to "wait and see," with periodic examinations and visits to the physician if new problems appear or changes occur. In most instances, the diagnosis becomes clear over time. This requires patience by both the person with symptoms and the physician, but if they agree that they will wait together, the patient usually accepts the situation, having been reassured that other conditions, such as a tumor, have been ruled out. In some instances, the problem later turns out to be something other than MS, often a mild, benign, or treatable condition. It is better to wait than to be prematurely labeled as having MS on the basis of unclear evidence, especially since that may result in MS therapy being prescribed. Also receiving a label may reduce the likelihood that the diagnosis would be re-assessed.

## The Outcome

When a person develops MS, she or he naturally wants to know what this will mean in the long term, relative to life, health, and family. Unfortunately, uncertainty and unpredictability are characteristics of the disease as well as of its pattern of symptoms and course. What we *can* say in general terms is that the outlook is improving year by year and will continue to improve, as the new therapies show they are better at reducing activity of the disease. Even before there was therapy to treat the underlying disease, the life expectancy of most people with MS had been extended close to the normal range as a result of the development of treatments such as antibiotics for bladder and kidney infections and better therapy for many of the complications of the disease. Newly available treatments for the underlying cause of the disease undoubtedly will change the long-term tendency for repeated attacks, progression, and disability, but we still have a long way to go. Research is proceeding rapidly and, although it will never be fast enough or great enough for those living daily with MS and its symptoms, we are heading in the right direction.

# CHAPTER 3

# What Is the Cause of Multiple Sclerosis?

**M**S has been known and studied as a distinct disease since the mid-1800s. However, the cause (etiology) of the disease remains unknown. There are many theories about the cause of MS, but the answer is still uncertain. Because the development of effective treatments depends on a better understanding of the disease, research into its cause is one of the most active areas of scientific exploration. Recent findings have brought us closer to an understanding of MS and have led to a series of new therapies and new approaches.

### Theories About the Cause of MS

Multiple sclerosis presents itself as symptoms involving the central nervous system: the brain, spinal cord, or optic nerves. The peripheral nervous system, the long nerves to the body and limbs, are unaffected.

Studies of the pathology in the central nervous system show evidence of an immune reaction occurring with patches or plaques of inflammation. In these plaques there is swelling of tissue, breakdown and loss of the myelin surrounding nerve fibers, and some damage to the nerve fibers, or axons themselves. As healing occurs some scar tissue can form in the area. There may be many such scars—called lesions—widely distributed in the central nervous system, thus giving rise to the disease's English name, multiple (many) sclerosis (scars). Immune cells, such as T and B lymphocytes and macrophages—normally seen in the bloodstream—are present in the lesions and are activated against central nervous system tissue. The major questions are what initiates the immune reaction to myelin, and what is it in the myelin that the immune reaction is directed toward? The information about the immunology in MS have been extremely important because the central nervous system normally is immune "privileged" and immune cells usually remain in the bloodstream outside of the central nervous system. In MS, however, such cells become activated against myelin and are able to penetrate the barrier between the blood and the nervous system—the blood-brain barrier.

Penetration of activated immune cells across the blood-brain barrier into the central nervous system triggers a further complex process of immune-mediated damage of myelin and underlying nerve fibers. As mentioned, when the myelin is damaged there is a disruption of the electrical and chemical signals responsible for nerve conduction from the brain and spinal cord to muscles and from sensory organs back to the brain and spinal cord. When nerve signals become slowed or blocked by this immune-mediated damage, the person can experience the neurological problems in balance, gait, vision, bladder and bowel control, numbness, pain, and other symptoms typical of MS.

### Tissue Abnormalities, Infections, and the Environment: Links to an MS Cause?

Many theories have been explored as to why the myelin of the central nervous system is attacked by a person's own immune system in MS, a so-called "autoimmune" (self-immune) attack. For example, it is possible that the myelin is not normal for some reason and the immune system reacts to it as "foreign," but so far studies have not shown that there is anything distinctly different about the basic structure of myelin in a person with MS.

In recent years it has been shown that the plaques of inflammation in the white matter are not the only areas involved. Sophisticated MRI studies as well as pathological studies have shown that areas of the brain that appear normal are actually not entirely normal and show subtle inflammatory changes as well. There are also changes in the grey matter. It appears that MS is more widespread than it would seem from the patches viewed on the MRI.

The possibility that an environmental toxin or even a dietary imbalance may be the cause of MS has been considered. Although toxic substances and diet can cause other nervous system problems, there is no convincing evidence that they are the cause of MS. Occasional reports have been made of "clusters" of MS, where more cases than might be expected in a town, neighborhood, or in a school class. Such reports have triggered studies to determine if such clusters are real or simply coincidence; and if real, to evaluate any environmental factors that might be involved. None, to date, has shown a direct environmental agent to be involved in the development of MS, and most seem to be random clusters, expected in a disease that is relatively common in the population.

For decades, studies of where MS exists in the world and where it is absent (the sciences of epidemiology and demographics) have suggested that some triggering factor in the environment might be related to the risk of MS. Data from studies of people migrating from one area to another with a different incidence of the disease suggest that such a factor probably acts before the age of 15 in order for the disease process to be triggered later in life. Although somewhat controversial, this finding has stimulated the search over the last half century as to what this trigger factor could be.

Many common and uncommon viruses have been proposed as causative agents for MS over the past several decades. Many of these proposals have been based on the presence of virus in tissues from individuals with MS or, more often, the presence of immune system antibodies against viruses in the blood. Evidence was often weak as the suspect virus was often only slightly more common than in the normal population. In recent years, technology has become more sophisticated, and such searches include the use of polymerase chain reaction (PCR) analysis to detect protein "footprints" in blood, cerebrospinal fluid, and tissue even if whole virus cannot be seen. In each case in which claims for causative or triggering infectious agents have been made, further study has failed to support the claim or at least failed to provide convincing supporting evidence. Ongoing work continues to focus on a few suspicious viruses. The human herpesvirus 6 (HHV-6), a common virus that causes roseola in infants, has been linked by some scientists to MS. A common bacterium, *Chlamydia pneumoniae*, which is responsible for "walking pneumonia," also has been linked to MS by some researchers, but original claims of a causative or triggering link for this bacterium have not held up. The Epstein-Barr virus, the cause of infectious mononucleosis, continues to attract attention as a possible trigger for MS. There is increasing information about a link with Epstein-Barr virus. A study of the brains of seven people with MS showed that in plaques there are high levels of an inflammation-stimulating chemical (interferon alpha) that helps the body fight viruses, and in the surrounding tissues there are immune B cells inactively infected by Epstein-Barr virus, but no evidence of an active viral infection. This raises the question whether the virus may indirectly stimulate MS disease activity.

Rather than focusing on a single infectious agent, many scientists now believe that individuals with MS have a heightened immune antibody response against a host of common and uncommon viruses and other infectious agents, and that past claims based on antibody responses against a specific virus are likely misleading.

There is increasing evidence that low vitamin D might play a role in the susceptibility to MS. As vitamin D levels are often lower in people living in regions more distant from the Equator, it could explain the increased incidence in the same geographic regions. Some studies have shown that in large groups, those who developed MS had lower levels of vitamin D than the rest of the group. There are studies in large populations of nurses in Britain and in military recruits in the United States with information that vitamin D may play a role. Also, the lower levels of vitamin D over the winter months would explain why more individual with MS were born in the months around May than in November, possibly related to a lower level of vitamin D in the pregnant mother over the winter.

With a new understanding of the importance of immunology in the MS disease process, many scientists have shifted their view of the role of specific viruses and other infectious agents in MS away from a direct cause of the disease and toward learning how an immune system response against an infectious agent may result in a later autoimmune disease. Increased attention has been paid to the possibility that many viruses, bacteria, and perhaps other pathogens could serve as a trigger for the autoimmune process that becomes MS.

There is a lot of research into possible risk factors for MS which might influence the development of the disease or the progression. Recently it has been found that smoking can influence both. It was noted that smokers or those subjected to passive (secondary) smoke have an increased risk of developing MS, and smokers progress to the secondary progressive stage of the disease faster than nonsmokers and have a greater risk of having more disability. It also seems that smokers do not get the full effect of the drugs that benefit people with MS. It was also noted that stopping smoking did slow the progression of the disease.

In spite of years of investigation into infectious or environmental causes for MS, there is little convincing evidence for either of these factors as a potential cause of the disease. However, claims still appear from time to time in the media or scientific literature of the "latest" cause of the disease, but these have so far turned out to have little merit. However, because a possible association between MS and such potential causes could be one of the unsolved mysteries of the disease, and we know there must be some kind of a trigger that initiates the disease in a predisposed person, these areas are still being explored. Until the cause of MS is discovered, rational, careful studies in these areas are still appropriate, and we must keep our minds open to all ideas.

## The Underlying Immune System Problems in MS

Research on the cause of MS since the mid-1950s has focused increasingly on the immune system function in MS and on the theory that MS is an autoimmune disease. Autoimmunity is by no means unique to MS. Diseases such as rheumatoid arthritis, systemic lupus erythematosus, juvenile-onset (type 1) diabetes (JD), scleroderma, myasthenia gravis, and others are autoimmune in nature. Many of these diseases share some important characteristics. In each, cells and/or antibodies of a person's own immune system attack and damage what appear to be normal tissues of a person's body. Most (but not all) such diseases share a tendency to be more prevalent in women than in men. (Juvenile-onset diabetes is an exception: Gender distribution is about equal between men and women and, in a few rare conditions, male predominance is seen.) All may be susceptible to treatment through a variety of routes that suppress or otherwise regulate immune function.

The evidence that the immune system is involved in MS is clear. First, people with MS seem to have clear-cut abnormalities in immune function compared with healthy individuals. These include, among other factors, evidence that specific white blood cells (T lymphocytes or T cells, and B lymphocytes or B cells) are present in the central nervous system that are primed to "recognize" and launch attacks against tissues of the nervous system, such as myelin and nerve fibers. In individuals with MS, there is clear and specific reaction of T white cells against proteins that compose central nervous system myelin. Also, B lymphocytes are involved and recent successful therapies have been directed to the B cells. Interestingly, it has been known since the mid-1990s that individuals *without* MS also have T cells that can react against myelin, but in such individuals these cells remain circulating in the bloodstream, separated from the central nervous system by the blood-brain barrier. In MS, the blood-brain barrier is broken or breached, allowing the immune cells to move into the central nervous system tissue and initiate their damaging effects. Breaks in the blood-brain barrier can actually be visualized with contrast-enhancing (gadolinium-enhanced) MRIs and other sophisticated imaging techniques.

An additional clue to the immune system's role in MS is the overrepresentation of cells and other immune system components that enhance immune responses in individual with the disease—so-called pro-inflammatory immune cells—and a relative underrepresentation of cells and immune mediators that suppress immune responses—anti-inflammatory cells. Most notably, in tissue from individuals with MS, immune system cells are found in active lesions of the brain and spinal cord. These immune characteristics are not normally seen in individuals who do not have MS.

Although immune system involvement in MS seems clear, evidence that the problem is *autoimmune* is difficult to obtain in humans. Actual proof of autoimmunity requires that immune system cells that cause damage in one patient be injected into a different, healthy patient and cause damage and disease there as well. Although this kind of experiment can be done in laboratory animals to prove autoimmunity, it obviously is not ethical to undertake such studies using humans, since such experiments would cause autoimmune disease in otherwise healthy people. In laboratory animals with a disease called experimental allergic (or autoimmune) encephalomyelitis (EAE), a model used to mimic the changes in MS, such experiments show that an autoimmune disorder can produce similar changes seen in MS lesions.

For this reason alone, EAE has proven to be a useful animal disease model to help understand human MS. While EAE is not MS, and laboratory animals are not humans, there are many similarities in clinical symptoms and central nervous system lesion immunological mechanisms in EAE in laboratory animals and MS in humans. EAE thus serves as a model for the study of MS, and in particular for studies on the very specific elements of immune function that might be involved in MS-like disease. EAE studies not only have contrib-uted to our understanding of immune problems in MS but also have been used productively to demonstrate a "proof of concept" for new immune therapies that might be used for human MS; and EAE stud-ies have led to some of the immune-modulating drugs that are used in MS today.

## The Role of Genetics in MS

That there is a genetic influence in MS has been known for a long time, based primarily on the observation that MS may occur in more than one member of the same family. We know that MS is not directly inherited, but it is increasingly clear that a complex set of genetic factors helps to determine who may be susceptible to MS and who may not. Observations that suggest a genetic factor in MS come from studies of many populations around the world.

First, approximately 20 percent of all individuals with MS have at least one additional family member, either in the same generation or in a different generation, who has or had MS. While 80 percent of people with MS appear to have no family history of other cases, this 20 percent rate of *concordance* (the occurrence of disease in more than one family member) suggests a genetic link or genetic influence. However, the concordance rate among family members is in itself not high enough to support a direct disease inheritance and, in itself, does not help us understand what genetic factors might be involved. Such concordance could happen, for example, simply because of a shared environmental cause or trigger for MS. However, results from a large-scale study in Canada in the 1990s indicated that the tendency for multiple cases of MS to occur in families is truly genetic and not due to other factors such as environment or diet, and there are many other studies verifying a genetic influence.

In families with more than one case of MS the risk of disease is still quite low, and even lower as the relationship becomes more distant. In the United States, about one in 1,000 people have MS; when a family member (parent, sibling) already has the disease, the risk increases to two to five per 100, depending on the degree of relationship. If one twin has MS, the risk is 30% in the other twin if the twins are identical, but only 5% (the same risk as siblings) if the twins are fraternal. This is strong proof of a genetic factor being involved. The fact that the other identical twin has only a 30% risk rather than 100% suggests there is some other trigger involved, as they are genetically identical.

There is evidence that the genetic risk is greater through the maternal line, and the risk is highest in mother to daughter, and lowest in father to son.

Beyond the reasonably frequent occurrence of MS in more than one family member, it also has long been known that there are ethnic or religious populations in the world that are *genetically isolated*— they rarely or never marry or bear children outside their own group and thus have developed a relatively restricted and unique gene pool. MS never or rarely occurs in some of these groups. Examples include such religious sects as the Hutterites in Canada and such ethnic groups as Eastern European gypsies. While living in areas where there is a relatively high incidence of MS, these groups seem to be protected from MS. Such genetically isolated populations are of great interest in disease research—not only those that seem to be "resistant" but also those in which disease may be prevalent. Such populations most likely have a more restricted pool of genes, raising the possibility that they can be used to more easily isolate disease-relevant gene factors. Studies on genetics have been undertaken in genetically isolated populations in locations such as western Finland and Tasmania and are currently underway in Iceland where scientists hope that new clues to MS genetics may be easier to obtain.

Related to this is the fact that there are racial differences in the incidence and even in the clinical appearance of MS. In North America, the disease occurs more commonly among white people than among African Americans, even in the same community, and the clinical symptomatology and severity of the disease may be different in these two groups. And there may be differences in how individuals of different racial backgrounds respond to MS therapies as well. Pure African Bantus virtually never develop MS, although whites living in the same part of Africa are susceptible. Importantly, genetic studies of African Americans with MS may yield important clues to MS genetics. African Americans often have a mixed genetic background—a combination of original African ancestral genes and white genes that have been inherited through white ancestors since the time of slavery in North America. Through "admixture" analysis of the genetic background of African Americans with MS, Africans who do not have MS, and whites with MS, it may be possible to more closely identify MS disease-related genes, and such studies are under way. Finally, MS is seen much less often in Asians, a clinical type somewhat different from that of whites. All of these factors point to a clear genetic influence on MS even if the disease is not directly inherited.

While such information might one day provide us with the ability to predict susceptibility, it cannot yet help us. The risk rates are low even within families in which MS already exists. Inheritance patterns in MS are extremely complex and poorly understood. Large genetic studies to search for common genetic factors that might underlie MS have been undertaken in the United States, Canada, the United Kingdom, Europe, and Australia, taking advantage of the existence of families with multiple individuals who have MS. From these studies, we have learned that no single genetic factor is responsible for MS or even dominant in the MS genetic picture. Rather, there are many genetic factors that might contribute to MS susceptibility. There is no current identified single gene, and there is not likely to be one, that can be said to cause MS, as has been shown for diseases such as Huntington's chorea, Duchenne muscular dystrophy, and cystic fibrosis. However, work is underway to identify genetic patterns that might allow prediction of susceptible persons in the future.

Genetic research in MS is among the most highly technologic areas of research today. With each year, new findings from the massive genetic research efforts are being applied to the study of MS. The description of the full human genome in the late 1990s helped to identify genes that make us "human" and set the stage for discovery of genes that might underlie specific human traits and specific human diseases. The human genome map has led to efforts in the first years of the twenty-first century to describe completely the human *haplotype* map—a description of the blocks of genes that tend to be inherited together from generation to generation. This so called "hap map" will greatly reduce the complexity of the search for disease-related genes in the human population. MS was among the first diseases to be studied by these technologies.

There is a genetic predisposition for MS but genetics cannot be the whole story. The fact that genetically identical twins are not always concordant for MS clearly indicates that some other factor, or "trigger," must be involved.

## So, What Is the Cause of MS?

Multiple sclerosis is, to be sure, a complex disease that is just beginning to be unraveled. There remains no known single initiating cause of MS, and it is likely that the disease is the result of a number of related factors. While symptoms come from problems in the nervous system, MS appears to be a disease of immune system function, most likely an autoimmune disease, which attacks the central nervous system. Although the disease is not directly inherited, there is a genetic susceptibility. It appears that a genetic pattern makes one susceptible to MS but many people may have the genetic susceptibility without getting the disease. A triggering factor, or a combination of factors may be needed, but so far no definite virus, bacterium, or other infectious or environmental agent has been identified. The ultimate consequence of the immune system problems in MS is the entrance of immune cells into the central nervous system, attack of myelin around nerve fibers, and eventual myelin and nerve fiber loss and scarring. The entire process results in the failure of nerve signals to operate properly, resulting in the well-known symptoms of MS.

# CHAPTER 4

# *What Treatment Is Available for Multiple Sclerosis?*

The medical management of MS is accomplished through a partnership of health professionals, the person with MS, and the family. In this chapter, we address both the symptomatic treatment and management of the disease course.

People often say that there is no treatment for a disease when what they really mean is that there is no "magic bullet," a simple cure that makes the disease go away, as penicillin may do for pneumonia. As with most medical diseases, there is yet no "cure" for MS, but there are many beneficial treatments and approaches that will help you cope with the challenges of MS. We are in an era in which there are agents that lessen the number and severity of attacks, the progression of the disease, the development of disability, and also reduce many of the symptoms of the disease. Each year things become more positive and hopeful as we see advances in diagnosis, treatment, symptom management, rehabilitation, assessment, classification, and understanding of the disease.

## *Resources*

One of the most important first steps in dealing with MS is to learn more about it. You need to know what you can do to stay healthy and to reduce the problems that may confront you and your family. You are in control of much that is important in managing this disease. The fact that you are reading this book shows that you are already taking charge of one of the first things over which you have control—being informed and educated about MS so that you can make better decisions and manage the challenges.

You should begin by getting in touch with groups that can provide you with information and support. The National Multiple Sclerosis Society (NMSS) in the United States and the Multiple Sclerosis Society of Canada (MSSC) are two such organizations that you can use as starting points. These organizations have up to date information sources and are there to support you. You can learn about ongoing research and important advances as they occur. These MS organizations and their local chapters have many pamphlets and educational programs on all the important aspects of the disease.

There are many books about MS. Some are excellent, and others are not. Some are by professionals who manage the disease, some are by individuals who have successfully adapted to its limitations, and some are by enthusiasts who are proposing some treatment that they are selling. Consulting one of the MS societies will help to keep a balanced view because the publications it recommends have been carefully reviewed for both accuracy and usefulness.

People with MS often hear of possible treatments from friends and the media, and it is often difficult to distinguish between those that are useful and those that are not (or those that may be harmful) and those that have scientific evidence from randomized trials to support the claims of benefit. We strongly recommend that you check any suggestions about treatments made by people other than your physician or nurse with reliable sources, including the MS societies or the books recommended in the Additional Reading section of this book.

## Types of Treatment

Treatments in MS can be grouped into different categories:

- Management of the acute attack
- Treatment of the underlying disease
- Management of symptoms
- Interventions related to emotional and social issues

### Management of Acute Attacks

When there is a change in symptoms over a few days or weeks, with the development of new symptoms or the worsening of old ones, the event may be a new "attack," or relapse, of the disease. It usually means that new patches of inflammation and demyelination are occurring in either new or old spots in the central nervous system—the brain, spinal cord, and optic nerves. These often are mild and cease after a few days or weeks and need no treatment. If your symptoms are severe or continue to worsen you may need to seek treatment. The swelling and inflammation in the plaques of demyelination can be reduced by high-dose intravenous steroids (methylprednisolone). Some schedules of treatment vary but a common practice is to administer 1000 mg of methylprednisolone intravenously over 30 minutes as an outpatient, and repeat this daily for three to five days. There may be variations in the total steroid dose, the number of days of treatment, and the time between doses, but all are characterized by a high dose over a short period. It is also possible to treat acute attacks with oral steroids, but it involves a very large dose of steroids, equivalent to the intravenous dose. The treatment is well tolerated by patients, although some may have trouble sleeping when they receive high doses of steroids.

Some people may begin to recover soon after steroid therapy has started, but for others, improvement may occur only slowly, even weeks after the treatment. As some spontaneous recovery is expected after most acute attacks, it sometimes is difficult to know how much was due to the treatment and how much would have occurred without it.

If there is mild numbness in a limb, dizziness, or some other symptom that is annoying but not limiting in any way, your neurologist may decide to wait and see if the problem clears spontaneously, as it often does. An attack that has stopped progressing and is improving may be allowed to clear on its own. High-dose steroids help people to recover from an attack somewhat faster, but since they might recover just as well with time, decisions about treatment must be made on an individual basis. The repetitive use of steroids can have long-term effects that include cataracts, osteoporosis, and weight gain; therefore, their use should be reserved for more serious attacks that are not clearing spontaneously. A rare but important complication is avascular necrosis of the hip that requires a hip replacement.

Although it is reasonable to rest when you have MS, especially during attacks, there is a tendency to rest too much and people who care for you will often over-encourage rest. You need some rest but there is little evidence that your MS will be worse with less rest. If you overdo rest you may actually feel weary and weak, and may stop work or neglect responsibilities when you are capable of continuing these activities. A reasonable approach is to develop a schedule that allows for a slower pace but allows you to manage despite the fatigue.

The best advice to people with MS is not "rest, with reasonable activity," but rather "stay active, with reasonable rest." The difference is in placement of the emphasis. Slow down and rest more when symptoms and fatigue are a problem or when an attack occurs, but stay as active as you can and increase your activity again when the symptoms are relieved.

## Treatment of the Underlying Disease

### When to Begin Therapy?

I believe there are two important concepts to keep in mind when you have been diagnosed with MS and therapy is being considered:

A. **Early is late**. This means that when you experience the first symptoms of MS, and feel it is early in the disease, there are usually indicators that the disease has been there for a long time, with evidence of changes that caused no symptoms. So it seems early, but it is really late.

B. **Treatment should start as soon as the diagnosis is confirmed**. There is a lot of evidence that the benefits of therapy are greater when started early. The object is to reduce the activity of the disease as judged by the clinical activity and the MRI activity, and preserve the brain's ability to repair itself and compensate for damage. There is a limit to the brain's healing powers and plasticity to compensate for damage, so treatment should start early to protect the brain. Another expression used by some neurologists is *"Time is brain,"* meaning the longer you wait, the more brain damage occurs.

### The Objective of Therapy

The objective of the current therapies for MS is to reduce the activity of the disease. The hope is to achieve a state where there is no evidence of disease activity (NEDA). This means no relapses, no progression of disability, and no evidence of activity on the MRI. Not all patients can achieve this with therapy, so the second choice is minimal evidence of disease activity (MEDA). These concepts are relatively new, and only possible because the therapies have improved and have greater effect, especially when used early.

*Disease-Modifying Therapies*

We now have available therapies that offer the promise of having an impact on the ultimate course of the disease. None of the currently available therapies will cure the disease, but these medications can reduce the number and severity of attacks and result in less progression and disability over the years.

The following therapies are approved by the Food and Drug Administration in the United States and Health Canada:

### Injectable medications

> Avonex (interferon beta-1a)
>
> Betaseron (interferon beta-1b)
>
> Rebif (interferon beta-1a)
>
> Copaxone (glatiramer acetate)
>
> Extavia (interferon beta-1b)
>
> Glatopa (glatiramer acetate)
>
> Plegridy (peginterferon beta-1a)
>
> Zinbryta (daclizumab)

### Oral medications

> Aubagio (teriflunomide)
>
> Gilenya (fingolimod)
>
> Tecfidera (dimethyl fumarate)

### Infused medications

> Tysabri (natalizumab)
>
> Lemtrada (alemtuzumab)
>
> Novantrone (mitoxantrone)
>
> Ocrevus (ocrelizumab)

They have been approved in many countries, and other agents will soon appear. Each country has a system of approval, so the list of approved drugs may vary in different countries. These agents have been approved for use in MS based on extensive clinical trials and review of the evidence of benefit and risk. Most neurologists make their decision as to which drug is appropriate for a given patient based on that individual's disease characteristics as well as the patient's lifestyle and preferences. The latest approved drug has been Ocrevus (ocrelizumab), which targets B lymphocytes, and is the first drug approved for the treatment of primary progressive MS.

There is good evidence that the drugs discussed in the following sections are helpful if they are used in the early relapsing stages of the disease, but evidence for their effectiveness if the disease changes to a progressive phase or has been progressive since the start is less clear. However, some recent studies in the progressive stages of the disease are showing promise.

It is important to have a good understanding of the expected benefits of these drugs because if there are greater expectations than the treatments can deliver, it would be easy to become discouraged and stop the drugs, even though they are helping. The expectation and hope is that, over time, you will be better than if you did not have the treatment, not that you will suddenly notice yourself improving or even that relapses and symptoms will cease completely.

The MS societies have information, guidelines, and consensus statements on the use of disease-modifying agents that are very useful to the person diagnosed with MS. The National MS Society has published the Consensus Statement of the National MS Society on the disease-modifying therapies. Further information can be found on their web page (www.nationalmssociety.org).

These drugs have been shown in randomized clinical trials to reduce the frequency of relapses, reduce the development of new lesions on the MRI, and show probable reduction in progression of the disease. The experience of MS neurologists is that these drugs are important in reducing the activity of the disease and improving the quality of life of MS patients. The therapy, however, has to be continued for years, as stopping therapy causes a return of activity to the pre-treatment level.

The Society recognizes that the factors that enter into a decision to treat are complex and best analyzed by the individual patient's neurologist. Initiation of treatment with an interferon beta medication or glatiramer acetate should be considered as soon as possible following a definite diagnosis of MS with active, relapsing disease, and may also be considered for selected patients with a first attack who are at high risk of MS (classified as the Clinically Isolated Syndrome).

The first disease-modifying therapies shown to modify the outcome of the disease were interferons. Beta interferons are naturally occurring proteins that are produced when the body reacts to a foreign substance or agent such as a virus. They belong to a class of molecules called *cytokines*, the hormones of the immune system. These cytokines are important regulators of the immune response to viruses and inflammatory conditions. Interferon beta seems to "calm" and modulate the reactions of the immune system, and is referred to as an *immunomodulatory agent.*

Natalizumab is generally recommended by the Food and Drug Administration for patients who have had an inadequate response to, or are unable to tolerate, other multiple sclerosis therapies.

Treatment with mitoxantrone may be considered for selected relapsing patients with worsening disease or people living with secondary-progressive MS whose symptoms are getting worse, whether or not relapses are occurring. It requires assessment for cardiac function and has a limited total dose that can be administered because of cardiac risks. It is used less now that there are other new and powerful therapies that can be used when someone is failing on other drugs.

The whole MS community has been waiting for years for an oral drug for MS to replace the repeated injections, and the first of these is fingolimod. It is easy to take, and tolerated well, but it was noted to cause a drop in heart rate with the first dose in many patients, raising concerns about more serious complications— as this is being written a number of sudden deaths with the first dose have been reported. This will now require further assessment of the safety of the drug and monitoring of every patient for hours after the first dose.

Patients' access to medication should not be limited by the frequency of relapses, age, or level of disability. Treatment is not to be stopped while insurers evaluate for continuing coverage of treatment, as this would put patients at increased risk for recurrent disease activity.

Therapy is to be continued indefinitely, except for the following circumstances: There is good evidence of lack of benefit; there are intolerable side effects; better therapy becomes available. All of these FDA-approved agents should be included in formularies and covered by third-party payers so that physicians and patients can determine the most appropriate agent on an individual basis. Unfortunately, in the United States there are some third-party payers who limit access to some of the drugs and thus regulate which drug their members may have. Movement from one disease-modifying medication to another should occur only for medically appropriate reasons.

None of the therapies has been approved for use by women who are trying to become pregnant, are pregnant, or who are nursing mothers.

### DRUGS APPROVED FOR THE TREATMENT OF MS

The following is a brief introduction to the variety of disease modifying therapies to give you a sense of the options available in the treatment of MS. The choice of the drug that best fits you, your disease course and characteristics, and your life style is a discussion between you and your neurologist.

### INJECTABLE THERAPIES

**Interferon beta-1a (Betaseron)**, a preparation of interferon beta-1b (8 million units, or 250 micrograms [mcg]), was the first medication to be approved for treatment of the MS disease process. Early studies of the drug were carried out on patients with established relapsing-remitting MS. They demonstrated a reduction in the number and severity of attacks, as well as a reduction of the number of lesions seen on the MRI brain scan. Longer term studies are showing some modification in the rate of progression of the disease as well.

The drug is self-injected under the skin every other day, using a technique similar to the way a person with diabetes uses insulin. It does cause some side effects, which usually are manageable and tolerable. These include mild flu-like symptoms after the injections, which can be relieved by simple analgesics taken before the injections. The flu-like symptoms almost always disappear with time. Local redness may occur at the injection site, which usually fades over the next week or so. Should side effects become a problem for you, your MS nurse will be able to suggest ways to help you manage them. About one in four patients will develop antibodies to the drug, and this may necessitate switching to a non-interferon drug such as glatiramer acetate (Copaxone), as the antibodies may decrease the effectiveness of the drug. There is increasing information indicating that those who started on Betaseron many years ago are showing long-term benefit from the drug, particularly those who started on the drug early in the course of the disease.

A generic form of interferon beta-1b has been recently available from Novartis as **Extavia**, which is an identical drug to Betaseron.

**Interferon beta-1a (Avonex)** a preparation of interferon beta-1a (6 million units, or 30 mcg), has also been shown to be safe and effective. It is administered weekly by intramuscular injection. Avonex is approved for the treatment of relapsing-remitting MS to slow the accumulation of physical disability and decrease the frequency of relapses. It has been shown to delay a second attack of MS if used soon after a first episode. This first episode is not sufficient to diagnose MS, and is called a clinically isolated syndrome (CIS). People who have had a positive MRI and one episode that looked like an MS attack (CIS) are said to be at risk for having MS. As discussed in Chapter 2, one of the criteria for labeling someone as having clinically definite MS is having had more than one attack. The MRI may sometimes show slight brain shrinkage (brain atrophy) even early in the disease, and this drug may slow or delay that process. It has the advantage of needing to be injected only once a week. It also has a low risk of antibody formation that may inactivate the effectiveness of the drug. However, some experts believe that higher dosed, more frequently administered drugs may be more effective. It is important to discuss this issue with your physician. Avonex is an intramuscular injection (similar to the flu shot) and has an injector to help give the injection.

**Interferon beta-1a (Rebif)** (44 mcg) is similar to natural interferon beta and is administered by the subcutaneous route three times a week, usually on Monday, Wednesday, and Friday, via a pre-filled syringe. This dose demonstrated reduced relapse frequency, slower progression in disability, and fewer lesions in the brain in patients with relapsing remitting MS. Since starting a disease-modifying therapy at a low dose and gradually increasing the dose over time tends to decrease side effects, a titration pack is available to facilitate this process. About one in four people may develop antibodies to the drug, which will require consideration of a switch to a noninterferon medication such as glatiramer acetate (Copaxone). To address this issue, a new formulation of Rebif, which has reduced development of these antibodies, may be available in the future.

**Peginterferon beta-1a (Plegridy)** is a pegylated form of interferon beta-1a. The process of pegylation allows for a longer half-life of the drug so it required less frequent dosing. It is injected every two weeks subcutaneously using a pre-filled autoinjector.

**Glatiramer acetate (Copaxone)** is not an interferon. Rather, it is a *substitute antigen* that mimics myelin basic protein, an important component of the central nervous system myelin sheath, a major immune target in MS. It is given at a dose of 20 mg subcutaneously daily by injection under the skin and is well tolerated by most people. Glatiramer acetate appears to inhibit the central nervous system immune reactions that are responsible for tissue damage and the production of MS plaques in people with MS. It has been shown to reduce both the number of attacks and the number of brain lesions seen on MRI in patients with relapsing-remitting MS, but the MRI and clinical parameters take some time to have effect. Side effects are minimal compared to the interferons because Copaxone does not cause the flu-like reactions often seen with those drugs. It can occasionally cause episodes of flushing, palpitations/tachycardia, chest pain, and dyspnea (difficulty breathing), but these are very infrequent and transient and often absent on the next injection. Injection site reactions may occur with glatiramer acetate and your MS nurse can provide you with help should they become a problem. A generic form of glatiramer acetate has been approved as **Glatopa**.

**Daclizumab (Zinbryta)** is a laboratory-produced monoclonal antibody designed to inhibit certain inflammatory functions of the T lymphocytes believed to be involved in the immune reaction in MS. It is injected subcutaneously each month (150 mg) using a prefilled autoinjector syringe. Because serious liver complications and some immune conditions can occur, liver tests are required before starting and during the course of therapy.

*ORAL MEDICATIONS*

**Teriflunomide (Aubagio)** is taken as a pill once a day, and in clinical trials has reduced the number of attacks of MS by a third, reduced new lesions on the MRI, and lessened progression in about a third of the patients. You should not take teriflunomide if pregnant or planning a pregnancy, and women of child-bearing age must use an effective means of birth control and continue it two years after stopping the drug. It lasts a long time in the body, perhaps as long as two years, so any risks may last that long. In the first months on the drug there can be nausea and hair thinning but this usually passes. Some elevation of liver enzymes may occur. Some blood tests for blood cell counts and liver function are done before beginning therapy, and then liver function tests every two weeks for the first six months and then every eight weeks on therapy. The drug seems to have an effect on MS by reducing both the T cells and the B cells.

**Fingolimod (Gilenya)** was the first oral immunomodulatory therapy approved for MS. Potential adverse events with this agent include novel complications such as a slowed heart rate after the first dose (patients are closely monitored for this), macular edema, and a low risk for severe infections. The slowed heart rate after the first dose can result in death so the patient has to be carefully monitored.

Results from the study of half of the patients who did the initial trial showed they had infrequent serious infections and a very low relapse rate. Patients who took fingolimod from the beginning of the study were more likely to be relapse free (61 percent) than on placebo. As experience grows, the risk—benefit ratio of this drug will become clearer. Some deaths have occurred, so at the time of this writing the safety of the drug is being reviewed.

**Dimethyl fumarate (Tecfidera)** is an oral medication for MS (120 mg twice a day for the first week then doubled to 240 mg twice a day as the maintenance dose). It works by reducing immune activity by decreasing the activation of T lymphocytes. Because some cases of progressive multifocal leukoencephalopathy (PML) have occurred, careful monitoring of the patients on therapy is required.

*INFUSED MEDICATIONS*

**Natalizumab (Tysabri)** is delivered by a monthly intravenous infusion. It is a monoclonal antibody against alpha4-integrin that is thought to inhibit white blood cells from getting into the central nervous system and attacking nerves. Shortly after this promising new agent was released for MS, having a striking effect on reducing attacks of MS, it was voluntarily withdrawn from the market by the manufacturer as a few patients developed a serious, and often fatal, central nervous system infection called progressive multifocal leukoencephalopathy (PML). Some but not all of the cases of PML had a history of taking another drug that would also affect the immune system so the combination was of particular concern. After a careful assessment, recognizing the risks, it was re-released, with the caution about additional drugs and for careful monitoring of patients under treatment through a restricted distribution program.

The drug has been an important addition to the options for therapy because of remarkable effectiveness in reducing attacks of MS by 70 percent and resulting in smaller, fewer, and in some cases no new MRI lesions. It is generally recommended for people who have not been helped by the other MS drugs. Of the patients who developed

PML, many were still alive but often with significant disability. The risk overall has been about one in a thousand in the first two years, but it should be noted that the risk increases the longer the person is on the drug, and in those who are positive for anti- John Cunningham virus (JCV) antibodies where the risk may be as high as eight in a thousand. The risk is also greater in those who have taken another immunosuppressant drug before going on natilizumab. If a person has all three of the risk factors (over two years on the drug, positive for JCV and prior immune suppressant drug), the risk may be as high as eleven per 1,000. In January 2012, a test for the JCVs was approved by the FDA (Stratify JCV Antibody ELISA test), which will be helpful in screening for this risk factor for the development of PML.

It has been noted that those who stop natalizumab have a return of the relapses and MRI activity within a few months.

PML is an opportunistic viral infection of the brain caused by the JCV. It usually results in death or severe disability. To avoid the risk of PML, a patient being considered for natalizumab therapy will be tested to see if the JCV is present and then, when on therapy, retested periodically to make sure the JCV has not developed.

**Alemtuzumab (Lemtrada)**. Lemtrada is a monoclonal antibody that binds to the antigen CD52 on immune cells but we don't yet completely understand its mechanism in MS, although it is likely the drug modulates the immune system through depletion and repopulation of lymphocytes. It is given by infusion for patients with relapsing-remitting MS. There is not enough information as yet to tell if the benefits and risks justify use in those under 18 or over 65, or in pregnant or nursing mothers. The usual pattern of infusion is over four hours on five successive days, and a year later an infusion daily for three days. There are many potential side effects during the infusions and they occur in most people but only a small number are serious. It is important for patients to be aware of the symptoms they might experience. The neurologist will monitor the patient for any evidence of autoimmune thyroid disorders, which can occur in one out of three people who receive the infusions. Also, patients will be assessed for immune thrombocytopenia (about two in a hundred risk for this), a drop in platelets in the blood, which can cause bleeding. About three in a thousand patients might get a glomerular nephropathy, a kidney disorder. A number of different infections may also occur as the immune reactions are altered, so these must be identified and treated.

**Novantrone (mitoxantrone).** Novantrone is an antineoplastic drug that is used in some forms of cancer, but has been found in trials to reduce progression in relapsing-remitting MS patients who have entered a secondary-progressive stage of the disease. It targets T and B cells and macrophages that are involved in the immune reaction in MS. It is administered by a intravenous infusion, and this has to be done with supervision as the drug can cause damage if it gets into other tissues. Because the drug can cause damage to the heart, assessment of the cardiogram and left ventricular ejection fraction is done before therapy and before each infusion. An infusion is given every three months. Because the risk of heart effects increases as the amount of drug increases, it is usually limited to a total dose ($140 \ mg/m^2$), which is usually the amount given over about two to three years. Cardiac assessments will continue after therapy to look for any late cardiac effects. Another risk is the development of leukemia, which might occur in one patient out of four hundred treated.

**Ocrelizumab (Ocrevus).** An important addition to the therapies for MS was the approval by the FDA in late March 2017 of Ocrevus. All the other approved therapies are for relapsing-remitting MS; this is the first drug for patients with primary-progressive MS (PPMS). The patients with PPMS have been waiting a long time for a drug that would help them. The drug is a humanized monoclonal antibody that binds to CD20 on the surface of B cells and causes a depletion in the population of B cells. It is given by an intravenous infusion, 300 mg initially, repeated in two weeks and the 600 mg every six months.

## Experimental Drugs

At present, several medications are under study and if the trials show acceptable benefit and safety, applications will be made to the FDA for approval for treatment of people with MS. This is a very detailed and rigorous process, aimed at both bringing new and better therapies and also ensuring protection for patients. In the next few years we shall see a number of new effective therapies for MS.

## Sequencing of Drug Therapy

MS drugs have different ways to interfere with the immune response that is producing the disease activity. Some reduce the activity of immune cells by altering their release of cytokines, and others may prevent the immune cells from getting into the nervous system. Others act by reducing the population of cells that are involved in the immune reaction. It might then seem logical to combine drugs to get combined effects. The problems are twofold: There are safety reasons as the risk of serious side effects is increased by combining drugs, and the costs would be prohibitive. The approach instead is one of sequencing. Your physician will help you select the initial therapy that seems appropriate for you, your lifestyle, and the activity of your disease. If there is a reason to move to another drug, the selection could be based on increasing the impact of the drug, which might bring increased risk.

## Vitamin D

There is increasing evidence that vitamin D plays a role in the risk of developing MS and in the disease activity. There is some evidence that deficiency of vitamin D in the mother during pregnancy might increase the risk of MS in the child later in life. Vitamin D has a known effect on the immune system and that might explain the relationship to MS activity. It has immunomodulatory function, modifying cytokines to a more anti-inflammatory profile. As a result of a number of studies linking low vitamin D to the risk of developing MS and to relapses of the disease, many have started taking vitamin D as a treatment before there is a definitive clinical trial to demonstrate a therapeutic benefit. However, it may be difficult to carry out such a large trial, and since taking vitamin D is safe and cheap, and does not require a prescription, it is often recommended for patients. There is early evidence that the MRI activity may be reduced by vitamin D therapy. The effect of vitamin D in studies seems to be greater in the white population and in women. The most effective dose is not known but many are recommending doses in the 1,000 to 5,000 IU range. The type of vitamin D may make a difference. A recent study indicated that it was difficult to increase vitamin D blood levels in MS patients using over-the-counter low dose chole-calciferol (LDC, unhydroxylated vitamin $D_3$) but high dose ergoc-alciferol (HDE, fungal-derived vitamin $D_2$) had a greater ability to raise vitamin D levels. Despite the safety of high doses of vitamin D (up to 10,000 IU have been taken by some patients without problems), it is reasonable to have serum levels of calcium and phosphorus periodically tested to make sure there are no serious metabolic disturbances.

### Stem Cell Transplantation

There are a number of studies underway to assess the results of autologous stem cell transplantation following bone marrow suppression in MS. The method involves taking stem cells from the person, then by immunosuppressant therapy the bone marrow is suppressed. Bone marrow function in making new blood components is re-established by giving the person back their own stem cells (autologous hematopoietic cell transplant [HCT]). In the many trials underway there has been remarkable reduction in the activity of MS. They had no further activity on the MRI, no relapses, and some patients show surprising improvement. This is important, as this is a very risky and expensive procedure with a 5 percent mortality. Initially only very advanced and rapidly progressive patients were studied, so the good results are impressive as this is a group of patients who have failed on other therapies. More recent studies, following the patients for 5 to 10 years after bone marrow suppression and stem cell transplantation, have shown impressive results. After five years, almost 70 percent of the patients had no evidence of disease activity—no relapses, no progression, and no new lesions on the MRI, fulfilling the criteria of NEDA (i.e., no evidence of disease activity). This procedure would never be a practical procedure for the many hundreds of thousands of MS patients, but we will likely learn very important information that will be used to develop other approaches that are more practical, safe, and effective. It already tells us it is possible to stop the disease at least for many years, and we will see if that is permanent as time goes on. The results after five and ten years in some patients are very promising.

This is not to be confused with "stem cell injections," which have been advertised on the Internet, offered by over 350 private clinics in the United States and many in other countries, but without the necessary randomized clinical trials to show if there is any benefit.

### Biomarkers

In the future, we hope to have ways to determine the risk of developing MS, the activity of the disease, and the response to therapy by tests that can be used to monitor patients. There is a lot of research seeking *biomarkers*, which are measures of biological activity, that assess biological indicators, so we can identify and monitor MS and the response to therapy. Currently we use clinical assessment and increasingly the MRI to define the level of disease activity, but in the future we hope to have blood tests that could be used to measure different aspects, and results assessed and therapy adjusted. It would be helpful to be able to have biomarkers that identify the risk of developing MS, of monitoring the progression and changes in the disease and what therapeutic approach would work best in each patient at different stages, and how well a medical therapy is working. Recently, Australian researchers are exploring changes in a pathway in the central nervous system activated by chronic inflammation called the kynurenine pathway, which may be a biomarker for the switch in patients from the milder pattern of MS to the more progressive form. Recently a biomarker, micro-RNA, has been found to be a way to assess the amount of inflammation and tissue destruction during the course of MS, so this may be an indicator of when and how to change therapy. This is a very promising area of research that could lead to more effective ways to classify patients, design specific treatment programs, and assess their status.

## Management of Symptoms

The most common symptoms of MS include numbness, fatigue, weakness, blurred vision, poor balance, bladder frequency and urgency, and difficulty walking. It is important to recognize that although a wide range of symptoms may occur with MS, a given individual may experience only some of them and never have others. Some symptoms may occur once, resolve, and never return. Because it is such an individual disease, it is not helpful—and may be misleading and frightening—to compare yourself with someone else, who often will have different symptoms, a different pattern of disease, and a different course.

### WEAKNESS

It is common for a person with MS to have symptoms of weakness in one or both legs. Initially this may be transient, lasting days or weeks during an attack, but in some people, weakness progresses over many years as a major symptom. Because the nerves in the central nervous system have important function in the motor control over muscles, patches of demyelination may affect these fibers and cause weakness in different muscle groups, most commonly in the legs. In some people, especially those who develop the disease after the age of forty, leg weakness and spasticity may be the only symptoms of MS, progressing slowly without any acute attacks.

It is common to develop weakness during an attack of MS, but sometimes weakness may be present all the time. The pattern of weakness can be asymmetrical, involving one limb or one side more than the other, or it can seem to be only in the legs. If it comes on in an acute attack, it is treated with intravenous steroids. If it is persistent, it is important for the neurologist to decide how much is related to weakness in the muscles, how much is due to spasticity or increased tone in the muscles, and how much is contributed by a change in sensation that makes the limbs seem more clumsy. If weakness is present, it is important to increase your level of exercise to strengthen the muscles. A physical therapist can help if you experience a lot of weakness, but if the weakness is mild, you can do an exercise program on your own. It is important to remember that any muscle can be strengthened. Just as "normal" muscles can be made stronger by exercise, weak ones also can be trained and strengthened by exercise. The muscles may not return to normal, but they will be stronger than they otherwise would have been, and that is always worthwhile.

If there is a lot of weakness in a limb, various aids, such as an ankle brace for foot drop or a cane, may be necessary to help with walking until improvement is seen. Foot drop usually is first noticed when "tripping" over your foot occurs, causing the tips of shoes on the affected side to become scraped or scuffed. If weakness persists after treatment with steroids, a referral for physical therapy may be arranged so that the problems can be assessed, an exercise program developed, and any immediate problems treated. You should continue a regular exercise program even after weakness has improved (see the section "A Note About Exercise" later in this chapter).

### SPASTICITY

A complex control of muscle movements normally allows some muscles to contract and others to relax when a movement is carried out. This normal pattern can be disrupted when nerves in the central nervous system are damaged by MS, resulting in the simultaneous contraction of many muscles, both the ones that help (agonists) and those that oppose the movement (antagonists). This causes the "tone" to increase in all the muscles, the limb to feel tight, and the limb movements to be slower and less smooth. It is more difficult and more tiring to walk with legs that have spasticity.

Spasticity can be reduced by exercise and by normal use of the muscles. It is important to perform stretching exercises of the spastic, tight muscles to prevent *contractures*, a state in which the tight muscle shortens. Each muscle should be stretched fully and held for a minute (see the section "A Note About Exercise" later in this chapter).

A number of over–the–counter muscle relaxants do not work well in MS and can have side effects. An effective medication for spasticity and the symptoms that it produces (spasms, cramps, pain, aching) is baclofen (Liorisol), which can be taken in different ways depending on the symptoms, their severity, and the person's tolerance to the medication. Because some people have painful spasms only at night and minor spasticity in the daytime, a nightly dose may be all that is needed. Others need relief from spasticity all the time, and a schedule of multiple doses a day is developed. Because all patients can reach a dosage level that seems too high, causing a general feeling of weakness and drowsiness, your doctor may start you with a very low dose, perhaps half a tablet (5 mg) twice a day, and slowly increase by adding a further half tablet every 3 or 4 days until symptoms are reasonably controlled. If symptoms are helped at a low dose, the dose will be held there. If you develop side effects when the dose is increased, the effects may be eliminated by skipping a dose and going back to the previous level. Baclofen is very helpful in reducing the spasms and pain sometimes associated with spasticity, but it is only somewhat helpful in improving function that has been limited by spasticity. The level that patients can tolerate is varied and some cannot tolerate even the lowest dose. This is unfortunate as the benefits are greater with higher doses. One way to get higher doses into the nervous system has been with the baclofen pump, which requires surgical insertion of an apparatus that injects baclofen into the cerebrospinal space. It can be effective in keeping the person mobile who is requiring aids to get around, but is complex, expensive, and only available where there is a system organized to provide the service.

Tizanidine (Zanaflex) is also an effective antispasticity agent that has effects similar to those of baclofen. It is especially effective for night spasms and sometimes is effective in reducing spasticity in patients who do not respond to other agents. Its use in combination with low doses of baclofen may produce an optimal antispasticity effect with fewer side effects. It has the benefit of not having the dose-dependent weakness seen with baclofen but has the disadvantage of causing fatigue in many patients. Since people with MS already have a lot of fatigue, adding a drug that might cause more fatigue is a problem. It can be minimized by slowly increasing the dose as this therapy begins.

Dalfampridine (Ampyra) was approved by the FDA in 2010 to improve walking speed in patients with MS, the first symptomatic drug approved specifically for MS. It is a potassium channel blocker and increases the conduction in demyelinated nerves. The usual dose is 10 mg twice a day twelve hours apart. In clinical trials, about one third of patients had a 25 percent improvement in their walking speed. The improvement is lost if the drug is stopped. It is interesting to note that the improvement was seen in all groups of MS patients including those with primary progressive MS.

### DISTURBANCES OF BALANCE AND GAIT

Disturbances of balance and gait are common in MS because they can be caused by changes in different parts of the nervous system. A person may notice that he or she does not walk or stand as steadily if experiencing incoordination, weakness in one or more limbs, numbness, dizziness, vertigo, or even visual problems. One of the most troublesome causes of gait disturbance is spasticity in the muscles of the legs. For some people, this is the most limiting problem of MS. Because so much of what we do involves being mobile, this problem causes the most disability and handicap in the disease over the lifetime of many (but not all) people with MS.

In many instances, difficulty in walking comes with the various symptoms of an attack of MS, improving or clearing as the attack settles down. In other instances, it is an ongoing problem. A person with MS may have few other problems except a gait difficulty that slowly increases over a period of years. This pattern is more common in those who develop the disease later in life.

Physical therapy can be helpful for gait difficulty, and a physical therapist can show you techniques of gait training, muscle strengthening, exercises, safety hints, and the use of mobility aids.

*A Note About Exercise*: Exercise is important for everyone, especially a person with MS. A program of range-of-motion exercises is one exercise program that you should do daily, or even more than once a day if your muscles are very stiff. Each joint is put through its full range of motion to keep it healthy and lubricated and to stretch and loosen the muscles that move the joints.

A simple exercise program that anyone can manage is the 10-10-20 exercise program, in which ten general exercises are performed, each for ten repetitions, for a duration of a twenty-minute exercise period. The ten exercises are general ones that improve overall fitness. They can be altered according to individual capacity and the need to overcome specific problems or weak areas. They can be individually designed by a physical therapist and modified as needed.

Swimming has a number of advantages, although it often is more difficult to arrange on a regular basis. Swimming exercises most muscles, and some movements and exercises can be done more easily in water because the water supports the body during movement. The water should be cool because most people with MS are sensitive to heat and may be bothered by exercises that increase body heat or by warm exercise rooms. Function may be improved just by cooling in a swimming pool. Although swimming in the ocean can have the same effect, waves can easily put you off balance.

Relaxation techniques are useful and improve the enjoyment and rewards of a regular exercise program. They involve methods of learning positive relaxation of the mind and body, deep breathing, and mental imagery, combined with alternating contraction and relaxation of various muscles.

An exercise program should be regular and enjoyable. Anyone can carry out a boring exercise program for a few weeks, but not for a lifetime—which is what we all need to do. That is why many basements have a corner with almost new exercise equipment gathering dust. Some machines look terrific, but they are not very enjoyable to use, and sometimes we think that it is the machines (or physiotherapists) that are going to make us strong. YOU do the exercises, not the machine.

Exercise programs that many people enjoy include swimming, mat exercises, walking, yoga, and tai chi, but you must think about the exercises that you would find most enjoyable and can imagine still doing regularly years from now.

### SENSORY SYMPTOMS

*Numbness:* The term *numbness* covers many alterations to the sensory system that affect sensation, particularly in the skin. People may experience numbness, but more often they feel tingling, pins and needles, burning, coldness, or other sensations that are difficult to describe. The disruption to the sensory nerves can be caused by damage to the spinal cord, the brainstem, or the brain itself.

Tingling and numbness are "normal" symptoms that virtually everyone has experienced (a leg falling "asleep," dental anesthesia, cold feet in the winter), but these common occurrences are due to pressure, anesthetics, or cold to a peripheral nerve in an arm or leg, whereas MS affects the myelin of the nerves (and sometimes the underlying nerves) in the central nervous system. It may seem as if the nerve in the leg (the peripheral nervous system) is affected in MS, but in fact the demyelination is in the central nervous system. Numbness most often is felt in the ends of the limbs, the feet and lower legs, or the hands, but it can seem to rise from the legs up to the upper abdomen. Sometimes the numbness seems to have a level, as if a belt of numbness were wrapped around the abdomen; it also may be painful, with decreased sensation below the level.

Although numbness often is only a brief annoyance, it can cause other problems if it persists or only partially clears. You may drop things when your hands and fingertips are numb, even light objects such as paper, because you do not know how tightly you are gripping them. Because feeling in your fingers is decreased, you may need to use your vision to help recognize things that you could identify previously with your fingertips. You may have trouble identifying objects in your purse or pocket because numbness can decrease your ability to recognize a comb or a coin by its characteristic feel.

You may not realize that good balance involves sensing information about the muscles and tendons in the limbs, which is carried to the nervous system by sensory nerves. If numbness is present in the legs, people use their eyes to maintain good balance, and tend to look down as they walk. On the other hand, they will have more difficulty if they look up or around, and if they walk on uneven ground or in the dark.

Numbness occasionally is accompanied by disagreeable sensations called *dysesthesias*, such as burning, "creepy-crawly" feelings, or sensitive skin (sensations similar to those felt when dental anesthesia is wearing off). These disagreeable feelings usually improve as sensation improves, but they sometimes require treatment. When numbness or dysesthesias occur as part of an acute attack, it usually improves with intravenous steroids. More persistent disagreeable sensations may be reduced by a tricyclic antidepressant such as amitriptyline (Elavil). This medication, although an antidepressant, has other beneficial effects and is useful in many pain syndromes as well as disturbing sensory problems.

Some changes in sensation are described as pain, which is discussed later in this chapter. One of these is the symptom of an electric shock–like feeling in the back or limbs on flexing the neck. This occurs when there is some inflammation in the posterior columns of the cervical spinal cord, and the bending of the neck stretches these inflamed fibers, causing them to fire. The symptom is called *Lhermitte's phenomenon*, after the French neurologist who described it. It often is transient, clearing when the inflammation abates, and can be made to clear faster with intravenous steroids.

*Facial Numbness:* A common and upsetting symptom in MS is numbness on one side of the face. However, this is a minor symptom that usually clears without treatment. You might have a tingling feeling or a numbness, often described as similar to dental anesthesia, that at times can involve the gums and tongue. Symptoms around the face are perceived as more disturbing to people than the same degree of numbness elsewhere, such as the foot or hand, but facial numbness often goes away in days or a few weeks. The neurologist may also find subtle differences to various sensations in the face on examination, of which the person is unaware.

*Vision Loss*: Several types of vision problems may occur in MS. *Optic neuritis* (sometimes called retrobulbar neuritis) is an episode of demyelination in the optic nerve behind the eyeball. Because it occurs in the nerve, a physician looking in the eye during the first episode may not see anything wrong. Later, some scarring may occur in the optic nerve, and it will look pale in the back of the eye, when seen by the doctor through a hand-held instrument called an oph-thalmoscope. High-dose intravenous steroids is the standard treat-ment when one eye or occasionally both eyes are affected. Symptoms include blurred vision, loss of peripheral or "side" vision, and one or more black or "blind" spots. Total loss of vision in one eye may occur in some instances, but this will usually improve with time. Optic neu-ritis sometimes also causes pain in the eye, which clears quickly when steroid treatment is begun. Vision returns more slowly. It is common for individuals with relapsing-remitting MS to have one or more epi-sodes of optic neuritis, although many people never experience this problem.

Another visual complaint people with MS may experience is a vague feeling that their vision is not as clear as it should be, even if a recent eye examination indicates vision to be normal. The problem may be with certain contrasts in the visual fields, or with color, which causes a mild change that usually is not detected on standard eye tests. When this occurs, text with sharp contrast is easiest to read. A related symptom is a decrease in vision associated with exercise (Uhthoff's phenomenon), which is probably related to an increase in body heat that affects nerve conduction. Vision returns when the person stops exercising and cools down.

Some people with MS experience double vision and complain that they cannot see well. Actually, the vision in each eye separately may be normal, but the eyes do not focus together. Although it is annoying, double vision usually clears on its own or responds to intravenous steroids. It is rarely a persistent problem and can be temporarily relieved by patching one eye.

Another problem with eye control that may be experienced as a visual problem is *nystagmus*. When your physician asks you to move your eyes in different directions, he or she is testing eye movements and control. Nystagmus is a regular fine jerkiness of the eyes that may occur when looking to the sides, which usually is not noticed by the patient. Sometimes the eyes operate differently in that situation, with one having more jerkiness than the other. This causes a sensation that the environment is moving (oscillopsia) or looks double when looking to the sides. In some people, the pupillary response to light is slowed, experienced as difficulty with bright lights, especially while driving at night. Glasses with photosensitive lenses usually compensate for this problem.

All that affects vision is not MS, and you should have regular eye examinations to see if you need glasses to correct the vision changes and eye problems that occur in all of us with age.

*Pain*: At one time, it was believed that pain was unusual in MS. We now know that pain, in one form or another, occurs in more than half of all people who have the disease. It may take the form of an aching in muscles, shooting pains, jabbing facial pain, or discomfort from burning, tingling, or other sensory changes. The first step is to determine the specific cause of the pain. Not all pain is the result of MS, so other problems must be considered. Since pain problems in MS have specific treatments, as does pain from other causes, it is important to identify the underlying cause.

The pain of spasms and cramps in the large muscles of the legs that occur when tone is increased by spasticity can be reduced by

> *Remember that not all symptoms in people with MS are due to the MS, as all the problems that occur in anyone else can also occur in the person with MS.*

Joint pain, back pain, abdominal pain, headaches, and other problems may be due to conditions that have nothing to do with MS and should be investigated and treated just as they would if MS were not present.

physical therapy, exercise, relaxation techniques, passive stretching, massage, and local cold. The pain associated with spasticity can often be effectively reduced with baclofen or tizanidine (Zanaflex).

*Facial Pain:* A type of nerve pain that can occur in the face, called *trigeminal neuralgia,* is characterized by a sharp, jabbing, knife-like pain, usually over the cheek and sometimes over the eye on one side. Although it can occur as an isolated syndrome in the elderly, it often indicates the underlying demyelinating process of MS in a younger person. Several types of pain occur in the face, including temporomandibular joint (TMJ) pain, tension headache, and migraine. If trigeminal neuralgia is the cause, it is treated with a group of medications that decrease the nerve firing. The initial treatment usually is carbamazepine (Tegretol), to which most people quickly respond well. In those few people who have unacceptable side effects, baclofen, diphenylhydantoin (Dilantin), gabapentin (Neurontin), or duloxetine hydrochloride (Cymbalta) is substituted.

A small number of people do not tolerate these medications, lose the beneficial drug effect over time, or do not respond to them. In such cases, a surgical procedure may be considered. It usually is done on an outpatient basis by a needle procedure through the face into the trigeminal (fifth cranial) nerve. This is usually successful. Trigeminal neuralgia associated with MS is due to the presence of a plaque in the connections of the fifth cranial nerve in the brainstem. Although it can cause severe facial pain, trigeminal neuralgia usually is successfully managed. It is not uncommon for the problem to return months or years after it has been controlled, but treatment can be restarted if it does.

*Hearing Changes:* It is unusual for people with MS to notice any change in hearing other than that seen in the normal population, but MS can on occasion cause a decrease in hearing. More commonly, a subtle change can be noted on specific testing of the hearing system, but without producing noticeable symptoms. Significant hearing change due to MS is rarely a problem and, when acute episodes of hearing loss do occur, full recovery can be expected.

## BLADDER AND BOWEL SYMPTOMS

*Bladder Control:* The most common symptoms of bladder involvement in MS are the need to urinate *often* (frequency) and the need to urinate *now* (urgency). If these symptoms are particularly troublesome, involuntary wetting (incontinence) can occur because of difficulty getting to the bathroom in time. Many people manage this by being aware of their symptoms and taking opportunities to urinate regularly. Markedly restricting fluid intake, which seems to be a logical method of dealing with the problem, is actually a bad idea; your kidneys and bladder need a continuous flow of fluids to excrete wastes and minimize the opportunity for infection.

If frequency and urgency are more serious problems and cannot be managed by simple measures, medications such as oxybutynin chloride (Ditropan), propantheline bromide (Pro-Banthine), tolterodine tartrate (Detrol), or flavoxate hydrochloride (Urispas) may control the problem. It is important to determine that urinary retention is not present before these medications are initiated. A number of problems with the bladder can occur in MS, each of which needs a specific approach to management. If simple measures and these medications are not sufficient to control the problem, a urologic assessment is needed to see if other approaches are required.

It is important to know that bladder problems are common in MS and that they can be managed with simple measures in most cases, but also that they can lead to serious complications if untreated. Urinary infection in men should always be explored further, and recurrent urinary tract infection in women also requires investigation. If burning or painful urination occurs, especially when the urine is cloudy and has a foul odor, you probably have a bladder infection and need to be in touch with your physician right away.

Bladder symptoms sometimes can be reduced by drinking about eight glasses (64 ounces total) of fluid daily, limiting citrus juices (orange, grapefruit, and tomato juices), and adding cranberry juice or cranberry tablets several times daily, which reduce infections.

*Bowel Control*: Bowel control problems (primarily constipation) are less common than bladder problems, and in most cases they also can be managed by simple methods. The first step is to maintain a regular bowel schedule. Try to have a bowel movement each day after breakfast because establishing a regular daily pattern avoids constipation and a tendency to irregular bowel movements as a result of inactivity. Each day take the time to sit and try at the same time—do not wait until you feel like going to the bathroom—to try to develop a regular reflex timing for bowel movements. Your diet should be high in fiber, including a serving of bran each day, and there should be adequate fruits and vegetables in your meals. Drinking enough fluid is also critical, as hard, dry stool is the most common cause of constipation.

Another factor in bowel health is exercise—this helps maintain good bowel function in everyone, but it is especially important when you have MS. Loss of bowel control is a more serious problem and can be managed by altering diet and some exercises, and in some cases medication will help. A consultation with a gastroenterologist may be needed if the bowel problems persist, especially if there is poor bowel control, because this problem can discourage a person from taking part in many social and family activities.

### OTHER SYMPTOMS

*Fatigue*: People with MS may notice two patterns of fatigue. One is a feeling of tiredness and weakness that occurs with increasing exercise or other physical activity. For instance, walking may be fine at the onset, but your legs may become increasingly heavy and tired after walking a long distance, with some dragging of the feet. Strength is recovered and you can continue again after sitting down and resting for a brief time.

Another kind of fatigue is a general feeling of exhaustion, which can be more annoying and limiting. This can be mild or severe, intermittent or continuous. You may experience this type of fatigue quite suddenly during a normal day, which may come over you like a wave, making it difficult to continue with whatever you are doing.

More commonly, a general fatigue is present no matter how much or how little you do. It may be aggravated by overdoing activity or getting less sleep, but it may be present even if you do nothing and have had a good night's sleep. When we ask people with MS to list the symptoms that bother them the most, fatigue usually is at the top of the list; it also is the most common.

Most people learn to modify their day in ways that allow them to manage fatigue, such as taking brief rests or even occasional naps. Others say that they cannot do this because of the nature of their work or responsibilities, and they push through the fatigue without causing any problems. It simply makes you tired to overdo it when you have fatigue; it does not worsen your MS. The most common problem from overdoing things is to be more tired. It is common for people to say they can push through their work or task but that they pay for this effort with several days of increased fatigue. Some find their fatigue occurs at the same time each day, which may allow for some restructuring of activities in work or other schedules to manage the fatigue better.

Most people with MS say that the fatigue they experience feels abnormal, unlike the normal tiredness that everyone experiences. Most neurological diseases are not associated with this pattern of tiredness, although a number of other autoimmune diseases do exhibit unusual fatigue. Because it is so "different" and so common in MS, it is surprising that it was not recognized as a characteristic symptom of MS until recently. If you are experiencing fatigue, it is important to take a careful look at your typical day. You are subject to the same fatigue from overactivity as anyone else and the fatigue you are experiencing may not be due to MS.

*Cognitive Impairment:* People with MS, sometimes even those with a new diagnosis, may experience difficulty remembering things, finding the right words, or concentrating. These problems might reflect *cognitive impairment*—problems with thinking and memory that occur in about 50 to 60 percent of people with MS, which are generally unrelated to disease duration or seriousness of other symptoms. Fortunately, most people do not have extensive difficulty, and compensatory activities can be introduced, such as establishing regular routines (e.g., always putting the house keys in the same place), relying more on written information (such as written driving directions), and using a day calendar to track important activities. Formal testing can be done to identify any problems you are having so that a management plan can be tailored to your needs. If you are concerned about cognitive function, discuss this with your MS doctor, nurse, or mental health professional so that the issue can be addressed.

*Tremor:* Everyone has some tremor (to see the normal physiologic tremor, put a piece of paper on top of your outstretched hand). Multiple sclerosis may be accompanied by different types of tremor, ranging from annoying to fairly disabling. There are a variety of approaches to controlling them, some of which people learn on their own. For example, bracing the forearm against the side or on a hard surface reduces arm and hand tremor. Another variation is to have a method of immobilization that is used for some specific task, such as writing, but is removed when the task is completed. Physical and occupational therapists may use *patterning*, repeating movements to make them smoother and more automatic. Adding weights to the limb may reduce tremor, and adaptive equipment can be useful.

Medication is only partially effective, and some of the drugs tried in the past seemed to give only limited assistance and caused side effects. Perhaps the only drugs that may have a significant effect are beta blockers such as propranolol (Inderal). Mild sedatives and tranquilizers may help, but they probably are only worthwhile when you have some other need for a sedative, such as tension or anxiety, that aggravate tremor. There are studies showing that selective injections of onabotulinum toxin-A can improve marked tremor. Although this can weaken the muscles injected, this was found to be mild and resolved in a few weeks. Stereotactic brain surgery has been used in selected cases, but this is unusual and carries significant risk.

*Vertigo:* Vertigo is the sensation that many people call "dizziness," but since that term can mean different things, it is necessary to explain exactly what you feel. Vertigo has the sensation of movement, whether it seems that the room is moving or turning or that *you* seem to be moving. If it is severe, the room seems to be spinning, or you may feel like you are tipping or falling or that the floor is coming up to meet you. This sensation usually is due to a disturbance in the vestibular system of the middle ear or its connections within the brainstem and brain. In MS, the problem most often is in the nerve connections in the brainstem. It usually is transient, lasting hours or occasionally weeks; it is unusual for it to last much longer. If it persists, it can be treated by stimulating the vestibular system or by suppressing the vestibular reflexes with medication. If the onset of vertigo is acute and lasts for many days, it can be treated by intravenous steroids, but it usually resolves by itself. When vertigo is worsened by movement, as it often is, paradoxically the problem can be reduced by purposely stimulating the vertigo. Thus, positional exercises can be done using a simple method on a soft surface such as a bed. The vestibular system is stimulated by falling onto the bed to one side three times (the vertigo lessens each time), then to the other side, and then backward. There often is a position of comfort when a person has vertigo, with fewer symptoms when lying on one side and more symptoms when lying on the other side, and with the head supported at a certain angle. Sedatives are helpful, as is diazepam (Valium), which suppresses the vestibular reflex.

Vertigo can be mild, experienced as a slight swimming feeling in the head. Mild nausea and poor concentration often are associated with this. Again, positional exercises and an exercise program are more helpful than sitting still, which is the natural tendency.

*Seizures.* Seizures are not common in MS but occur in about 6 percent of patients. They usually are effectively treated with common anticonvulsants such as phenytoin (Dilantin) or carbamazepine (Tegretol). An unusual type of "seizure" is a localized spasm that is more like a major muscle spasm than an epileptic seizure and often occurs on one side of the body. Such spasms also respond to medication such as carbamazepine.

*Facial Weakness.* Facial weakness can occur suddenly in MS, although it is uncommon. When it does happen, especially early in the course of the disease, it may resemble Bell's palsy, a benign form of acute facial palsy that often follows a viral infection. Both Bell's palsy and the facial weakness of MS respond to steroids. In MS, no treatment may be needed if the weakness is mild or is already rapidly improving on its own.

## *Summary*

MS brings with it many uncertainties about the future. However, what is certain is that MS is treatable, with many new therapies on the horizon. You have every reason to be optimistic about your future and the promise of better treatments to come. Be sure you have the best health care team for your needs, then work closely with them, and your MS society, to maintain the highest possible quality of life.

# CHAPTER 5

# Unconventional Medicines and Multiple Sclerosis

People who are recently diagnosed with MS often look to unconventional and alternative medicines in the hopes of finding something that might be helpful for their disease or their symptoms. There are hundreds of these therapies available from health food stores, on-line, or from therapists. How can you find information that is reliable about so many products and procedures, and evidence about whether a product or therapy is effective and safe? There is great variability in the quantity and quality of information about these therapies, sometimes coming only from the person selling the therapy, but in others there may be clinical studies allowing you to judge the claims. Also, some are cheap and others expensive. Some are safe and others have known serious side effects and complications. Consequently, it is especially important to be knowledgeable and cautious in this area.

This chapter provides background information about unconventional medicine, strategies for evaluating unconventional therapies, and MS-specific information about unconventional therapies that are popular or are particularly relevant to MS.

## Definitions

*Unconventional medicine* is a term that is surprisingly difficult to define. Part of the difficulty is that many different terms are used. In addition to *unconventional medicine*, other frequently used terms include *alternative medicine*, *complementary medicine*, and *integrative medicine*. These are often referred to as CAM, for complementary and alternative medicine, referring to treatments that are not part of standard medical care. One of the more commonly used terms is *unconventional medicine*. This is sometimes defined as therapies that are not typically taught in medical schools or generally available as standard care in hospitals. However, this definition is awkward because it states what unconventional medicine *is not*, as opposed to what it *is*. Also, this definition is a "moving target" because it depends on the medical traditions of the country in which it is used, and in some countries, including the United States, many medical schools now offer courses in unconventional medicine. Also, if something unconventional can be shown to be effective it may then become standard care.

There are many other definitions of unconventional medicine. One definition that is more precise, but also more complex, is provided by the National Institutes of Health (NIH). There is a branch of the NIH that provides information and research on CAM called the National Center for Complementary and Alternative Medicine.

In the NIH definition, unconventional medicine is subdivided into categories. These categories, with representative examples, include:

- Biologically based therapies: Dietary supplements, diets, bee venom therapy
- Mind-body therapies: Guided imagery, hypnosis, meditation
- Alternative medical systems: Traditional Chinese medicine, ayurveda, homeopathy

- Manipulative and body-based therapies: Chiropractic, reflexology, massage

- Energy therapies: Therapeutic touch, magnets

Other terms refer to the way in which the therapies are used. Unconventional therapies that are used instead of conventional medicine are known as *alternative medicine*, while unconventional therapies that are used in conjunction with conventional medicine are called *complementary medicine*. An even broader term, *integrative medicine*, refers to the combined use of conventional and unconventional medicine.

There have been many studies of the use of CAM in the general population and in people with MS. In studies in several countries, it has been found that about one half to three fourths of people with MS use some form of unconventional medicine, usually in conjunction with therapies recommended by their physicians. In other words, the unconventional medicine is used as *complementary medicine*.

## Evidence for the Safety and Effectiveness of Therapies

Before using an alternative therapy it is important to get information on what evidence there is for its effectiveness and also its risks. Often the claims of benefit and safety commonly come from personal stories or from people selling the remedy, but without any published clinical trials or convincing scientific evidence.

Statements that things are "natural" are insufficient to guarantee either benefit or freedom from side effects. That a therapy has been around a long time, even centuries, is also not assurance of benefit. Bleeding was used a therapy for thousands of years until some of the earliest clinical trials showed it was not helpful and even harmful in some patients. Different types of evidence may be available to determine the safety and effectiveness of unconventional as well as conventional therapies. Information about a therapy may be based on personal stories, theoretical arguments, experimental studies, or clinical trials of people with MS. When reviewing information about a therapy, it is important to determine the strength of available evidence. Some CAM literature does not distinguish between the various levels of evidence and may make very strong recommendations on the basis of weak evidence.

Ideally, for any therapy, whether conventional or unconventional, there should be scientific evidence for the claimed benefits, and clear evidence for the risks.

People with MS who are interested in CAM should use a careful and thoughtful approach that is similar to that used for conventional therapies for which the evidence is limited. It is important to obtain unbiased MS-relevant information, evaluate the safety and effectiveness of the therapy, and discuss the therapy with your physician or other conventional health care provider. If a therapy is pursued, there should be a plan for monitoring for an expected response. If that response does not occur, the therapy should be discontinued and other approaches considered. It is important to use caution, realize that the safety and effectiveness information about most CAM therapies is limited, and recognize that there is a certain degree of risk in pursuing any CAM therapy.

## Using Complementary and Alternative Medicine

It can be reasonable to use CAM in some circumstances, such as taking a treatment that seems safe for mild fatigue or mild muscle stiffness, or for symptoms for which conventional medicine has no effective therapies or only partially effective therapies. On the other hand, a serious disease such as MS should not be treated initially or exclusively with CAM therapies when there are effective therapies supported by clinical trial evidence of safety and benefit.

Some CAM books make erroneous claims about MS, some of which are potentially dangerous. One frequent misunderstanding is that because MS is an immune disease, it should be treated by stimulating the immune system with dietary supplements. This is incorrect. MS is an immune disease, but it is characterized by *excessive and abnormal* immune system activity. As a result, agents that have been proven to be effective in MS generally *decrease or modulate* the immune system activity.

Features of some CAM therapies that should raise concerns:

- "Secret ingredients," or little objective information about safety or effectiveness
- Extremely strong claims about effectiveness, such as claims that a single therapy is effective for many different conditions
- Use of "testimonials" in which individuals make strong claims about effectiveness

There are common misconceptions about dietary supplements, which include vitamins, minerals, and herbs. Some supplements are claimed to have therapeutic effects and no side effects, which is not true. Supplements, especially herbs, are similar to medications and contain chemicals that may produce beneficial effects but may also cause side effects. Also, it is sometimes claimed that "more is better," especially with vitamins and minerals, which can be not only incorrect but dangerous. Finally, it is sometimes stated that "natural" compounds are safe and beneficial, but some can be toxic, especially if taken in high doses, and many can have harmful interactions when taken with other medications.

## Unconventional Therapies Relevant to MS

For some individuals, the thoughtful use of CAM therapies, especially in combination with conventional medicine, may allow for an individualized treatment plan and provide hope, control, and a sense of empowerment. The remainder of this chapter provides MS-relevant information about CAM therapies that have been specifically studied in MS, are used commonly in the general population or by people with MS, or raise specific safety concerns.

*Acupuncture and Traditional Chinese Medicine*

Acupuncture is one component of traditional Chinese medicine (TCM). Other components include traditional Chinese herbs, nutrition, exercise, stress reduction, and massage. TCM is based on a theory of body function that is very different from that of Western medicine. Specifically, it is believed that energy, or *qi*, flows through fourteen major pathways, or *meridians*, on the body. There is also a balance of opposites, which are known as *yin* and *yang*. According to TCM, disease occurs when there is disturbance or disharmony of energy. With acupuncture, thin, metallic needles are inserted in specific points on the meridians. It is believed that the insertion of acupuncture needles alters the flow of energy in such a way that it produces therapeutic effects.

There is limited information about *acupuncture* in people with MS. There have been a number of small and poorly designed trials to assess acupuncture in the treatment of MS but these have not been definitive enough to indicate effectiveness and acupuncture is not recommended in the treatment of MS. In fact, the theory of acupuncture is that it might stimulate the immune system, and there have been suggestions that it may worsen MS. There is better evidence for benefit of acupuncture in pain, and it may have a place if the MS patient is seeking relief of pain rather than treatment of the MS. Acupuncture is usually well tolerated, especially when it is done by a well-trained acupuncturist. Sterile needles should be used to avoid infections, including hepatitis and AIDS. Acupuncture is moderately expensive, especially as it often involves repeated treatments. When done by a well-trained therapist it is low risk.

The safety of *Chinese herbal medicine* has not been well characterized, especially in people with MS. There is a theoretical risk of worsening MS with immune-stimulating herbs, which include Asian ginseng, astragalus, and maitake and reishi mushrooms. In addition, one herb that mildly suppresses the immune system, thunder god vine (*Tripterygium wilfordii)*, may produce serious side effects, including death. Chinese herbal medicine is a low-to-medium cost therapy, but with some risks and uncertain benefit.

## Marijuana (Cannabis)

For years, it has been claimed that marijuana, also known as *cannabis*, is an effective treatment for MS. Marijuana, which is still illegal in many countries, contains compounds known as cannabinoids. These compounds, which include tetrahydrocannabinol (THC), produce specific biochemical effects in the body. Marijuana may be smoked or ingested. There are prescription medications that contain cannabinoids. In the United States, THC is available as dronabinol (Marinol). In Europe, Canada, and Australia, a synthetic form of THC is available as nabilone (Cesamet). An oral spray form of cannabis (Sativex) is approved in Canada for treating MS pain.

Cannabinoids exert several biological effects that, on a theoretical basis, could be therapeutic for MS. First, they bind to proteins in the central nervous system that suppress excessive nerve cell activity. This could result in a decrease in pain and muscle stiffness (spasticity). Also, cannabinoids bind to another type of protein on immune cells and mildly suppress the immune system. It is possible that cannabinoids could be beneficial in the course of MS but this has not been proven in clinical trials. It has some benefit in the treatment of pain and spasticity in MS.

There are mixed results in studies. In several surveys of people with MS who have smoked marijuana, symptoms commonly reported to be improved include pain, spasticity, depression, and anxiety. Importantly, surveys such as this are not rigorous enough to provide definitive evidence for effectiveness. Actual clinical studies of the effects of smoked or oral marijuana on MS symptoms are of variable quality.

Significant risks are associated with smoking marijuana, including nausea, vomiting, sedation, increased risk of seizures, and poor pregnancy outcomes. Driving may be impaired for up to 8 hours after smoking marijuana. High doses of marijuana may impair heart function, decrease reaction time, and produce coordination and visual difficulties. Chronic marijuana use may cause heart attacks, impair lung function, cause dependence and apathy, and increase the risk of cancer of the lung, head, and neck. An apathy syndrome develops in some chronic users. There is evidence that it may worsen schizophrenia and depression. Many patients do not like this as a form of therapy as it makes them feel "stoned" and they wanted pain relief, not to feel these other effects. Needless to say, there are legal problems if marijuana is used where the laws prohibit its use. It is legally available to MS patients for pain and spasticity in Canada, and steps toward legalization of marijuana are being taken, as in many U.S. states. Smoked marijuana and prescription medications containing cannabinoids are of low-moderate cost. Marijuana, where it is legal, has been used for some symptom relief of pain and spasticity, and may have some benefit for MS. The benefit is still unclear and under study.

### Chiropractic Medicine

Chiropractic medicine is one of the most popular forms of CAM in the United States, with over 60,000 practitioners. Chiropractic medicine is based on the concept that the nervous system plays a critical role in health and that many diseases are caused by abnormal pressure of bones on the nerves in the spine. There are within chiropractic two groups—those who adhere to the original concepts and those who add newer ideas and other approaches to their practice.

Chiropractors believe that misalignments of the bones of the spine cause abnormal pressure on the nerves that travel from the spinal cord to the muscles and organs of the body that results in impaired muscle and organ function. Spinal manipulation techniques, known as "adjustments," are thought to normalize bone positions and restore normal function.

There are no well-designed studies that document that spinal manipulation or other chiropractic methods can alter the disease course in MS. Isolated clinical reports have described improvement in some MS symptoms with chiropractic treatment, but there are no systematic clinical studies of chiropractic treatment for MS symptoms.

Chiropractic treatment is generally well tolerated, but complications of manipulation can occur, and some are serious. One of the more common adverse effects is aching muscles, which may be present for one to two days after manipulation. A rare, but serious, complication associated with neck manipulation is stroke when arteries in the neck are damaged. Very rarely, low back manipulation may cause compression of the nerves of the lower spine (cauda equine syndrome). Pregnant women, people taking anticoagulant medications, and people with spinal bone fractures, spine trauma, significant disc herniations, bone cancer or infection, severe osteoporosis, and severe arthritis should avoid chiropractic therapy. Importantly, since chiropractors are not as well trained in diagnosis as physicians, people with serious diseases or conditions should be evaluated and treated by a physician and should not substitute chiropractic medicine for conventional medicine. Chiropractic therapy is of moderate cost but can be higher if a long course of therapy is carried out.

### Cooling Therapy

Cooling therapy is a form of CAM that is unique to MS. It has been known for years that changes in body temperature may significantly affect MS symptoms. Specifically, small increases in body temperature ($32.9°F$, $0.5°C$) may worsen symptoms, while small decreases may improve symptoms. Consequently, various cooling methods have been developed. These methods range from simple techniques, such as drinking cold liquids and staying in air-conditioned areas, to complex methods, such as using specially designed cooling suits. Cooling suits may be *passive* or *active*. Passive garments use ice packs for cooling; active garments use circulating coolants.

Beneficial effects of cooling garments have been noted in several clinical studies. Unfortunately, some of these reports are preliminary and most of the studies have been small and not rigorously conducted. Among these studies, improvement in fatigue is frequently seen. Other symptoms showing transient improvement include leg weakness, spasticity, difficulty walking, bladder dysfunction, sexual difficulties, visual changes, speech difficulties, cognitive difficulties, and incoordination. The results of the most rigorous cooling study in MS showed by objective measures that cooling was associated with mildly improved walking and visual function. By subjective measures, cooling improved fatigue, strength, and cognition. Cooling garments may be especially well suited for those who are most heat sensitive.

The use of cooling garments is usually well tolerated. Some people feel uncomfortable when cooling begins, and some cooling suits are cumbersome, particularly the active circulating suits that require attachment to a motor to keep a coolant circulating. Some people with MS have a paradoxical sensitivity to cold, in which case cooling may actually *worsen* symptoms. This is by a different mechanism, as cooling can further tighten the muscles that are stiff and spastic.

Costs of cooling are dependent on the method used. Simple techniques are of low cost. Passive cooling garments are of moderate cost. Active cooling devices are expensive.

### Dental Amalgam Removal

Removal of dental amalgam has been proposed as a treatment method for MS. For more than 150 years, cavities have been filled with dental amalgam, which is composed of mercury as well as silver, copper, tin, and zinc. Amalgam is currently used in about 80 to 90 percent of tooth restorations.

Although some have argued without convincing evidence that the mercury in dental amalgam might be related to the cause of MS on the grounds that if some mercury were absorbed it could damage the nervous system or its presence could generate electrical activity. There is no convincing evidence that mercury or the presence of dental amalgam has anything to do with causing MS, so there is no reason to remove the dental fillings. Paradoxically, removal of mercury fillings may increase the blood levels of mercury.

Studies of trace metals in MS using a Slow Poke Atomic Reactor showed no abnormal levels in MS patients and no difference from a normal control group. Dental amalgam removal as a treatment for

MS is not supported by multiple professional organizations, including the National Multiple Sclerosis Society of the United States. Removal of dental fillings is moderately expensive but not recommended.

## Dietary Supplements

A wide range of compounds is included in the category of dietary supplements. Vitamins, minerals, and herbs are commonly used supplements. Other diverse compounds, including amino acids, hormones, and enzymes, are also classified as dietary supplements. In this section, dietary supplements that are popular or are relevant to MS are addressed.

### Antioxidants

Free radicals are chemicals that may injure cells in the body through a process known as *oxidative damage*. Antioxidants are compounds that can decrease oxidative damage. Commonly used antioxidants include selenium and vitamins A, C, and E. Other compounds in the antioxidant category include alpha-lipoic acid, inosine, uric acid, coenzyme Q10 (CoQ10), grape seed extract, pycnogenol, and oligomeric proanthocyanidins (OPCs). Antioxidants are sometimes specifically marketed as a treatment for MS.

There are two major reasons that antioxidants could be considered in MS. First, it could be theorized that free radicals may be involved in the pathology of MS by damaging the myelin around nerves if free radicals were released by immune cells. Also, the nerve fibers themselves, the axons, are damaged in MS through a degenerative process that may involve free radicals. Indeed, some studies indicate that oxidative damage is increased in experimental allergic encephalomyelitis (EAE), the animal model of MS, and in tissue from people with MS.

Specific studies of antioxidants in MS are very limited. Studies in EAE indicate that antioxidants may decrease disease severity. Recent studies have shown that alpha-lipoic acid and uric acid are effective in mice with EAE. Clinical studies in people with MS are currently being conducted with alpha-lipoic acid and inosine, a compound that is converted to uric acid.

Since many antioxidant compounds activate immune cells that are already excessively active in MS, further stimulation by antioxidants could potentially worsen the disease. Whether this occurs and is clinically important in MS has not been investigated and remains a theoretical risk.

The safety of many dietary supplements, including antioxidants, has not been determined in women who are pregnant or breastfeeding. Supplementation with antioxidants is a low-cost therapy.

### *Cranberry and Other Supplements Used for Urinary Tract Infections*

People with MS are prone to bladder difficulties, including urinary tract infections (UTIs). There is a long-held belief that cranberry juice and related products might prevent recurrent infections but recent studies in susceptible populations such as nursing home residents did not show any benefit over a placebo. The ideal clinical trial with cranberry has not been done in MS patients but there is little reason to believe it would be more beneficial in MS patients. There is also little evidence for two other UTI-related dietary supplements, vitamin C and bearberry.

Cranberry is inexpensive and generally well tolerated. Cranberry tablets are less expensive than juice. Cranberry may interfere with blood-thinning medications, such as warfarin (Coumadin). Long-term use of high doses may increase the risk of kidney stones and may cause gastrointestinal discomfort, loose stools, and nausea. There is insufficient information about the safety of cranberry in women who are pregnant or breastfeeding.

### *Echinacea and Other "Immune-Stimulating" Supplements*

Echinacea and several other dietary supplements are known to activate the immune system, leading some therapists to suggest that MS patients should take echinacea and other dietary supplement.

This is a potentially dangerous concept because MS is character-ized by increased immune activity and compounds that stimulate the immune system could worsen the disease. However, many dietary supplements and herbals said to stimulate the immune system actu-ally do not have any effect on the immune mechanisms so probably do not help or worsen MS.

The immune system effects of some dietary supplements have undergone limited investigation in test-tube or animal experiments. These studies have investigated components of the immune sys-tem that are excessively active in MS. Activation of these cells has been produced by echinacea and several other dietary supplements, including:

- Herbs: Alfalfa, Asian ginseng, astragalus, cat's claw, garlic, maitake mushroom, mistletoe, shiitake mushroom, Siberian ginseng, stinging nettle
- Vitamins and minerals: Antioxidant vitamins and minerals (see the preceding section on "Antioxidants"), zinc
- Melatonin

Based on scientific evidence, these compounds pose theoretical risks to people with MS.

### Ginkgo Biloba

Ginkgo biloba usually refers to the extract that is derived from the leaf of the *Ginkgo biloba* tree. Among herbs, ginkgo is one of the most extensively studied and one of the most popular. There are sev-eral effects of ginkgo that might suggest a use in MS. Ginkgo has anti-inflammatory and antioxidant effects. Also ginkgo was thought to improve cognitive function in people with Alzheimer's disease, although clinical trials have not borne this out.

Ginkgo has undergone limited investigation in MS. Ginkgo and related compounds decreased disease severity in some, but not all, studies in the animal model of MS.

Although a small study suggested it might be helpful in reducing MS attacks, a larger and more rigorously conducted trial failed to show any benefit. Thus, it does not appear to be effective for MS attacks. There are no convincing studies of ginkgo for other benefits in MS such as reducing the course of the disease or improving cognitive function, and there is growing concern about the side effects and dangers of ginkgo.

Ginkgo is usually well tolerated in low doses. It may have a blood-thinning effect and thus should be avoided in people who have bleeding disorders, or who take antiplatelet or anticoagulant medication, or are undergoing surgery. It can provoke seizures and should be used with caution by those with seizure disorders. It may also cause dizziness, rashes, headache, and gastrointestinal complaints, including nausea, vomiting, diarrhea, and flatulence. The safety of ginkgo in women who are pregnant or breastfeeding is not known. Most medicinal ginkgo is made from the leaf; in some counties the seeds are used, and these are much more dangerous. Ginkgo is inexpensive.

### St. John's Wort

St. John's wort is not a treatment for MS but is sometimes used by patients who are suffering from symptoms of depression, and depression is a relatively common symptom in patients who have MS. It is so named because it blooms around the time of the feast day of St. John the Baptist (June 24). The red pigments in its buds and flowers are associated with the blood of St. John the Baptist.

Some small studies suggested that St. John's wort had benefit in milder depression, but there was no greater effect than a placebo in a large study. There is no evidence that St. John's wort is effective for treating severe depression. It is unclear how the effectiveness of St. John's wort compares to that of the newer antidepressants known as selective serotonin reuptake inhibitors (SSRIs), such as fluoxetine (Prozac), paroxetine (Paxil), and sertraline (Zoloft).

Although St. John's wort is usually well tolerated, there are several important factors related to its use. People who are concerned they may have depression should not attempt to diagnose and treat this condition on their own. St. John's wort may worsen MS fatigue or increase the sedating effects of some medications. St. John's wort may cause a sensitivity of the skin and nerves to sunlight ("photosensitivity"), especially in those who are fair skinned. It should be avoided by women who are pregnant or breastfeeding because of possible side effects. Finally, St. John's wort may alter the levels of multiple drugs, including anticonvulsants, antidepressants, heart medications, blood-thinning medications, and oral contraceptives. St. John's wort is inexpensive.

### Valerian

People with MS are prone to sleep disorders. Valerian, an herb that has been used for more than 1,000 years, may be helpful for treating insomnia. The mechanism by which valerian might produce its actions is unclear.

Several clinical studies of variable reliability have suggested that valerian is effective for treating insomnia. Valerian is also sometimes claimed to be effective for depression and muscle stiffness (spasticity). However, due to limited clinical studies, its effects on these conditions are not known. A review of nine studies of valerian on sleep by the National Center for Complementary and Alternative Medicine at the National Institutes of Health concluded that the results, some negative and some positive, were too variable to be conclusive about whether valerian was effective in the treatment of sleep disorders.

Valerian is generally safe. It may cause sedation, which may worsen MS fatigue or increase the sedating effects of some medications. The safety of long-term use and use during pregnancy or breastfeeding has not been established. Valerian is inexpensive.

### Vitamin $B_{12}$ (Cobalamin, Cyanocobalamin)

Supplements of vitamin $B_{12}$, also known as cobalamin or cyanocobalamin, are sometimes claimed to be effective therapies for MS.

Vitamin $B_{12}$ is essential for maintaining normal nervous system functioning. Almost all people get enough vitamin $B_{12}$ from their normal diet and need no additional supplements. Exceptions are people with pernicious anemia, who cannot absorb $B_{12}$, and rarely strict vegans whose diet is so limited that they do not get enough natural $B_{12}$ in their diet. People with vitamin $B_{12}$ deficiency, like some people with MS, have injury to the optic nerves and the spinal cord. For these and other reasons, it is sometimes concluded that vitamin $B_{12}$ supplements could be effective MS therapies but there is no convincing supportive evidence.

The mechanism by which nervous system injury occurs in MS is different from that associated with vitamin $B_{12}$ deficiency. In addition, most people with MS have normal vitamin $B_{12}$ levels. For people who have normal vitamin $B_{12}$ levels, there is no evidence that vitamin $B_{12}$ supplements provide any significant beneficial effects.

Vitamin $B_{12}$ supplements are usually well tolerated. It can be taken by oral tablets or wafers, but in pernicious anemia must be taken by injection. Rarely, vitamin $B_{12}$ may cause diarrhea, rashes, and itching. Vitamin $B_{12}$ is inexpensive.

### Vitamin D and Calcium

There is a lot of research on the possible role of vitamin D in the potential cause, treatment, and prevention of MS. A large conference on vitamin D and MS evaluated the current evidence and the studies necessary to answer many questions.

Vitamin D and calcium have multiple actions in the body, including an important role in maintaining bone density. Vitamin D and calcium are relevant to people with MS because people with MS are at risk for developing osteoporosis and a less severe form of decreased bone density known as osteopenia. In addition, vitamin D and calcium are involved in the immune system function in a way that could be therapeutic for people with MS (see Chapter 4).

A possible therapeutic effect for vitamin D in MS is suggested by several studies. In the animal model resembling MS, disease severity is worsened by vitamin D deficiency and improved by vitamin D supplementation. A recent observation that will have implications for therapy trials is that the protective effects of vitamin D in the animal model of MS seemed to be in the females but not the males, suggesting that estrogen may be essential to the protective effect.

Epidemiologic studies indicate that the use of vitamin D supplements is associated with a decreased risk of developing MS, and those with low blood levels of vitamin D are at greater risk of MS than those with higher levels. This was found in a large British nurses health study and also in a study of U.S. veterans, and there are more recent supportive studies.

Unfortunately, there is very limited clinical trial information about vitamin D as a treatment of MS, although such studies are currently being designed and a few are already underway. There are short-term studies suggesting some reduction in relapses and in fewer new lesions on the MRI with vitamin D therapy. Although vitamin D research is taking many interesting directions, a large randomized clinical trial is difficult to arrange as so many people are now taking vitamin D, which is so easily available. It will be difficult to keep strict control over a large population of patients in the two groups, treatment and placebo, over a number of years.

No one knows what the dose should be, but larger and larger doses are being tried, often in the 2,000 to 5,000 IU range. A study of tolerance to high dosage showed that MS patients could tolerate a course of 40,000 IU, then lowering the dosage to 10,000 IU daily, without much difficulty. The concern would be with prolonged therapy as we do not know the overall risks of long-term treatment with high doses in MS populations.

In reasonable doses, vitamin D and calcium are usually well tolerated. Calcium may interfere with the absorption of some medications (antibiotics, thyroid medication, osteoporosis medication) and minerals (iron, magnesium, zinc). In high doses, vitamin D and calcium may cause multiple side effects. Vitamin D and calcium are inexpensive and available without a prescription.

## Diets

Many diets have been proposed as effective MS therapies. For many of these diets, there is no clear underlying rationale or clinical evidence to support their use in MS. Diets for MS that are not supported by a strong rationale or clinical data include allergen-free diets, gluten-free diets, pectin-restricted diets, fructose-restricted diets, severely sugar-restricted diets, and diets that reduce or eliminate processed foods.

On the basis of scientific, epidemiologic, animal model, and clinical trial studies, there is suggestive evidence that diets that are low in saturated fats and high in polyunsaturated fatty acids (PUFAs) may have a therapeutic effect in MS. PUFAs include omega-3 and omega-6 fatty acids. Omega-6 fatty acids include compounds known as linoleic acid and gamma-linolenic acid. Examples of omega-3 fatty acids include eicosapentaenoic acid (EPA), docosahexaenoic acid (DHA), and alpha-linolenic acid (ALA). The first PUFA-enriched diet that was extensively studied in MS was the Swank diet. Subsequently, several MS clinical studies evaluated the effects of supplementation with omega-6 and omega-3 fatty acids.

### The Swank Diet

In the 1940s, Dr. Roy Swank developed a dietary approach to MS that was low in saturated fat. With this diet, saturated fat intake is decreased to 15 grams (g) or less daily, high-fat dairy products are excluded, frequent fish meals are recommended, and 10 to 15 g of fluid vegetable oil and 5 g of cod liver oil are added to the daily diet.

Dr. Swank reported on his group of treated patients over many decades, suggesting their rate of MS attacks was decreased by 70 percent relative to the attack rate prior to entering the study. Unfortunately, there was no control group to compare these results, and no indication of how those who dropped out of the study fared, so it is difficult to know if these patients would have done the same without the dietary change. Also, over time, the number of attacks of MS is expected to come down. However he did note that compared to untreated MS patients in the literature, his patients had less frequent attacks, less progression of neurological disability, and decreased mortality. These beneficial effects were greatest in those who adhered strictly to the diet and those who were mildly affected or were early in the course of the disease. Although these findings were encouraging, it needed to be confirmed with a blinded randomized clinical trial, as his patients were not selected randomly, there was no placebo group, and the patients and the physician were not "blinded" as to who was on treatment versus on placebo, with follow-up of all patients, including those who drop out of the study. Due to these and other shortcomings, this study is not rigorous enough to provide definitive conclusions about the effectiveness of this dietary approach. It is recognized that a long-term, blinded dietary study with a control diet group is very difficult to perform. In the 1980 three studies were done and two suggested some benefit on reducing attacks and an analysis of all three together suggested some benefit on attacks and disability in the mildest cases of MS. A subsequent rigorous trial did not show a statistically significant benefit, but a trend toward benefit in disability progression.

This Swank diet is usually well tolerated. Long-term adherence to the diet may not be possible because the recommended food is not appealing. Due to the decreased meat intake in the Swank diet, people who use this dietary approach should be certain that their protein intake is adequate. Although cod liver oil, one component of this diet, is generally safe, it may rarely cause adverse effects. Cod liver oil may have a blood-thinning effect and should be used with caution by those who take aspirin or anticoagulant medication, are undergoing surgery, or have bleeding disorders. Diabetics should also use cod liver oil with caution. Finally, cod liver oil contains relatively high concentrations of vitamin A, which may be toxic in doses greater than 10,000 IU. The Swank diet is inexpensive.

### Supplementation with Omega-6 Fatty Acids

Supplementation with omega-6 fatty acids is an approach that increases the intake of polyunsaturated fatty acids (PUFAs). Most studies of omega-6 fatty acid supplementation have used sunflower seed oil or evening primrose oil. Other dietary supplements that contain omega-6 fatty acids include flaxseed oil, borage seed oil, black currant seed oil, and spirulina (blue-green algae).

As noted for the Swank diet, epidemiologic studies indicate that a high intake of PUFAs may be associated with a lower risk of developing MS. There are other findings that support the use of a diet enriched in omega-6 fatty acids. Some, but not all, studies have shown that the blood levels of PUFAs are decreased in people with MS. In addition, scientific studies show that in the body PUFAs are converted to compounds that have anti-inflammatory effects and immune system–modulating effects that, on a theoretical basis, could be therapeutic for MS.

In the animal model of MS, disease severity is worsened by deficiencies in omega-6 fatty acids and lessened by supplementation with omega-6 fatty acids. In people with relapsing-remitting MS, three placebo-controlled clinical trials have evaluated supplementation with omega-6 fatty acids as part of the low PUFA diet already mentioned. As mentioned an analysis of these diet-supplement studies showed a benefit over the placebo groups in the milder groups of MS, but no effect in those with greater disability. In studies of people with progressive MS, omega-6 fatty acid supplementation has not been effective. Evening primrose oil, a dietary supplement that contains an omega-6 fatty acid known as gamma-linolenic acid has not produced therapeutic effects in people with relapsing-remitting or progressive disease.

Supplementation with omega-6 fatty acids is usually well tolerated. The safety of long-term supplementation with omega-6 fatty acids has not been well studied. A concern has been raised that linoleic acid supplementation may increase the risk of some forms of cancer, but this has not been proven. Since supplementation with PUFAs may cause vitamin E deficiency, supplementation with vitamin E may be necessary. Evening primrose oil, and perhaps other gamma–linolenic acid–containing supplements (black currant seed oil, borage seed oil, spirulina), may rarely provoke seizures. Also, gamma–linolenic acid–containing supplements may have blood-thinning effects. Omega-6 fatty acid supplements may increase triglyceride levels and thus should be used with caution by people with elevated triglycerides. One specific supplement, borage seed oil, may contain liver toxins. The safety of black currant seed oil has not been well studied. Spirulina products may contain heavy metals, bacteria, and other contaminants. The safety of omega-6 fatty acid supplementation in women who are pregnant or breastfeeding is not known. Supplementation with omega-6 fatty acids is inexpensive.

### Supplementation with Omega-3 Fatty Acids

This approach increases the intake of omega-3 fatty acids, which include eicosapentaenoic acid (EPA), docosahexaenoic acid (DHA), and alpha-linolenic acid (ALA). EPA and DHA are present in relatively high levels in fish, especially fatty fish such as salmon, Atlantic herring, Atlantic mackerel, bluefin tuna, and sardines. Dietary supplements containing EPA and DHA include fish oil and cod liver oil. Rich sources of ALA include flaxseed oil, canola oil, and walnut oil.

The rationale for this approach is similar to that outlined for the Swank diet and supplementation with omega-6 fatty acids. In addition, immunologic studies indicate that, among the polyunsaturated fatty acids (PUFAs), the omega-3 fatty acids exert the most potent anti-inflammatory and immune-modulating effects. Also, omega-3 fatty acids appear to be important in forming and maintaining myelin, a part of the nervous system that is injured in MS.

Studies of omega-3 fatty acid supplementation in the animal model of MS are limited and conflicting. The most rigorous clinical study of this approach was a placebo-controlled trial of fish oil in people with relapsing-remitting MS. There was a trend for the treated group to show less disease progression, fewer attacks, and decreased attack duration, but these findings were minimal and not statistically significant. Therapeutic effects were noted in two uncontrolled studies, one with cod liver oil, calcium, and magnesium, and the other with fish oil, other dietary supplements, and dietary advice. A small study evaluated omega-3 fatty acid supplementation in combination with interferons or glatiramer acetate. People were treated with their MS medications along with either fish oil plus a very low-fat diet, or with olive oil and a low-fat diet. There was a trend for improved physical and emotional functioning in those taking fish oil. Both dietary interventions were associated with a decrease in relapse rate.

Fish oils are certified as generally safe for use by the U.S. Food and Drug Administration. The long-term safety of other omega-3 fatty acid supplements is not known. Increased dietary intake of ALA may increase the risk of prostate cancer. Although fish oil supplements generally do not have a significant amount of mercury, some fish, such as shark, swordfish, and king mackerel, do contain relatively high mercury levels. Fish and flaxseed oil may have a blood-thinning effect. Fish oil may impair lung function in those who are aspirin sensitive. High doses of fish oil may increase blood sugar levels in diabetics. High doses of flaxseed oil may produce cyanide toxicity. There are potential side effects that are specifically associated with cod liver oil (see the discussion of the Swank diet). For women who are pregnant or breastfeeding, the safety of omega-3 fatty acid supplements, including fish oil, is not known. Supplementation with omega-3 fatty acids is inexpensive.

## Other Types of Therapy

### Feldenkrais

Feldenkrais, a type of bodywork, teaches comfortable and efficient body movements. It is claimed to improve multiple symptoms and to provide therapeutic effects for people with MS. The retraining of movements with Feldenkrais is believed to increase the efficiency and comfort of body movements. This is claimed to improve walking stability, increase strength and coordination, and decrease stress.

Feldenkrais has undergone very limited investigation in MS and other conditions. In one small study, twenty people with MS were treated for eight weeks with either Feldenkrais or sham sessions. The treated group had significantly decreased stress and a trend for decreased anxiety relative to the sham group. This study was not rigorous enough to be conclusive.

Feldenkrais is generally safe and of low-moderate cost.

### Guided Imagery and Relaxation

Guided imagery, also known as *imagery* or *visualization*, is a relaxation method, often used in combination with other relaxation methods, such as progressive muscle relaxation. It is claimed to be effective for treating a variety of symptoms including anxiety, depression, and pain. In guided imagery, an individual creates mental images that have specific effects on the body and mind.

In one published study of thirty-three people with MS, it was found that anxiety was decreased, but these methods had no effect on depression or other MS symptoms. Guided imagery and relaxation are usually well tolerated. Relaxation may cause or worsen muscle stiffness. Imagery may cause fear of losing control, anxiety, and disturbing thoughts, and so people with psychiatric conditions should use it with caution. Guided imagery is inexpensive.

### Hyperbaric Oxygen

Hyperbaric oxygen (HBO) treatment is a form of oxygen therapy in which a person breathes oxygen under increased pressure in a specially designed pressure chamber. The oxygen content of the blood increases with the use of HBO that results in an increased amount of oxygen in different body tissues. HBO is an accepted treatment for a limited number of specific medical conditions, including carbon monoxide poisoning, burns, severe infections, gas gangrene, and decompression sickness (due to deep-sea diving). Unfortunately, there is no accepted evidence to support the use of HBO in MS. Although there was an initial trial that suggested some benefit, this has not been borne out in subsequent trials. Many clinical trials were conducted and found that HBO did not produce beneficial effects in people with MS. Two large independent reviews of all studies of HBO in MS concluded there is no therapeutic effect of HBO in people with MS and that HBO should not be used to treat MS. In addition, the Cochrane Collaboration, which conducts reviews of clinical trials, concluded that on the basis of current evidence further studies of HBO in MS are not justified. Despite the negative conclusions, the initial enthusiasm for HBO therapy resulted in numerous pressure chambers being placed in clinics, and this procedure is still available.

HBO is usually well tolerated. Reversible, mild visual symptoms may occur. Rarely, HBO may cause serious side effects, including seizures, collapsed lungs, pressure injury to the ear, and cataracts. HBO is expensive.

### *Magnetic Field Therapy (Electromagnetic Therapy)*

There are two main forms of this therapy: static, permanent magnets and pulsed electromagnetic fields. Static magnetic therapy involves the use of magnetized devices such as bracelets, belts, and mattress pads. Although these devices are widely available and sold for many different conditions there is no evidence or accepted rationale for their use.

Pulsed electromagnetic field therapy, which has been more extensively studied in MS than static magnets, uses devices that produce pulsing, electromagnetic fields at a specific frequency. In one MS study, devices with a strong, pulsing magnetic field were placed on the spine. In other studies, small devices with weak, pulsing magnetic fields were placed on the legs on specific acupuncture points.

In four placebo-controlled clinical trials of pulsed electromagnetic therapy in MS three of these have involved weak magnetic fields, and one involved strong magnetic fields applied to the spine. In the study of strong magnetic fields applied to the spine, spasticity was found to be significantly decreased in the treated group compared to the placebo group. In the three studies with the weaker devices, beneficial effects on spasticity and improvement in pain, bladder function, hand function, fatigue, and quality of life were found in some studies. Given the variable findings and lack of rigor in some of these studies, further investigation is needed to clarify whether this therapy has any definite beneficial effects.

Short-term use of magnetic field therapy is usually well tolerated. The long-term effects of this treatment have not been investigated. Treatment with a strong magnet on the spine may produce dizziness and a band-like sensation around the torso. The weaker devices may cause headaches. Pregnant women and people with pacemakers or other electronic medical devices should consult with their physician before using these devices. Devices with a weak magnetic field are of low-moderate cost. Devices with a strong magnetic field are for experimental use and are not generally available.

### Massage

Massage, one of the oldest forms of treatment, is a form of bodywork in which soft tissue is manipulated with pressure and traction. The common forms of massage in Western countries are derived from Swedish massage, which was developed by a Swedish physician in the nineteenth century.

In one study of massage therapy, twenty-four people with MS were assigned either to a control group that received "standard medical care" or to a massage treatment group that received standard medical care in combination with twice-weekly, in-home massage therapy. Relative to the start of the study, the treatment group exhibited less anxiety and depression after the first massage session and improvement in self-esteem, body image, "image of disease progression," and social functioning at the end of the five-week study. The results of this study are promising but not definitive. Larger studies with more well-matched groups and more rigorous study design are needed.

Massage is usually well tolerated. Minor side effects include headache, lethargy, and muscle pain. More serious side effects, such as bone fractures and bleeding into the liver, are possible but rare. Massage should be avoided or used with caution by people with the following conditions: clotted blood vessels (thrombosis), burns, skin infections, open wounds, bone fractures, osteoporosis, cancer, pregnancy, and heart disease. Massage is readily available and of low-moderate cost.

### Reflexology

Reflexology is a type of bodywork in which manual pressure is applied to specific areas. These areas, which are usually on the feet but may also be on the hands and ears, are thought to correspond to specific organs and distant parts of the body. It is believed that pressure at specific reflexology sites improves energy flow to the corresponding body parts. This improved energy flow is claimed to improve health.

In one controlled study of reflexology, seventy-one people with MS were treated for eleven weeks with either reflexology or non-specific massage of the calf area. Relative to the control group, the people treated with reflexology exhibited significant improvement in paresthesias, urinary symptoms, and spasticity. Larger and more rigorous studies with lower dropout rates are needed.

Reflexology is generally well tolerated. Mild side effects include fatigue, foot pain, and changes in bowel and bladder function. Reflexology should be avoided or used with caution by people with bone or joint conditions of the feet and by those with other foot conditions such as gout, ulcers, and vascular disease.

### Tai Chi

Tai chi is a traditional Chinese martial art that has been practiced for centuries in China. There has been recent interest in tai chi in some Western countries. Tai chi is characterized by a series of body postures that are linked by slow, graceful movements.

In one study, nineteen people with variable levels of MS disability were enrolled in an eight-week tai chi program. At the end of the program, there was improvement in walking speed and muscle stiffness, as well as in vitality, social and emotional functioning, and ability to carry out physical and emotional roles. Another study of sixteen people with MS used the tai chi principle of "mindfulness of movement," which involves developing moment-to-moment awareness of movement, breathing, and posture. Relative to the control group, which received "current available care," the treated group did not improve in balance but did improve in multiple MS-associated symptoms, as assessed by patients and by their relatives. Relative to pre-treatment, the treated group improved in balance. Larger and more rigorous studies are needed.

Tai chi is usually well tolerated. Mild side effects include strained muscles and joints. It may worsen MS-related fatigue. It should be avoided or used with caution by those with severe osteoporosis, acute low back pain, significant joint injuries, and bone fractures. Tai chi is low-moderate cost.

### Yoga

Yoga is a mind-body approach that was developed in India thousands of years ago. It is derived from the Sanskrit word for *union* and is meant to unite the mind, body, and spirit. In *hatha yoga*, one of the more popular forms of yoga, the three main components are breathing, meditation, and posture.

In spite of yoga's popularity in some countries, there are very limited clinical studies of its effects in MS and other diseases. There is one well-designed, controlled trial of yoga in MS. In this six-month study, sixty-nine people with MS were randomized to a control group that received no intervention or to groups that were treated with conventional exercise or yoga. Relative to the control group, the yoga and conventional exercise groups had significant decreases in fatigue on the basis of two different measures. There were no consistent effects of yoga or conventional exercise on cognitive function or mood. It is not possible to determine whether yoga's effects on fatigue were due to the result of the yoga itself or resulted from other factors, such as a placebo response or benefits from being in a social setting.

Yoga is generally safe. In the clinical trial of yoga and MS, it was not associated with any serious adverse effects. Difficult postures or vigorous exercise should be avoided or done with caution by pregnant women, people with significant heart, lung, or bone conditions, or people with heat sensitivity, fatigue, and decreased balance. Yoga is a low-cost therapy, especially when it is done in groups.

### Angioplasty of Neck Veins

In 2009 Dr. Paolo Zamboni presented a small, uncontrolled study of sixty-five patients that had what he called chronic cerebrospinal venous insufficiency (CCSVI), with narrowing or obstruction of neck veins he postulated would cause back pressure and reflux of blood into the nervous system. The treatment would then be to unblock the abnormal veins by a balloon inserted by catheter through the venous system. The balloon would be blown up to expand the vein, and then withdrawn. He had assessed the neck veins of normal people and a group of patients with other neurological conditions and said all MS patients had CCSVI, but none of the normal people or those with other neurological conditions. This caused great media attention and excitement in the MS community. There were immediate calls for this treatment to be made available.

Neurologists have been skeptical because there were no randomized clinical trials to substantiate the benefits and safety of the procedure and many studies soon after have failed to demonstrate the claims of Dr. Zamboni. There was also concern that Dr. Zamboni's claim was that early relapsing-remitting MS patients showed benefit, but those with secondary progressive or primary progressive MS did not benefit, the latter two groups were most of the patients who went for this therapy.

No study since has shown the dramatic results in the test or treatment that he showed. A Buffalo study shortly after Zamboni's initial presentation showed that only half of the MS patients had some evidence of obstruction in their neck veins, indicating half did not have this. More puzzling, almost half of the people with other neurological disease had some venous obstruction in their neck, and one out of four normal people had some obstruction to neck veins. This raised questions about whether it was a real disorder or not. Other studies showed that the positioning of the patient could alter the results and show obstruction, when another position did not. Also, later studies showed that evidence of some obstruction was less common at the beginning of the disease and more common later, suggesting it may be the result of having MS rather than a cause of the disease. Part of the Zamboni theory is that venous obstruction would cause increased pressure in the venous system within the brain and spinal cord, but a study with ophthalmodynamometry did not show any difference in the venous pressure in the central nervous system in thirty MS patients and thirty normal people.

Studies from England, Germany, Canada, Sweden, and the United States raised questions about the CCSVI concept as the studies did not show much difference between MS patients and normal people when neck veins were assessed by different procedures. Many clinical research groups feel the apparent neck obstruction is a reflection of how the studies are done, not a real obstruction, and that CCSVI is not a real condition. Also, the weight of evidence from many studies shows that patients often say they feel better but there is no objective evidence that their condition is measurably improved. In fact, a study from Texas suggested the MRIs had more lesions in the group who had the neck procedure performed compared to the sham-placebo group. There are many things to be learned about the CCSVI story. It seems clear that CCSVI is not the cause of MS, and many not even be a condition.

In the midst of all this confusion, conflicting results and unanswered questions, we are seeing claims by patients that some of their symptoms, especially fatigue, "brain fog," limb coldness, and numbness, may improve after having the procedure. Studies are being completed to answer further questions about diagnosis, treatment results, and follow-up results. It has been shown that many of the veins collapse after the procedure and the apparent benefit is lost. The current procedure often fails and the patients have a return of their symptoms after some months. To prevent the vein from collapsing, a stent could be put in, a procedure often used in arteries for coronary disease, but putting stents in veins has many risks and complications. In an artery the stent will stay fixed as arteries get smaller beyond the stent. In veins the stent can get loose as veins get bigger beyond the stent, and clotting around the stent is common as blood flow is slower and under less pressure than in arteries.

The major questions for patients and neurologists will only be answered by a large and well-designed randomized clinical trial that assesses a large range of subjective and objective measures of symptoms, MRI and neurological outcomes. Many such trials are now underway and others are in the design stage.

Carrying out clinical trials takes large numbers of patients and a large control group, and takes a long time if the trial is to demonstrate clinical symptoms and disability. Patients who were excited about the idea of CCSVI were frustrated by the length of time it would take to get the answers and wanted the therapy available before adequate randomized clinical trials, which are required before any drug would be approved for therapy. Unfortunately, this has resulted in a tension between patients and the clinicians, MS organizations, and even governments who were portrayed as delaying their ability to get the procedure.

It is expensive and the amount depends on the country where it is being done, travel, and follow-up. There are known risks and complications, including collapse of the veins, clotting, stroke, and death. The detailed degree of risk is uncertain as many of the centers do not conduct follow-up studies.

# CHAPTER 6

# *Practical Guidelines for Living with Multiple Sclerosis*

There are many things you can do to stay as healthy as possible, take control of your life, and cope with the challenges that MS may bring. The disease should not be in control—*you* are in control of your life, your attitudes, your relationships, your approach to problems, your interests, and your activities.

This chapter discusses some things you should do and some things you should not do. For example, you should get more information about MS; you should make sure you have an opportunity to ask questions about the disease; you should exercise; you should try to live a normal, active life, adapting to any limitations; you should work to improve your relationships; you should express a positive attitude; and you should have regular medical assessments.

There are things you should not do. Do not withdraw from life and friends; do not stop exercising; do not expose yourself to a hot environment; do not try every treatment that you hear about without first getting reliable information about the scientific evidence, possible benefits, and side effects; and do not feel ashamed or diminished because you have MS.

## *Where Can I Learn More About MS?*

Many things are known about MS, and many advances are being made. There are many unanswered questions, but it is important to learn more about the questions that are being asked by researchers and the theories that are being tested.

One of the best initial sources of information is the Multiple Sclerosis Society, which can be accessed through their website in each country. They can be contacted directly as well. In the United States, call 800-344-4867 to reach the National MS Society; in Canada call 800-268-7582. Other sources of information are the Multiple Sclerosis Association of America (MSAA; www.msassociation.org) at 800-532-7667, and the Multiple Sclerosis Foundation (www.msf .org) at 800-225-6495.

## *What Should Others Know About MS?*

It is important for your family, friends, and coworkers to understand MS. Initially you may feel that you do not want others to know that you have MS. That is understandable, but it is essential to tell the people you love, and others when necessary, so that they can understand and help you deal with the disease. Most people with MS are pleased and surprised at how supportive and understanding others are when they are informed. Many people may have guessed that something was wrong but did not know what to do or say. Until they know the truth, employers may not understand your need to take time off or to rest, and they may think you are not working well. Decisions to inform should be made on an individual basis, but, in general, disclosure is a good idea.

Once family and friends are aware of your diagnosis, they might benefit from literature that would allow them to better understand MS.

In particular, your family should understand your symptoms and problems so they can be helpful and supportive. This is not possible if they are unaware of your MS and how it makes you feel.

## Who Can Answer My Questions?

It is important to have your concerns addressed and your questions answered. Often people are afraid that they might ask too many questions or that their questions might not be clear. Make a list of the questions you want to ask. Bring the questions to your physician or nurse on your next visit or call the MS Society. You probably will find that they are questions most people ask and that they are not new to the staff. If there is no clear answer to a question, it is important to find that out as well. Each new piece of information will add to your overall understanding of MS.

## What Can I Learn from Other People Who Have MS?

People with MS soon learn that it is a common neurological disorder and that there are many others in their community who have the same disease. It often helps to talk to others who share the challenges and problems of coping with MS, but there are some cautions.

> *You cannot compare yourself with others in terms of the type of disease, the course, or the symptoms. Multiple sclerosis is an individual disease, and you probably will find that the features of your MS are quite different from those of the next person.*

It may seem puzzling that there are so many individual patterns for the disease, but that is actually fairly common in other diseases as well. The variety of symptoms of MS is great, so the variations in individuals are great as well.

One way that people with MS can benefit from each other is in self-help or support groups. These take various forms, but they usually are small groups that meet in homes or in community facilities to talk about and better understand MS. The object is always to take a positive approach and to take control over everything that you can manage so that you can help yourself and others. The MS Society has information on support groups and MS centers often sponsor them. It is important to select a group lead by someone who truly knows MS and can make your experience with the group a positive learning one. A group without direction and without a positive focus can be a negative experience.

## When Is Information Not Helpful?

Misinformation is not helpful and can cause much trouble and distress, not to mention wasted time and money. If someone says that mercury in dental fillings causes MS, check it out from those who know—staff at the MS Society, someone in the MS clinic in your area, or your physician—but do not go to the dentist and have your fillings removed. If someone tells you that ginseng cures MS, check it out. If someone says there is a doctor in a clinic somewhere who has a cure for MS, call the MS Society, not your travel agent. Although there is good information on the Internet, there are some sites and chat rooms that provide misinformation. It is sometimes hard to see which are reliable and which are not. So choose your Internet sources wisely and always question what you read.

## What About My Activities?

People with MS should lead normal and active lives within the limitations of their symptoms. This means that we encourage activity more than rest and staying active and involved rather than withdrawing and dropping out. We want people to remain productive and working. It is understandable that symptoms and problems may make this harder for you, taking more time and energy, but it is still better to do it than not to do it.

People with MS are happiest and at their best when they live as normally as possible and carry out the activities they enjoy. There are no absolute limitations—if you feel like walking in a march, running a race, or climbing a mountain, and do not have symptoms and problems that limit you, go for it! Unfortunately, MS does cause symptoms that may limit activities to some extent. It requires adjustment so that you can continue to do as much as you can, in the time you need, and in the way you can manage. If you work at managing your problems, coping with any limitations, and keeping a positive attitude, not only can you do many of the things in life you want to do, but also you may accomplish much more than others without MS, as they often do not use these positive skills to deal with life.

## What About Exercise?

Simply put, exercise is good for everyone. When the diagnosis of MS is made, you should set about getting yourself in the best shape that you can, both mentally and physically, in order to manage any challenges that come with the disease. We all benefit from regular exercise, and it is even more important for the person with MS. If fatigue is a problem, you should arrange your exercise for times when fatigue is less bothersome, schedule it in periods with breaks, or redesign the type and pattern of exercise so that you can still do it.

In general, the best exercise is one that you enjoy so that you will continue to always do it, not just because it is good for you. Exercise should be a lifetime habit for all of us, including people with MS, even if the exercise program needs to be modified at times. Try to involve others in exercise as well. Exercise programs in the community have a tendency to motivate you to participate regularly; they also have an enjoyable social aspect.

## Can I Overdo It?

Many MS patients worry that overdoing things might cause attacks of MS and worsen the disease. Friends and family often tell MS patients to rest most of the time. This is not good advice.

There is no evidence that exercising or even overdoing work and activities have any deleterious effect on MS. True, it may make you feel tired for the next day or so, but there is no evidence that it worsens your MS. Some people "push through" their fatigue, which also may make them tired the next day but does no long-term harm.

It might be tempting to blame over-activity for the development of a new attack of MS or a new symptom, especially if it happened a day or a few days later, but a careful accounting of strenuous events, stressful events, and the occurrence of attacks would show that this is probably coincidental. Do not worry about activity; be reasonable, keep active, and do what you can.

## *How Much Should I Rest?*

Because fatigue is a major problem for many people with MS, a reasonable balance between maintaining your normal activities and taking brief rests is appropriate. People usually find their own balance of activity and rest, and in this way they keep up their activity, work, and other responsibilities.

It is important to recognize that the fatigue in MS is not "normal" tiredness that follows too little sleep or a long, hard day though people with MS are not exempt from that kind of tiredness as well. When you are experiencing fatigue, it is important to take the time to examine all that you are doing in a day to see if what you expect of yourself is reasonable. The fatigue in MS is usually felt as different from the normal fatigue everyone experiences; it is unrelated to the amount of sleep and activity. It can occur in waves and may seem overwhelming at times. If you are experiencing MS fatigue, examine the hour of the day and change your schedule so that you are not doing the most important things when you know that fatigue is greatest. Adapting the level of activities is often successful, and some medications also may be helpful (see Chapter 4).

Do not rest too much. *Activity* is a more important watchword than rest in MS.

## What About Stress?

Everyone experiences stress in their lives, and being given a diagnosis of MS is certainly stressful. Having to see yourself and your life in a different light, with greater uncertainty, is stressful. But marriage, raising children, doing our jobs, and the "daily-ness" of life also bring stress. The central point is not whether stress is present in your life (it almost always is), but your response to it. People can, and do, react differently. Some see stress as a problem to be solved. Some respond emotionally, collapsing in tears, becoming depressed, or lashing out angrily at others. Some are initially upset, but then set about overcoming or dealing with the stress. Others do not believe it is possible to deal with it and give up. It is not the stress; it is our reaction to it that makes the difference.

When people react to stress in a nonproductive way, they often state that anyone would react the same way. That isn't true because in the same situation, different people respond differently. Fortunately, by analyzing such events, you can learn how to react more positively. It is not easy and sometimes requires counseling, but a person who reacts ineffectively to stress can learn how to respond better. It does mean that you must recognize that your responses could be more productive before you can work at it or seek help.

## Can I Develop Better Coping Skills?

We all have certain patterns of coping. Some of us react more intellectually to problems and stresses, while others react more emotionally. Most of us have a combination of the two; it is the balance of intellectual problem-solving responses and emotional responses that is important.

It is natural to feel upset when something stressful happens. However, it is not normal for that to be the only response. There is a point at which we must think clearly and objectively about what the stress is all about, how we can analyze it, and how we can most effectively deal with it. That combines the appropriate emotional and problem-solving aspect. You can improve these coping skills by improving their components. When a stressful event has passed, you can analyze how well you responded—whether your emotional response was appropriate and balanced, and whether the steps you took were the most effective ones to deal with the problem. Such analysis often gives you a different perspective, particularly if it is done in an honest fashion and enables you to see how you could respond more effectively the next time.

## How Can I Maintain a Positive Attitude?

The most important factor in dealing with MS—or any challenge in life—is a mature, positive, and good-humored attitude whenever possible.

Some people struggle harder than others. There is no question that a positive attitude is of great importance because a negative person cannot tolerate very much adversity. MS does not make you positive or negative; you already had an approach to life before you developed the disease. MS can challenge your approach, your positivity, and your good humor, however, so it is important to make an even greater effort to overcome difficulties in a way that makes you feel good and improves your relationships. People like to be around those who are positive and good humored. We can understand those who are negative and turn their frustration on others, but they do not manage well, are more unhappy, and do not learn to take control of the things they can manage.

It is important to practice being positive and good natured and cheerful. That may sound false, but when you smile and talk in a positive manner, you feel better and others feel better. Attitude is so important and you can practice seeing things and speaking in a positive manner. It will change how you see your world and your situation.

## What About My Relationships?

Good relationships are important to us all, and they become even more important when we have difficult challenges to overcome. In taking control of your health and your future you should strengthen your relationships. It may seem simplistic, but it actually is one of the most important things you can do. It has a positive effect on you when you do everything you can to improve your relationships with your spouse, your children, your family, your friends, and everyone with whom you come in contact. Our relationships with others are central to our happiness and state of well-being, and it is rewarding to continue to improve them. There is a large body of research evidence showing that better outcomes in MS are related to a strong support system of family, friends, and caregivers.

## Should I Tell People I Have MS?

It is natural that you may have felt uncertain about telling people— even your family or close friends—when you first were told that you have MS. It is hard to recognize that something about yourself has changed, and it is worrisome to think that it might affect your relationships and how people regard you. Eventually you will come to recognize that you are still the same person, that the people who love you will continue to love you and support you, and that others generally are understanding and helpful. Sometimes they may try to be too helpful, as most people don't want relationships to change. All of these feelings plus some embarrassment about "having an illness" make many people want to hide the diagnosis. They think, "maybe if I pretend the problem doesn't exist, it won't exist."

It is a good rule to be honest and open in our relationships and interactions. Of course, like all health matters, the fact that you have MS is a private and confidential matter, so who you confide in is a personal choice. It is common to keep the information within a small circle initially, especially because everything may be calm and stable for many years. A problem begins to develop when symptoms cause difficulties that are visible to others, but they have not been made aware that you have a health problem. At that point, others may wonder, worry, and speculate about what is happening, and their speculation can be more harmful than the truth.

It also is worth considering that people feel excluded and not trusted when they are kept in the dark yet know that something is being kept secret. There are some instances when keeping a medical problem a secret can be a serious offense or can cause serious problems.

For example, you cannot lie about having a medical problem when answering questions on insurance forms or other official documents. There are only a few instances when it is proper to ask such questions, but in such instances, you must answer truthfully.

### *What Happens When It Is Hot?*

Most, but not all, people with MS find that they are heat sensitive. They notice that they become weak or dizzy, or even feel sick, in a hot bath, on a hot humid day, or in a warm environment. They also notice the opposite—they feel better and function better when it is cooler, when they are swimming in cool water, or when they move from a warm room to a cool room.

Remyelinated and partially damaged nerve fibers may function less well when body temperature is elevated and, conversely, the nerves function better when temperature is lowered. This tends to be a transient phenomenon that does not produce a lasting effect. However, it can produce marked weakness, and people often describe themselves as feeling like a "dishrag" or "wiped out" on a hot day. This response to heat was once the basis of the *hot bath test*, which was used as a test for MS before modern diagnostic tests were available. Although it is suggestive of MS, it is not accurate enough to be an important test.

You may wonder whether becoming weak in a hot environment will make the disease worse, but the phenomenon is transient and disappears as soon as you cool off. We do recommend that you avoid a warm environment whenever possible because you will feel less well, function less well, and have more symptoms when it is very warm. Air conditioning often is required in summer months to maintain reasonable temperature control and is considered medically necessary for tax purposes (a letter from your physician is needed). Cool drinks are also helpful—get in the habit of carrying one with you. The fluids will help your bladder and bowel function as well. Cooling scarves and other cooling equipment may be helpful as well (see Chapter 4). Avoid sunbathing, saunas, and hot tubs.

## Should I Change My Diet?

The dietary approach to the management of MS has a long history. It is difficult to perform clinical trials on diets, but there was interest and some suggestion of a positive response from studies of diets that are low in animal fats (essentially a low-cholesterol diet) and with a supplement of a vegetable oil such as sunflower seed oil or evening primrose oil. A few of these studies showed some positive benefit but one large study showed no benefit. There also was some suggestion that people with early and mild disease benefit the most. Many people use the simple approach to diet of lowering the amount of animal fat and supplementing it with a vegetable oil because it is a healthy diet and everyone in the family can potentially benefit from it. Many more complex diets have been recommended in MS, which have little logic or justification and are so complicated that people give them up after a short time (see the discussion on diet in Chapter 5).

The most important points are to stick to a balanced, healthy diet, maintain normal weight, and limit your intake of animal fat. This is a good dietary recommendation for everyone.

## Should I Sleep More?

How much sleep you need is based on your own normal pattern. Some people require eight or nine hours a night, whereas others require only five or six hours. The average is seven and one-half hours of sleep, and the measure of effectiveness is how rested you feel in the morning. You should not change your sleep pattern because you have MS. Since fatigue is a major problem for many people, there is a tendency to think that you will be less fatigued if you sleep more.

However, even with normal or greater sleep hours, you will still tend to feel tired during the day if fatigue is due to MS. Surprisingly, over-sleeping often makes people feel more tired. It is worth remembering that many factors can decrease the quality of sleep, including alcohol and many drugs.

## *What If I Need Surgery?*

The answer to this question is simple. If you need surgery and there are good indications for surgery, you should have it. If you do not need surgery, you should not have it. This is a good rule whether you have MS or not. There does not appear to be any increased risk to people with MS who undergo surgery. In the past, there was concern that the stress of surgery might precipi-tate MS attacks, but the number of attacks of MS that occur in those circumstances is the same as that which would be expected in an average population of people with the disease, and no more. This is in keeping with the previous point that there is little evi-dence that stressful events precipitate attacks of MS, whether they involve surgery, anesthesia, trauma, or major life events. The most important rule is to be assured that surgery is truly indicated and necessary.

## *Is Pregnancy a Risk?*

The relationship between MS and pregnancy has been carefully studied. Pregnancy does not increase the incidence of attacks of MS and in the final trimester, the number of attacks is reduced. Studies indicate that the likelihood of an attack of MS decreases by up to 70 percent during this period. However, there are more attacks in the six months following delivery than would be expected in a six-month period (see discussion of hormones during pregnancy in Chapter 10). Those episodes should be treated and managed like any other epi-sode of MS. Pregnancy has no long-term effects on disability or dis-ease progression.

Two other aspects of pregnancy and child rearing must be considered. First, there is a small, but real, genetic risk for MS in a family— about 5 percent for a first-degree relative. This is greater than the risk in the normal population, but it clearly is low. More significantly, raising a child is a life-long responsibility, and people with MS must recognize that their health during the time that they will need to carry out this responsibility may be uncertain. For example, one cannot predict health status in ten or fifteen years. This probably is the major factor that governs the decision about having a child. Recognizing the risks and problems, each couple must determine for themselves as this very personal decision.

## *Will MS Affect My Sex Life?*

Because MS affects the central nervous system and the nerves that control various functions in the body, the complex and sensitive control system for sexual function also can be affected. Early in the disease there may be no physical effect on sexual function, but the enjoyment of sex may be affected by your emotional state. Worries, depression, or altered feelings about yourself can affect your relationship with others and the normal emotions associated with sexuality. Thus, sexual function may be affected by psychologic factors, and this possibility needs to be considered. More often there is a physiologic basis for the difficulties, seen in conjunction with bladder and bowel symptoms. For men, the most common problem is achieving or maintaining an erection, which can be helped by medication such as sildenafil citrate (Viagra), tadalafil (Cialis), avanafil (Stendra), or vardenafil (Levitra, Staxyn). Women may experience decreased vaginal lubrication, which can be accommodated by synthetic lubricating products, such as Astroglide or K-Y Jelly. Never use petroleum jelly (Vaseline). If you experience sexual problems, talk with your physician or health care professional and do not suffer in silence. There are informative pamphlets from the MS societies on sexuality in MS.

## *What About Driving?*

Driving is only a problem when symptoms or limitations make it risky or unacceptably difficult. Vertigo, double vision, or a temporary loss of vision would not permit you to drive safely. Problems with leg weakness, spasticity, or incoordination limit rapid and accurate use of brake and accelerator pedals and make driving unsafe. It may be possible to return to driving when symptoms improve, but it is wise to depend on the assessment of your physician when there is any question about this. Most rehabilitation facilities can assess whether a person can drive safely.

When a problem is more long standing and renders driving unsafe, it may be possible to adapt the controls on the vehicle to allow a person to drive. The most common adaptation is to covert foot pedals to hand controls.

Although a person may be anxious to continue driving and willing to take some chances, feeling that they are "all right to drive," greater consideration must be given to others who may be at risk, including passengers, pedestrians, and other drivers.

## *Should I Move?*

Some people with MS ask if it would be helpful if they moved to another area because they have read that the incidence of MS varies in different parts of the world, that it is more common in temperate climates, and that it is rare in very hot climates, such as near the Equator. The answer is no. In fact, they might find the heat a problem because it tends to make people with MS feel worse. We also believe that the geographic patterns of MS incidence probably have other explanations, and have had the effect earlier in life. There is no evidence that moving to another area once you have the disease will help.

## *Will I Be Different?*

It is natural to wonder how MS will change you. Young people see themselves as healthy and perfect and do not visualize themselves with a serious and chronic disease. When you are given a diagnosis of a medical condition, it is natural to begin to think of yourself differently, and you may have to readjust your self-concept. You are still *you*, but it requires you to see that a different element has entered your life. Many things change as you go through life—some good, some not so good. What is necessary is a positive approach to challenges and determination to move ahead. This may be easier said than done so don't feel guilty if your doctor suggests some counseling to get you started and give you support.

## *What About Other Questions I May Have?*

This chapter could not possibly cover all the questions you may have, but covers some of the most common questions I hear from patients. You will have many more, and they should be asked of your physician, other health care professionals, or staff at the MS Society. It is always better to ask a question even if you are uncertain about exactly how to ask it or if you think it sounds "silly" than to wonder or worry in silence.

We recommend the book *Multiple Sclerosis: The Questions You Have, The Answers You Need* as a more detailed guide to many of your questions (see Additional Reading).

# CHAPTER 7

# Coping with Multiple Sclerosis

B eing diagnosed with MS can create turmoil in every area of a person's life. In some ways, life will never be quite the same again. Even in the absence of impairment, the worry—or effort to camouflage worry—is always there. The diagnosis often precipitates a roller coaster ride of emotions. The time following diagnosis can be challenging and confusing. This chapter helps you to bring perspective to the emotional turmoil and helps you think about ways to ease the distress and continue with your life.

## The Crisis of Diagnosis

People have a variety of reactions when they are given a diagnosis of MS. Some experience a combination of fear and confusion when first confronted with the news. These feelings may be quickly replaced by denial, a refusal to believe that this could possibly be happening. "There must be some mistake!" is a common reaction to the diagnosis, often followed quickly by feelings of anger and resentment. Lisa's story provides an example of some of these feelings. When asked about her initial experience with the diagnosis of MS, Lisa (then 19 years old), replied:

> *I was having a multitude of symptoms that I didn't understand, such as numbness in my feet. I was having trouble feeling the ground when I was walking. I couldn't see very well out of my left eye—it was almost like looking through an oily film. A whole bunch of odd things were happening that I didn't understand. When I finally got the diagnosis, I was really scared. I didn't know what MS was or what would happen to me. I was afraid of the whole thing.*

> *Later I was angry—very angry. Then I decided there was no way I could really have this disease. In fact, my parents and I were second-guessing the doctors—going from one to another asking what was wrong with me. All I could think of was that can in the grocery store that you throw your loose change into—you know, the one with the picture of someone in a wheelchair. It was probably a good year before I even started to accept the fact that I have MS. There was no way I could have it—I'm too active and I do so many things. And I can't stop doing them.*

The diagnosis actually brings a sense of relief for some people, especially those who had disturbing but vague symptoms for a long time, sometimes years, but were given many explanations that didn't seem to provide an adequate explanation. After being told it was due to stress, a pinched nerve, or some vague condition, it is a relief to finally know the answer. They knew there was something wrong, and the lack of an explanation, or feeling doctors must think "it is all in my mind," was more stressful than having a diagnosis. There may also be a sense of relief if the person was worried about something worse, such as a brain tumor. Another sense of relief can come from now knowing how to deal with a definite answer.

Jim, who was diagnosed with MS in 2004 after a frustrating search for some answers, spoke about fear and relief at finally learning his diagnosis:

*It took me a year to get a diagnosis. I was scared to death when I heard "MS." I didn't even know what MS was. But I was also relieved. When you're used to not having a label for all the strange things that are going on and suddenly the problem is identified for you, that alone is a relief— all this finally has a name.*

Regardless of the initial emotional response, the diagnosis of MS creates a crisis for the individual and the entire family. The person who has been diagnosed may experience a sense of isolation despite efforts of family members to offer support. Lisa mentioned this experience:

*Even though people wanted to help, I was the one who had to learn to live with it and had to learn what I needed to do to live with it. You have to make your choice of how you're going to live your life. You have to do it because it's your disease and nobody can do it for you or make it go away.*

Family members are also immersed in their own concerns about their loved one, but also about the future and the impact that MS will have on their lives. The positive aspect of this type of crisis (if you can even imagine one) is that it provides an opportunity to assess future plans and a powerful motivation to take actions that support those plans. There is an opportunity to affirm the values and strengths of the individual and the family and all the good things that remain intact in spite of MS. In order to go forward, it is important to know that you can successfully move through the difficult emotions and continue to pursue your goals and dreams. A professional counselor—such as a psychologist or social worker—can be a helpful ally to the person with MS and family members in working toward a positive outlook for the future.

## The Adjustment Process

The initial reactions to the diagnosis of MS often give way to a feeling of sadness related to the addition of a serious chronic illness to one's identity and self-image. Chronic illness forces each person to confront the frailty and vulnerability of the human condition in a personal way. There is also the concern that there may be a negative attitude by society to people with a chronic disease. This process involves grieving for your former self-image and integrating the realities of MS into one's identity. Sadness, anger at the disease, and self-absorption also might be experienced during this time.

Grieving is necessary for a person to move forward, just as it is following the loss of a loved one. Unlike the grieving we associate with the loss of someone, the grieving process in chronic illness tends to ebb and flow of symptoms and physical changes over time. Grief may be postponed, but usually not completely avoided. Sometimes these feelings may be channeled inappropriately, such as anger at one's spouse or children or at health professionals who cannot cure the illness. It is important for everyone involved to understand this grieving process and to show understanding and support.

The period of intense grieving may last from a few weeks to several months, with gradually diminishing intensity. As it subsides, at least for the time being, one can again begin to focus on and enjoy special relationships and daily activities. Ideally, there is a gradual acknowledgment of the permanence of MS in one's life, while maintaining a sense of continuity between the past and the future as well as a commitment to maximizing the quality of life.

Depressive feelings may occur as part of the initial grieving process or in response to subsequent changes or losses imposed by the illness. Over the course of the disease, however, individuals with MS are at greater than average risk for depression. Often the person can get through this, particularly when they clarify their understanding, become more positive about how they are going to move ahead and deal with any issues. It is important, however, to recognize when this is not working and the person stays in a state of depression that is affecting his or her life and normal functioning, and therapy with counseling or medication may be necessary. Symptoms of significant depression include ongoing and pervasive sadness, loss of interest in or enjoyment of important activities and relationships, feelings of hopelessness and despair, sometimes including suicidal feelings or thoughts, and changes in sleeping and eating patterns. Family members may notice some of these changes and point them out to the doctor when they accompany the person at their next visit to the doctor. Intervention is recommended if any of these symptoms continue for an extended period of time or seem to be worsening. It is important to realize that relief from depression is readily available. Seeking help for this problem demonstrates an understanding of its significance, not personal weakness or deficiency.

Jim comments on his experience with depression:

*I was pretty depressed, so I went to see a psychologist. She was connected with a rehabilitation facility, so her primary interest was working with people who are chronically ill or disabled to help them find comfortable ways of living and thinking about themselves. It was a perfect match because that's just what I needed at that point.*

One hallmark of MS that is most troubling and challenging for patients is the unpredictability of the disease course and the uncertainties related to future ability/disability. That sense of control you had over your life is shaken. Questions that almost everyone faces include: What symptoms and impairments might occur? When will new symptoms appear? When will they go away Or will they go away? Amy, who was diagnosed eight years ago, addressed this issue:

*I think not knowing what will happen is the hardest thing for people when they're diagnosed with MS. They totally freak out and wonder, "what's this disease going to do to me?" They have to realize that what happens to someone else is not necessarily going to happen to them. And if it does, well, you will have to deal with it.*

Flexibility is a key element in living with the unpredictability of MS. Goals need to be assessed and revised, with a "plan for the worst, hope for the best" outlook. A college student named Leslie was pursuing a career in horticulture, which necessitated spending a fair amount of time in greenhouses. Her early symptoms included heat sensitivity, with temporary blurred vision and extreme fatigue when she was exposed to warm temperatures. Although this problem remitted, any future recurrence would have prevented Leslie from performing her job. After careful thought, she switched to teaching, an occupation that heat sensitivity and other possible MS symptoms would not prevent her from continuing. Similarly, the purchase of a new home should involve consideration of issues of mobility and accessibility. Many people with MS are not significantly bothered by problems with walking. However, since mobility impairment is a problem at some point for many people with MS, it is simply good planning to consider this possibility when choosing a home, even while being reasonably optimistic that serious walking difficulties will not occur.

## Resilience

The ability to overcome adversity and loss and come back even stronger, having learned from the experience is called resilience. Everyone experiences adversity in life, the loss of a loved one, failure in business, loss of a job, or breakdown of a marriage. The hope is that the person can at some stage step back, examine the situation, and reconfigure life, having learned some lessons.

Anyone is capable of this, but particularly those who have a positive personality, have a positive sense of themselves, a tendency to evaluate circumstances realistically, manage strong emotions, are effective at solving problems, and communicate well with others.

Some of the most prominent successful individuals are winners because they failed so many times (Steve Jobs, Winston Churchill, Oprah Winfrey, Thomas Edison, Michael Jordan, and Martin Luther King, Jr.). They were upset by the losses and failures, but could reassess their situation and come back stronger.

Managing the stresses and losses also requires you to be in the best general health, so have regular exercise and sleep, and mental relaxation. It requires you to be honest in your evaluation of yourself, your circumstances, and the options. It is helpful to have good communication with family and friends.

At the time of a stressful event it is tempting to feel there is no way to deal with it. Examine your responses and how you could have done things better. Don't make excuses or justify behaviors, but think about improving a better outcome for you and for others. Practice being positive. Examine and work at the positive things in your life. Don't dwell on things you can't do, but what you can do. Practice being more understanding and forgiving as resentments and anger sap your energy and make it hard to be happy and positive as you strive for a positive recovery from a difficult time.

## Coping Strategies

Coping strategies reflect an individual's personality and attitudes and the way the individual interacts with people and events. By adulthood, personal strategies have been selected and refined through an unconscious process; most of us do not consciously choose and evaluate our coping mechanisms. How we respond to issues in life is, to a great extent, developed early in childhood, but we can modify our responses if they are not helpful or constructive. We can assess how we deal with people, stresses, and life issues honestly and critically and accentuate the good patterns and train ourselves to modify and reduce personal reactions that are unhelpful and negative. The following are examples of two types of strategies.

### Denial

Denial is ignoring or minimizing the seriousness of the situation. Intermittent denial may be useful in the early stages of adapting to MS because it enables people to deal with the immediate symptoms they are experiencing without having to contemplate all the possible problems that may occur in the future. Denial is *not* useful if these potential problems are ignored when making important life-planning decisions such as buying a home or making career decisions. One of the most serious consequences of continued denial is avoidance of treatments, as intellectually people know they have MS but emotionally deny there is really anything wrong.

Denial can also interfere with obtaining optimal health care. A denial of a well-established diagnosis of MS can lead to a search for any other possible explanation resulting in unnecessary tests, unnecessary surgery, and delays in therapy that should be started early in the disease.

*Intellectualization*

Intellectualization is focusing on available factual information to the exclusion of feelings and other psychological issues. A certain amount of intellectualization makes it possible for people to learn about the disease, assess its impact on their daily lives, and make use of their problem-solving abilities to meet the challenges imposed by MS. Intellectualization becomes excessive when it consumes enormous amounts of energy; some people expend so much effort collecting and analyzing information that they have little or no energy left to deal with their emotional reactions to the disease or with the feelings and reactions of those around them.

Looking at these two examples, the strengths and weaknesses inherent in some coping strategies can be seen. Denial is useful in allowing a person to get on with his or her life, but it is detrimental if it interferes with obtaining optimal treatment or with life-planning issues. Intellectualization is useful in obtaining essential information, but it is harmful when it is used as a means to block feelings about the disease that should be expressed. At the same time refusing to learn anything about the disease can be equally problematic. One needs to be able to address symptoms that may be due to MS and report them to their doctor to be addressed. The blocking of emotional awareness and expression can interfere with long-range coping efforts.

Interpersonal difficulties may arise when two people who live together and must cope with MS have conflicting coping styles. A person who copes by talking through feelings and events or by reading all the literature on MS may encounter resistance and even anger from a partner who is trying desperately to maintain denial as a way of dealing with the disease. In some situations, counseling is useful to help a couple or family members recognize each other's coping styles and provide mutual support.

## Educate Yourself About MS

People with MS have indicated in National Multiple Sclerosis Society surveys that information about the disease and its effects is their most important need. Education about MS is available through a number of sources, primarily MS health care providers and the U.S., Canadian, and other national MS societies (see the Resources chapter). Keep in mind, however, that adults can choose to learn in a variety of ways and may choose to do so in different settings or at different times. For some, devouring every available piece of written material is the most desirable strategy. These individuals compare different sources of information, analyzing and sorting varied opinions, to create a personal perspective. The result is a sense of "ownership" of the information and its gradual integration into personal philosophy and decisions about day-to-day activities. Other people prefer a group setting that provides opportunities for the immediate testing of new ideas and feedback from peers and/or professionals.

Such group educational programs are widely available through the U.S., Canadian, and other national MS societies. The National Multiple Sclerosis Society in the United States has a mail program called "Knowledge Is Power" for people who have been recently diagnosed with MS. The program consists of a series of modules on topics of interest sent on a predetermined schedule to people who request this service. This mail series can be obtained by calling 1-800-FIGHT-MS. These publications are also available in Canada (416-922-6065). The Multiple Sclerosis Association of America and the Multiple Sclerosis Foundation also have excellent booklets of information that they make available for the asking. Each of these organizations has websites with good, unbiased information to access on the Internet as well. You'll find their web addresses in the Resources chapter.

Another component of the educational process relates to reports of possible treatments or "the cure" for MS. Given the variability and unpredictability of the illness over time, it is not surprising that diverse therapies have been heralded as having a significant impact on MS. When symptoms remit—as they frequently do quite naturally over the course of the disease—whatever treatment or activity is being used at the time is given credit for the improvement. Since dramatic improvement and long periods of remission are common occurrences in MS, even without any therapy, it is important to be prudently skeptical when evaluating therapies that claim to be of benefit. Only those treatments that have been evaluated for safety and efficacy in carefully designed and controlled scientific studies provide documentation of benefit. Other therapies are "experimental," meaning the benefits and risks have not yet been fully determined. There are also many suggested therapies, generally outside the usual medical interventions and called "complementary" or "alternative" therapies, that should also be carefully evaluated (see Chapters 6 and 11). Some of these claim a boost to the immune system and are not appropriate for people with MS, who already have an overly active immune system. Any non–physician-prescribed therapy that claims to reduce MS disease activity or any therapy that claims to cure MS should be avoided. Chapter 6 addresses unconventional therapies as does *Complementary and Alternative Medicine and Multiple Sclerosis* by Allen Bowling (see Additional Reading). Chapter 11 addresses the importance of clinical trials to clarify the safety and benefits of any potential therapy for MS.

## *Choosing Your Health Care Providers*

The choice of health care providers is a critical decision relative to long-term management issues. People with MS generally have a normal or nearly normal life expectancy, and management of the disease is a lifelong process. The physician who manages the symptoms and disease course will interact with the other physicians involved in your health care, such as your internist, gynecologist/obstetrician, cardiologist, or any other medical specialist whose services you might require during your lifetime. Members of your chosen health care team will also provide you on an ongoing basis with information that you will need to make important life decisions relating, for example, to job choices, family planning, or the selection of an MS treatment option. Choose your health care providers carefully. Investigate your physician's board certification (neurology, family practice, or internal medicine), experience with MS, hospital or medical center affiliation, and reputation in the community. In most cases, you will need to have a relationship with an internist or family physician to monitor your general health and serve as your "primary care provider," and a neurologist to manage your MS. It is important to remember that though it is easy to blame MS for anything that happens to you after your diagnosis, MS does not exempt you from any other health problems. The local chapter (United States) or division (Canada) of the Multiple Sclerosis Society, can suggest physicians in the community who have experience in the management of MS or, if none is available locally, they will identify MS specialists within the broader geographic region.

## Support Networks

Family and friends provide the major support for the person with MS. Their caring and concern are vital, especially during the difficult times following diagnosis or when a flare-up of symptoms occurs. A "sorting out" of friends and relatives may be necessary because not all people with a close relationship are able to be supportive in the same way. One person may be comfortable listening to concerns and providing emotional support, while another may find it easier to assist with more concrete activities, such as a ride to the doctor's office. Unfortunately, some friends may not be able to deal with chronic disease. Another friend or relative may be a great problem solver, helpful in finding solutions or identifying resources in troublesome situations.

At the same time, a person's ability to help should not be too narrowly or rigidly determined, especially without discussing it with him or her. It is important for all those who provide support to know how important their contributions are to the person with MS.

People with MS may find it especially helpful to talk with others who have the disease. This interaction will help to demonstrate that people with MS do indeed continue productive and satisfying lives despite the intrusion of the disease.

Many chapters of the National MS Society have "peer support" programs that train selected individuals with MS to be helpful to people who have questions about the disease. They are available to answer questions, discuss issues, and relate their personal MS successes and failures. In some areas, the peer is available for a telephone conversation; in other areas, the person may also be available at the local MS center on certain days. Amy commented on her experience with a peer support person:

> *Having that one-on-one interaction, having someone to talk to who understands, who has gone through similar experiences—that was really important to me. She was a source of strength and kept helping my self-image to stay in shape.*

Some people find a group setting most helpful because they can benefit from the experiences of a number of people with MS. Group members also feel good about the group interaction and support, which is much like a family support network. In an MS support group, MS temporarily feels "normal" because it is the common experience of all members. This normalization of MS is extremely supportive of the overall adjustment process. Instead of feeling isolated, the person in a support group sees MS as one component of a full and diverse life, which can be managed with an understanding of the disease, support of family, friends, health professionals, and peers with MS. Some support groups are led by a counseling professional such as a psychologist, or social worker, or MS nurse while others are "self-help" and are led by one of the group members.

To find a support group near you, or perhaps a telephone group, call 1-800-FIGHT-MS in the United States and 1-800-268-7582 in Canada. If you receive your care in an MS center, there may be support groups associated with your center.

## Wellness Orientation

In contrast to a *disease orientation*, which focuses on minimizing the impact of the chronic disease on all aspects of your life, a *wellness approach* looks at achieving the positive state of maximal health despite the presence of a chronic illness. Wellness is a balanced state of positive well-being in mind, body, emotions, and spirit. This model encompasses interpersonal relationships as well as relationships with the environment, the community, and society in general. The wellness orientation is comprehensive in its promotion of mind-body unity within the individual, as well as integration of the individual within the community and society as a whole.

A practical example of a wellness orientation is the practice of aerobic and general conditioning exercises, which have an orientation different from that of traditional physical therapy designed primarily to address disease-imposed impairments. Nutritional programs designed for general health (e.g., the prevention of heart disease and certain forms of cancer) go beyond traditional dietary measures that target specific MS-related problems such as constipation and urinary infections. Practices such as yoga, meditation, mindfulness exercises, and tai chi also fall within the wellness concept. Stephanie comments on her experiences, focusing on wellness behaviors:

> *I learned to practice breathing exercises and meditation when I have a stressful day. Even when waiting in a line I can make my body relax for a few minutes. I also am careful about having a healthy diet. After school I either spend a half hour in the pool or take a walk if the weather is good. I think I have learned to enjoy life and pay attention to things that were not as important to me than before I was diagnosed with MS.*

In following a wellness approach, you can improve your general health and sense of wellness. MS may still cause symptoms and problems, but these are better managed by people who are physically and mentally stronger.

Some people fall guilty if they practice a healthy life style and still experience an attack of MS, feeling they should have tried harder, not missed that exercise session, or fallen off their diet. It is important to take responsibility for ways to keep yourself healthy but you are not responsible for the natural events that occur in the disease. Assuming this kind of personal responsibility for disease progression is both harmful and self-defeating. Your energy—emotional and otherwise—is better channeled into pursuing wellness, always recognizing that the goal is an overall improvement in general health rather than control of the disease process.

People who struggle to control their MS sometimes feel that they are losing the battle or "giving up" if they begin to use an assistive device. These devices actually extend your abilities by conserving energy, promoting safety, and reducing effort. For example, those who fatigue easily or struggle to be ambulatory with a cane or crutches will find that their activities become severely limited. All their energy is used simply to get from one place to another, leaving little or no effort to do or enjoy whatever activity had been planned. Struggling to get to the supermarket may mean that there is no energy left to shop. People with MS should use whatever techniques, tools, or devices are available to maximize and extend their activities and opportunities. Someone who is comfortable walking for short distances may choose to use a motorized scooter on a trip to an amusement park, shopping mall, or museum. A worker in a large office who normally uses a cane might also choose to use a scooter to conserve energy and enhance productivity. The effective use of assistive devices is an important extension of the wellness philosophy. They should be seen as a means of maintaining a full, productive, and enjoyable life rather than as symbols of defeat.

## Children with MS

Although MS is considered an adult disease, it is estimated that there are between 10,000 and 20,000 children and teens with MS, or pre-MS symptoms, in the United States. This relatively uncommon situation presents special challenges to the family.

Establishing the diagnosis of MS in a child or teen can be fraught with even more difficulty than with an adult. The child is generally seen by a pediatric neurologist, who may not be accustomed to seeing this disease in children. In addition, there are non-MS conditions in children that make it difficult to sort out. As a result, months or years may go by before a diagnosis is established. Once a diagnosis of MS is made, issues for the child and family are also different. Parents worry about how they might have contributed to this diagnosis (not at all), and about the future of their child with a chronic disease, who will most likely outlive them. There is also the concern about normal childhood and teenage development and milestones. How will peers react, what about educational goals, and what will be the impact on critical social relationships?

The U.S. National Multiple Sclerosis Society has established six regional "Pediatric MS Centers of Excellence" that provide services unique to this population, and there are MS centers that address children's needs across Canada as well. Patients are assessed by a team who know the issues related to MS in younger people. In recent years there had been a lot of research on children with MS so it is not an unusual situation for the staff in MS centers. Rehabilitation, psychosocial, and other professional services are available through each of these centers, as well as care coordination.

Perhaps one of the most important areas for these children/teens is intervention with school personnel. Whether care is sought from one these centers or elsewhere, contact with the school is often critical. Most children with MS can and should continue with their normal schooling. The Society's six pediatric MS centers have staff to facilitate this, and the National Multiple Sclerosis Society chapters can provide additional help.

Also, the National Multiple Sclerosis Society and the Multiple Sclerosis Society of Canada have a multifaceted program to support families in this situation, which includes information, networking with other families, and telephone counseling.

## Cultural Sensitivity

Disease is regarded differently in different cultures, so this may cause people with MS to experience different attitudes. Some cultures regard disease as a biological issue, but others may feel it is a weakness, or one's own fault, or due to a curse, or because of bad actions or sin. How others regard MS can profoundly affect how a person experiences the disease. Changing cultural beliefs is very difficult but patients, caregivers, and health professionals should be aware of how this can impact the lives of people with MS. It also can impact therapy, as the attitudes of different cultures to disease is reflected in their views on treatments as well.

## Parting Thoughts

Amy relates her personal philosophy:

> *If I had never had MS, I would never have traveled the way I did. I took a year off after I was diagnosed and traveled all around Europe. I decided I was going to do things while I could because I didn't know when something might be taken away from me. And I think one thing I've learned from MS is to do the things I can. It's a lesson for everyone. We should all live each day to the fullest, because we never know when something might happen to take it away.*

Jim relates what gets him through:

> *I would say that I have a lot of support from my family and friends. That probably helped me through. I had quite a few conversations, talks,*

*heart-to-heart discussions with different people, and that helped me quite a bit. Also, I'm somewhat religious and that helped.*

Mary speaks about giving up denial:

*I have this disease, I have done nothing to deserve it, and there is nothing I can do about having it. I just have to begin to take each day, one at a time, do my best, and accept whatever comes. The sheer honesty of admitting that I have an illness is a great weight off my mind. I am more attentive to details in my life, and more willing to do what my body tells me to do, instead of fighting against it. I have found a new calm I had not known before.*

A religious or spiritual orientation has been linked with successful coping in a number of studies. It seems that religion helps some people find meaning in their illness, or at least put it into a meaningful context. Amy also refers to spirituality, as well as her own personal characteristics, as a support:

*Since I grew up in a single parent household, I always had to draw on my own resources. So I worked really hard on that—and on my own sense of spirituality. I just had to—I've always depended on myself. I've always demanded a lot from myself and I guess I just drew it from within.*

Amy refers to a key aspect of the coping process—a person's inner strengths. With an adult-onset disease, coping strategies have already been tested in other areas, creating a base on which to build. These strengths surface as the sense of crisis recedes. Amy has more advice for dealing with MS and with life in general.

*Another thing is to laugh—to have a sense of humor. Don't take things so seriously. If you don't have a sense of humor, it's all for naught, you know. Life is too short. It can just really drag you down if you let it—you can't let that happen. Just try to take things one day at a time. One day at a time and "slow is fast enough," you don't really have to be in that much of a hurry. Take your time and take it easy and don't be afraid to ask for help.*

When you have MS, hope is so important. Hope is justified. When we look at the history of MS in the early years in Chapter 1, and then look at the rapid changes occurring now in research, in the understanding of the disease, and in the remarkable development of increasingly effective MS drugs in the last few decades, we can see a positive future ahead.

# CHAPTER 8

# Employment Issues and Multiple Sclerosis

Many of us spend the majority of our waking hours at work and have a serious personal investment in and commitment to employment-related activities. Sometimes our self-image and identity are closely tied to our occupation or professional status. One of the first questions asked when getting to know someone is, "What kind of work do you do?" From a practical perspective, our income allows us to purchase goods and services to maintain our lifestyle and plan for the future. Work that is not associated with direct financial remuneration—such as parenting, homemaking, and volunteer activities—also contributes to our definition of self. These activities, however, *will* have a financial impact if they must be replaced by the paid work of others. Given all of these factors, it is not surprising that anything that potentially threatens the ability to continue employment or other productive and rewarding activity generates concern and anxiety. A diagnosis of MS certainly presents this kind of distressing situation.

The good news is that most people who discover that they have MS can and should continue working. The drugs approved for treatment of MS may help you to continue your employment status, although this factor has not been systematically studied.

Exacerbations may interfere with your usual work activities, but these episodes usually occur only on the average of about one a year or less in the early years of the relapsing-remitting form of the disease and decrease as time goes on. We see fewer relapses with earlier treatment with approved MS drugs. Progressive MS may require some changes in work activity, but disease limitations usually appear at a slow enough pace to allow for necessary modifications. It is important to be open with your employer about changes or adaptations you need in the work environment or routine that will allow you to continue to be fully productive. Employers already have made changes that are linked to prevention of disability, such as ergonomic desk chairs and hands-free headsets for the telephone. When put in this context, it likely will be easier for your employer to understand the benefit to productivity and the win-win situation for both of you.

When you receive a diagnosis of MS you may need to assess how this could affect your employment if symptoms occur. Usually for many years, people with MS carry on with their activities and employment as they are doing well, especially on treatment. Even attacks of MS symptoms are usually short in duration and with a good outcome in the early years. If symptoms remain, some adaptation at work may be necessary.

These factors are mentioned only to indicate that some adjustments may be needed in the workplace but are usually successful, and most people at work are understanding and supportive. If you have questions, discuss the situation with your employer or other staff members. Speak with others who have successfully managed MS and/or with a counselor who is experienced in helping people with MS think through the important issues related to employment.

## Myths About MS

A number of myths or false beliefs make adjustment to MS more difficult. These misconceptions are held not only by a segment of the general public but also by an alarming number of health professionals who do not have extensive experience with MS and/or are unfamiliar with the professional literature. Some of them have a direct impact on the work experience. They include:

- **Stress.** At various points in the history of MS, stress was thought to worsen the disease and escalate the disease process. Scientific studies have examined this issue in detail, and results remain unclear about the role of stress in both the onset and the progression of MS. Advice to quit working, get help to care for children, and curtail volunteer activities is misguided if it is based only on the diagnosis of MS. Specific symptoms may have an impact, but they need to be evaluated individually and carefully because problems may be self-limited or responsive to symptomatic therapy.

- *Activity.* It was formerly believed that physical activity was detrimental to people with MS. The directive was to "take it easy," stop all physical exercise, and rest as much as possible. Bed rest was the primary recommendation for this erratic and unpredictable disease. The major public figure to challenge this notion was Olympic ski medalist Jimmie Heuga, who could not accept a life of inactivity. We now know that Jimmie was right and that activity and exercise are actually beneficial to the well-being of people with MS. It follows that work-related activity should not be curtailed unless dictated by specific, long-standing symptoms that have not responded to therapy.

- *Incapacitation.* Before MS was routinely recognized in its early stages and in mild cases, the common belief was that it would inevitably, and usually quickly, lead to serious disability that would interfere with the ability to perform daily activities, including employment. This is not true—most people with MS can often remain active and involved for many years.

## Disclosure

The decision to communicate—or not to communicate—the diagnosis of MS in the workplace is complex and important and deserves careful consideration. Disclosure when interviewing for a new job poses different issues from disclosure when you already have an established position.

It is important to be aware of both legal and practical considerations whether you are seeking a new job or maintaining a current one. In the United States, people with disabilities are protected by the Americans with Disabilities Act (ADA), which became law in 1990. The definition of "disability" is complex, but may encompass MS regardless of whether symptoms are present. This is due to the possible perception of a disability. The employment section of the ADA states that individuals with disabilities who are covered under this law (a) have a mental or physical impairment that substantially limits one or more major life activities; (b) have a history of such an impairment; or (c) are perceived as having such an impairment. A diagnosis of MS carries such a possible preconception since an employer could potentially discriminate based on the association of MS with disability. The ADA prohibits employers from asking about or considering a diagnosis or general limitations in hiring and promotion decisions and only allows questions about ability to perform key components of the job. The ADA does offer the individual the option to request reasonable accommodations in order to perform those essential functions of your job. The challenge is that in order to tap into these protections under law, you would need to disclose that you have a disability and that it does affect one or more major life activities and that the accommodations you are requesting will assist you in effectively and efficiently completing the essential functions of your job. Determining who is the best person to disclose to, the best time to disclose, deciding what to say, and relating disclosure to accommodations are key things to be thinking about. It is important to identify the essential or key elements of your job because non-essential functions may potentially be delegated to or traded with other employees.

In a similar manner, Canadians are protected by the Employment Equity Act (Bill C-64) passed in 1995, which replaces the previous antidiscrimination legislation. This legislation seeks to eliminate employment barriers experienced by women, aboriginals, and visible minorities, as well as people with disabilities. Among the areas of concern that prompted this employment legislation was the severe underrepresentation in the workplace of people with disabilities.

Over time this has begun to change. Both the private and public sectors are covered by Bill C-64. The Act makes use of the Canadian Human Rights Tribunal (called the Employment Equity Review Tribunal when hearing employment equity cases). It also confirms the mandate for Human Resources Development of Canada to conduct research, provide labor market data, and administer programs to recognize outstanding achievement in employment equity. Both appeal procedures and enforcement measures are addressed.

In addition to legal considerations, people with MS are often concerned about health insurance, life insurance, and disability insurance. A prospective or current employee needs to explore policies relative to diagnosis of a chronic disease or occurrence of disability. "Preexisting condition" clauses must be carefully investigated, as well as "caps" (lifetime limits on expenditures for a particular condition or for an individual's total medical expenses) and related categories that potentially limit the availability of medical and health services because of MS or another chronic condition. These factors may or may not be disclosure related, depending on prior documentation of diagnosis and extent of information required for ongoing insurance coverage (see Chapter 9: "Financial and Life Planning").

The noninsurance, nonlegal aspects of working with MS often are more difficult to assess and address. Such considerations include anticipated employer and fellow employee support or lack of support, possible growth freeze if limitations are perceived by the employer, and personal emotional investment in efforts to acknowledge or deny issues related to MS. Colleagues, including supervisors, often rally to support a fellow worker with a health problem. In the case of MS, fund-raising teams have sometimes been created to support the individual who has been diagnosed through National Multiple Sclerosis Society events such as the "Walk" and "Bike Tour." Disclosure relieves the stress of covering up real needs and concerns and mobilizes team spirit and support.

You also need to disclose in order to request necessary accommodations. An accommodation may involve a change in scheduling, a parking space closer to the building entrance, or an office closer to the bathroom. Occasionally, equipment or a structural change such as a ramp may be needed. This is less often the case but usually is accomplished with minimal effort and cost when dealt with directly when the need is first identified. Many employers will permit and make it possible for you to work from home one or two days a week, an accommodation particularly helpful to someone bothered by fatigue.

An employer is required to make arrangements to help an employee perform "essential job functions." These accommodations must be "reasonable" in that they must be affordable and must not impose undue hardship on the employer.

There also are compelling reasons not to disclose: subtle or not so subtle pressure to resign, to accept lesser job responsibilities, or not to apply for promotion or expanded responsibilities. People have reported a "dead-end" feeling if a supervisor has clearly communicated lack of support for further advancement.

## Resources

You probably do not need this information now and may never need it. However, you should be aware that such information exists at the time of diagnosis so that you can obtain appropriate assistance at the first sign of difficulty and avoid larger problems altogether.

Modest effort early on can prevent serious situations later and support your smooth career development.

Literature is available from the National Multiple Sclerosis Society in the United States (1-800-FIGHT-MS, www.-national mssociety.org) and the Multiple Sclerosis Society of Canada (NMSS; 416-922-6065, www.mssociety.ca/). Several publications are particularly helpful: *ADA and People with MS* by Cooper, Law, and Sarnoff, which is available as a download from the NMSS, details your protection under law in an easy-to-read style. Another downloadable brochure *The Win-Win Approach to Reasonable Accommodations* by Roessler and Rumrill, provides a practical guide to obtaining workplace accommodations and covers employment protections under the ADA and disclosure issues. You can also find *Should I Work? Information for Employees*, which gives a general overview of employment issues that might concern people newly diagnosed with MS, *Information for Employers*, and *A Place in the Workforce*, on the NMSS's site.

Every state has a vocational rehabilitation office; the phone number can be obtained through the telephone directory or information assistance, or online at www.jan.wvu.edu/sbses/-vocrehab .htm. If you look in the blue government pages of the telephone book under "State Government," this agency may be listed under one of the following headings:

- Department of Vocational Rehabilitation
- Department of Rehabilitation
- Department of Human Services
- Department of Social Services
- Department of Social and Rehabilitation Services
- Office of Vocational Rehabilitation

Each chapter of the National Multiple Sclerosis Society has a designated person who can address common employment issues. This "employment advisor" may be a trained chapter staff or volunteer in the community who is familiar with employment concerns of people with MS. This person will be able to address your questions and refer you to other employment resources and agencies.

In 2005, the National Multiple Sclerosis Society created the Career Crossroads: Employment and MS program. This program comprises a workbook and video/DVD that addresses common employment issues including disclosure, accommodation strategies, legal rights and responsibilities (ADA, FMLA), insurance issues (HIPAA, COBRA), and resources. Chapters may offer this training periodically, and the format may vary from chapter-to-chapter.

Some important resources include:

- Job Accommodation Network (JAN):

  1-800-526-7234, www.jan.wvu.edu

- JAN ADA Information Line:

  1-800-ADA-WORK (1-800-232-9675)

- ADA&IT Technical Assistance Centers:

  1-800-949-4232, www.adata.org

- Equal Employment Opportunity Commission (EEOC):

  1-800-669-4000, 1-800-669-6820 (TDD), www.eeoc.gov

- U.S. Department of Justice ADA Information Line:

  1-800-514-0301, www.ada.gov

The U.S. and Canadian MS societies have a general program for people recently diagnosed with MS called "Knowledge is Power," which can be accessed by calling 1-800-FIGHT-MS in the United States (www.nationalmssociety.org) and 416-922-6065 in Canada (www.mssociety.ca). Society chapters also have periodic educational programs for people recently diagnosed with MS and their families and include issues relative to employment. Some Society chapters have job retraining programs for people who need to make career changes in order to be able to continue working.

# CHAPTER 9

# *Financial and Life Planning[1]*

One part of dealing with MS is managing your money and planning wisely for the future. Just as your MS symptoms are not exactly like someone else's symptoms, your financial situation also is unique. Now more than ever, you will need to take a clear look at your income, assets, debts, benefits, and other resources. This is something that you and your partner or family will probably need to do together.

At first glance, getting a good handle on your finances may seem overwhelming. If you give yourself some time and have a little patience, however, you can accomplish this step.

*When I was first diagnosed with MS, I asked "Am I going to die?" The doctor said that, yes, someday I would die—but not from MS. That was more than 30 years ago. Since then, I've had my ups and downs, but I'm*

[1] Modified with permission from *Adapting: Financial Planning for a Life with Multiple Sclerosis* produced by the National Endowment for Financial Education.

*still around, I still love life, and I've always managed to find a way to pay for the things I need.*

—Leslie, diagnosed in 1980

## Getting Organized

An important first step is to gather the following materials. It is helpful to make copies and put them in labeled file folders in one location that you can get to easily.

- Birth certificate
- Checking and savings account information
- Durable power of attorney document (establish one if you do not have one)
- Employee benefits information
- Insurance policies (life, health, disability, and long-term care)
- Investment account information
- Loans, including credit card statements
- Marriage certificate
- Military records
- Mortgage/deed of trust
- Social Security card
- Tax returns
- Titles (e.g., auto, house)
- Will

## Professional Advisors

It is important to include the names and contact information of your professional advisors with your financial file folders.

| ADVISOR'S NAME | PHONE NUMBER |
|---|---|
| Accountant/tax preparer | |
| Financial planner | |
| Insurance agent | |
| Lawyer | |
| Others | |

## Taking a Financial Inventory

Review your MS symptoms to see if any of them may lead to additional expenses. For example, you may need to pay for regular massages to lessen muscle stiffness, or buy an air conditioner to keep your home cool because of sensitivity to heat. The spending plan worksheet (see the worksheet in the section "Developing a Spending Plan") also can help you estimate your monthly income and expenses.

Next, write down an estimated value of everything you own and the dollar amount of your debts. You'll want this information as you plan for future expenses or apply for any benefits that are based on financial need. As you do this estimate, take into consideration the Internal Revenue Service's definitions of value (go to www.irs.gov) and consider obtaining a professional appraisal of valuable assets, such as your home, artwork, jewelry, or other collectibles. Your accountant or other financial advisor can guide you.

## Using a Health-Expense Spreadsheet

Another step you or a loved one can take is to create a health-expense spreadsheet, which should list items such as:

- Dates of doctor visits, hospital stays, or other treatments
- Charges for medical services, prescriptions, and medical supplies
- Portions of expenses covered by a health care plan

- Amounts and dates that you paid for health care services and any remaining balances
- Dates any deductibles were met, if applicable

Software programs can help you create a spreadsheet and will even do the math for you. If you do not own a computer, you can create a spreadsheet in a notebook or use the one provided in the section "Reviewing Your Health-Care Plan." Remember to keep copies of your supporting paperwork: doctor bills, health insurance statements, canceled checks, and bank statements in labeled file folders.

Realize that mistakes can happen when medical claims are processed. Even though these mistakes usually are unintentional, they can be costly. Check with your health care plan to see if it will share savings resulting from any errors you find in medical bills. Take careful notes while in the hospital or receiving treatment, and check the bill against your notes.

If you find possible billing errors, first try to resolve them with the doctor's or hospital's billing office. Next, get in touch with your health insurance company.

If the matter remains unresolved, contact your state's consumer protection office or insurance regulatory agency to file a complaint. Look in the blue pages of the phone book.

## Reviewing Your Health Care Plan

As soon as possible, review your health care plan, so you will know what the plan will cover, what is excluded, and what your out-of-pocket expenses may be. Having this information will help you plan for anticipated medical expenses and strengthen an appeal on a claim if you believe it was denied incorrectly.

Health care plans can be difficult to read and understand, but there are people who can help you. Check the back of your health care card for phone numbers to call for information about your plan. If your health care plan is provided through an employer, someone in the employee benefits department may be able to answer your questions.

## Health-Expense Spreadsheet

| DATE OF SERVICE/ MEDICAL PURCHASE | CHARGES | AMOUNT/ DATE PAID BY HEALTH CARE PLAN | AMOUNT/ DATE PAID BY ME | DATE DEDUCTIBLE AND/OR COINSURANCE MET | DATE OUT-OF-POCKET LIMIT REACHED |
|---|---|---|---|---|---|
| | | | | | |
| | | | | | |
| | | | | | |
| | | | | | |
| | | | | | |
| | | | | | |
| | | | | | |
| | | | | | |
| | | | | | |
| | | | | | |
| | | | | | |
| | | | | | |
| | | | | | |
| | | | | | |
| | | | | | |
| | | | | | |
| | | | | | |

When reviewing your plan, determine if it is a major-medical plan or a managed-care plan, such as a health maintenance organization (HMO), preferred provider organization (PPO), or point-of service plan (POS). Pay particular attention to information about copayments, coinsurance, deductibles, preexisting condition exclusion periods, lifetime maximums, and prescription drugs. These topics are discussed in the following sections.

### Copayment

Most managed-care plans require you to pay a small amount, called the copayment or copay, each time you visit a health care provider within the plan's network. The amount of the copay may change annually. If your plan also has a deductible, the copay will not count toward it. Major-medical plans and some major medical-type benefits under managed-care plans do not have a copay.

### Deductible

A deductible is the amount you must pay each year before a major-medical plan pays any expenses. For example, if your health care plan has a $500 deductible, you must pay the first $500 of covered medical costs before the plan begins to kick in. If the treatment is not covered by the plan, the cost for that treatment will not count toward the deductible. Managed-care plans, such as a PPO, HMO, or POS, may have a deductible if they permit care from out-of-network providers. Review your plan to determine which provisions apply to the provider you want to use.

### Coinsurance

Coinsurance is the portion of a health care expense that you pay in addition to the deductible (when these provisions are part of your plan). A typical coinsurance provision says that after the deductible is paid, the health care plan pays 80 percent of covered charges for a treatment. You pay the other 20 percent. The percentage is your coinsurance amount. Plans vary as to the amount they expect you to pay.

Most plans have a "stop-loss," "breakpoint," or "out-of-pocket" limit. This is the maximum amount you will have to pay per person, or per family, each year. For example, an insurance company may have a stop-loss of $5,000. After you have paid $5,000 in deductible and coinsurance payments, the insurance company will pay 100 percent of covered expenses for the rest of the year. Check your plan for details.

### Covered Expenses

Regardless of the amount charged by a provider, a plan will only cover certain treatments for certain amounts. Make sure you know what your plan considers a "covered expense," and if your health care provider will accept the plan's payment or will bill you for any amounts not covered by the plan.

### Pre-existing Condition Exclusion Period

A pre-existing condition is a medical problem you had before you joined a health care plan. With a pre-existing condition, you may have to wait a period of time before the plan will cover that medical condition. This length of time could be three months, six months, or one year. As a rule, a group health plan cannot make you wait more than one year unless you did not enroll in the plan when first offered, in which case the waiting period may be as long as eighth months.

Under the Health Insurance Portability and Accountability Act (HIPAA), you will not have to meet a pre-existing condition exclusion period under a new plan if:

- You have had medical coverage for eighth months before changing to a new plan.
- You already have met a pre-existing condition exclusion period under a previous plan.
- You have not been without health care coverage for more than sixty-two days in the last twelve months.

### Lifetime Maximums

Health care plans usually limit how much they will pay for health care through a "lifetime maximum benefit." When the limit is reached, the health care plan no longer pays for medical care. There also may be a limit for a single illness, injury, or condition, or an annual limit on certain medical services or equipment.

### Prescription Drugs

Drugs for MS can be expensive. Plus, you likely will require other medications to manage symptoms. Even if your health care plan offers prescription drug coverage, you may have to pay part of the cost of these medications, so it is important to plan for this expense.

You can start by finding out whether the medications you need are covered by your health care plan. This information is available in the plan's "formulary," which is a list of drugs the plan will cover. Many health care plans cover some of the drugs that have been shown to modify the course of MS. What is on the formulary of your plan may make the selection of the immunotherapy for you.

If you are having difficulty paying for your medications, consider the following options:

- The companies that manufacture the major disease-modifying drugs may offer prescription drug assistance programs. Each program has its own qualifications. Begin by reading *Comparing the Disease-Modifying Drugs* (updated 2016), published by the National Multiple Sclerosis Society (www.nationalmssociety.org).

- Information about other prescription drug assistance programs for people with limited resources can be found at www.pharma.org. Several states also have prescription drug assistance programs.

- Talk to your doctor about prescribing a less expensive drug or helping you apply for a prescription drug assistance program.

- Shop for the best price and the best pharmacy. Compare local prices with mail order or online pharmacies, including delivery charges. If you decide to use a mail order or online pharmacy, choose one that requires a written prescription from your doctor. Be careful about using foreign pharmacies because of the importance of ensuring that the product you order is genuine, of the right strength, and uncontaminated.

- If you are a veteran, you may qualify for Department of Veterans Affairs (VA) health benefits, which include prescription drugs. You must enroll to receive benefits.

## Family and Medical Leave Act

The Family and Medical Leave Act (FMLA) of 1993 requires employers with fifty or more workers, and all public/government employers, to provide up to twelve weeks of unpaid leave a year to eligible employees coping with certain family or medical situations. You can take the leave in small increments or all at once to care for yourself or an immediate family member, with the guarantee that you can keep your job and your health care benefits. Generally, the employer may decide whether FMLA time can be taken in installments.

To be eligible for FMLA leave, an employee must:

- Work for an employer that is covered by FMLA
- Have worked at the company for a total of twelve months
- Have worked at least 1,250 hours during the past twelve months

Employers may require employees to provide medical certification supporting the need for a leave due to a serious health condition affecting the employee or an immediate family member. In addition, when intermittent leave is needed for medical treatment, the employee must try to schedule the treatment so as not to unduly disrupt the employer's business.

## Short-Term Disability Insurance

You may have disability insurance through your employer or on your own. The insurance might pay you a benefit if you experience either a short-term or a long-term disability that prevents you from working.

Keep in mind that even though an exacerbation is temporary, it can be disabling. Short-term disability insurance can help you through these times. With short-term disability insurance, which usually is available only through an employer, you can qualify for benefits within a few days or weeks of becoming disabled. The benefits can stop after a varied number of months, depending on the policy. Typically, you will be paid about 40 to 60 percent of your wages. You must report the benefit as taxable income if the employer paid the premiums for the insurance.

## Job Changes and Health Care

One of the most important job benefits an employer can offer is a health care plan. Because MS is a lifelong condition, carefully consider the health benefits provided by an employer before accepting a position. Or, if you currently work for a company that does not offer a health care plan, you may want to look for a new job that has health care benefits.

In addition to COBRA, the HIPAA, also known as the Kennedy-Kassebaum Act, provides protection to individuals with a pre-existing condition when moving to a new health plan. HIPAA limits exclusions for pre-existing conditions and prohibits discrimination against employees and dependents based on their health status. This law guarantees that most workers with pre-existing conditions can move from their former group health plan to their new employer's plan without a break in coverage. For more information on HIPAA, go to www.dol.gov/pwba.

Don't ask to see the benefits package during the first interview, but when offered a job, ask to review the package before giving an answer. When reviewing the health care portion of the employer's benefits package, pay particular attention to the:

- Waiting period
- Pre-existing condition exclusion period
- Plan benefits and your costs

# Taking Control of Finances

## *Developing a Spending Plan*

The best way to know how much money you need to live on every month is to make a spending plan. Consider making several copies of the spending plan worksheets so you can use them throughout the year, or whenever your financial situation changes.

### STEP 1: IDENTIFY YOUR INCOME

| MONTHLY INCOME WORKSHEET | |
|---|---|
| **SOURCES** | **PER MONTH ($)** |
| After-tax wages | |
| Tips or bonuses | |
| Child support | |
| Alimony/maintenance payment(s) | |
| Unemployment compensation | |
| Social Security or Supplemental Security Income | |
| Retirement plan(s) | |
| Private disability insurance payments | |
| VA benefits | |
| Public assistance | |
| Food stamps | |
| Interest/investment income | |
| Other | |
| | |
| | |
| | |
| | |
| | |
| | |
| | |
| **Total Income:** | |

## STEP 2: LIST EXPENSES

| MONTHLY EXPENSES WORKSHEET | |
|---|---|
| SOURCES | PER MONTH ($) |
| Mortgage or rent | |
| Utilities (heat, electricity, and water) | |
| Telephone, cell phone, Internet provider | |
| Groceries | |
| Transportation (bus fare, car payment, gas, repairs) | |
| Insurance (cost per month for car, home, health, and life insurance) | |
| Housekeeper/gardener, etc. | |
| Prescription drugs, medical supplies and equipment | |
| Treatments or therapies (massage, exercise classes, alternative treatments, supplements, etc.) | |
| Doctor/dentist bills | |
| Home adaptations or improvements | |
| Clothing/uniforms | |
| Child care/child support payments | |
| Alimony/maintenance payments | |
| Loan/credit card payments | |
| Entertainment (movies, eating out, etc.) | |
| Miscellaneous (e.g., classes, gifts, vacations, pet care) | |
| Donations | |
| Taxes | |
| Savings/retirement plan contributions | |
| Other | |
| **Total Expenses:** | |

## STEP 3: COMPARE INCOME AND EXPENSES

| | |
|---|---|
| Write down your total monthly income (from Step 1). | $ |
| Write down your total monthly expenses (from Step 2). | $ |
| Subtract expenses from income and list amount here. | $ |

## Looking at Investments

You may have money in a 401(K) or other retirement plan, or have other investments. It is a good idea to periodically review where your money is invested. The challenge is to find the right balance between the financial risk you can tolerate and the need for your money to grow.

If you currently are putting money into an employer-provided retirement plan, try to continue doing so. This is one of the best ways to save for your future—and you get special tax breaks. In addition, employers often match all or part of the money you save in the plan. Put at least enough money into the retirement plan to qualify for matching dollars from your employer.

## Hiring a Financial Professional

If you decide to hire a financial planner to review your finances, ask the Multiple Sclerosis Society to refer you to professionals who have worked with people diagnosed with MS. The National Multiple Sclerosis Society in the United States has developed a partnership with the Society of Financial Professionals called the Financial Education Partners, which will provide volunteer professionals to meet one-on-one with people with MS. Be sure to call the Society at 1-800-FIGHT MS about this opportunity. In addition, the following organizations can provide names of financial planners near you:

- American Institute of Certified Public Accountants, Personal Financial Planning Division, www.cpapfs.org
- Financial Planning Association, www.fpanet.org
- National Association of Personal Financial Advisors, www.napfa.org
- Society of Financial Service Professionals, www.financialpro.org

## Setting Aside Money for Unexpected Expenses

Many financial experts advise putting aside enough money to cover your bills for three to six months. This money can help if you lose your job or face other unexpected costs. Because you are dealing with a chronic disease, try to save enough money to cover six months of expenses.

The money you set aside for unexpected events should be placed in an account that you can get to easily. Consider the following options:

- *Savings account.* Savings accounts are easy to open and offer quick access to your money. While they pay only a small amount of interest, savings accounts at banks, savings and loans, and credits unions are safe investments.

- *Money market account.* You often need $1,000 to $10,000 to open a money market account. You may earn more interest on this type of account than with a savings account, but you may have limited access to it. In addition, depending on where you open a money market account, it may not be insured by the federal government. Be sure to ask.

- *Roth IRA.* Even though IRA stands for Individual Retirement Account, you can use a Roth IRA as a way to set money aside for emergencies. Unlike a regular IRA, you can withdraw the after-tax money you put into a Roth IRA without paying a penalty or taxes. However, generally you *cannot* withdraw any interest the account earns until age 59½ without paying a penalty. You are not taxed on any of the money you withdraw from a Roth IRA provided that you withdraw the money after age 59½, and the Roth IRA has been in existence for at least 5 years. However, if you become disabled, and distributions are made because of your disability, you do not have to meet the age 59½ rule for distributions of earnings to be income tax free.

To learn more about saving, investing, and personal finance, ask your librarian to recommend several good books. One great book on financial planning for all of those living with a chronic condition or disability is *Estate Planning for People with a Chronic Condition or*

*Disability* by Martin Shenkman, CPA, MBA, JD. This is not a book aimed only at people who have money; it will take you through living wills, determining how much life insurance your family needs and other financial matters. Or you can take a look at the following websites: Alliance for Investor Education, www.-investoreducation.org; American Savings Education Council, www.asec.org; Investment Company Institute, www.ici.org; or National Endowment for Financial Education, www.nefe.org.

# CHAPTER 10

# *Research in Multiple Sclerosis: The Search for Answers and the Link to Treatments*

Research in MS can help uncover fundamental knowledge of the disease's cause, the underlying mechanisms involved in the disease process, and its relationship to other disorders. This information is essential for developing safe and effective therapies. Indeed, the secret of acquiring effective ways to manage, prevent, and cure the disease will depend on a vigorous international research effort.

The first systematic studies of MS began in the mid-1800s by outlining the characteristics of the disease to separate it from other neurologic conditions. Physicians kept records on people with MS to show the various patterns of the disease, the pathological changes, and the response to treatments. It has evolved now, more than 150 years later, into a specialty area of basic and clinical research that incorporates virtually every discipline of modern medical science and biotechnology, ranging from clinical and community studies to the most up-to-date molecular laboratory techniques, genetic technologies, population studies, socioeconomics, psychology, and the application of randomized clinical trials to test new therapies.

Scientific research is a specialized discipline. Scientists are trained not only in their area of specialty research but also in the discipline and principles of scientific inquiry. Scientific research is driven by theories or hypotheses that then need to be challenged and tested using controlled laboratory or clinical techniques that have the greatest likelihood of providing meaningful answers. A *hypothesis* is a tentative assumption, usually developed through early observational study that can be proved or disproved by scientific investigation.

It has been said that the hardest part of science is asking the right question. The question has to be asked clearly so the hypothesis can then be stated in a way that also makes it clear how to test it.

Although there are many hypotheses in MS research, a great deal of investigation is currently directed at four major concepts about the disease and its cause (see Chapter 2):

1. It is a disorder resulting from an immune reaction in the central nervous system.
2. It occurs in genetically susceptible individuals
3. it is triggered by some other factor (infectious? environmental? other?).
4. It results in immune system–mediated inflammation and loss of the myelin and underlying nerve fibers of the brain and spinal cord, causing neurologic symptoms and the associated socioeconomic problems.

## Research in Immunology—Uncovering the Root of the Disease

While MS is recognized as a disease of the brain, spinal cord, and optic nerves (the central nervous system), it is widely believed that

MS is caused by an immune system disorder that causes damage to central nervous system tissue. This disrupts the normal activity of the part of the central nervous system controlling movement, sensory perception, thinking, and emotional functioning.

The immune system of the body is complex and crucial to protecting us from attacks by a variety of threats such as bacteria, viruses, parasites, and other foreign substances that pose a threat. The immune system can identify that the foreign factors are different from our own body proteins, tissues, and cells. When something goes wrong and the immune system attacks its own tissue, it is called an auto-immune disease.

The immune system consists of the bone marrow, spleen, thymus, and lymph nodes. The bone marrow produces white blood cells, called leukocytes. The spleen contains many white blood cells that fight infection and foreign substances. The thymus gland is the place where T lymphocytes mature and help destroy infected or cancerous cells. The lymph nodes produce and store cells to fight infections. There are T and B lymphocytes that produce antibodies and help destroy infected or cancerous cells. Leukocytes are white blood cells that identify and eliminate infectious agents. There are also a host of regulatory substances that circulate in the blood called *cytokines* and *chemokines*, and many other key players.

Normal immune function protects the body from injury and disease caused by infectious agents—such as bacteria, viruses, and parasites—by mounting an attack against the "invaders" and clearing them from the body. Because our immune systems and our tissues and organs are all part and parcel of ourselves, our immune system recognizes our cells as "self." Thus, normally our individual body tissues are usually protected and not subject to attack by our own immune system. This "self-protection" is rooted in the identical genetic make-up of each person's immune system and other organs and tissues: The identical genetic background signals that the individual's tissues are a normal part of the body and should not be considered to be foreign invaders.

Sometimes, however, this innate protection goes awry and a person's own immune system begins to attack his or her own body tissues and organs as though they were foreign. Most scientists believe that this process may be the underlying cause of MS. The disease is the result of an abnormality in which a person's own immune system fails to distinguish foreign invaders from normal tissues in the body. As a consequence, the immune system attacks apparently normal body tissues as well as foreign invaders, resulting in inflammation and tissue damage that is often permanent.

Understanding immune function in the disease has helped to reveal important information on what happens in the disease and has allowed researchers to tailor new therapies that target specific aspects of the immune reaction. This is the basis of the disease modifying therapies (DMTs) available for MS patients today. We are now in a position to marshal this growing body of vital information about immune system function and dysfunction into the development of a new generation of therapies for MS.

## Animal Model of MS: Experimental Allergic Encephalomyelitis (EAE)

In addition to human studies, immunological research in MS has been aided by animal models that have many of the immunological and pathological features of MS. It is *experimental allergic encephalomyelitis* (EAE), a laboratory-induced autoimmune disease of the brain and spinal cord in rats, mice, guinea pigs, and nonhuman primates. Studies of animal models for MS have greatly facilitated our understanding of basic immune system function and what goes wrong in autoimmune diseases. We recognize that EAE is not MS but studying the immune changes in EAE has been useful in understanding how the nervous system can be damaged by an immune reaction.

Because MS involves the immune system, physicians have used powerful drugs that modify immune function by decreasing the growth and proliferation of immune cells. Many such therapies that have been tested for MS—drugs such as cyclophosphamide and azathioprine and procedures such as total body or total lymphoid irradiation—have global or widespread immunosuppressive effects, potentially leaving a treated patient open to a variety of infections and complications. This complication has made these therapies of questionable value in terms of *risk versus benefit*. Even while recognizing that some of these agents might be able to help control the disease process, the risks of serious short-term complications and long-term risks such as malignancies, has limited their acceptance and use. Pinpointing the exact immune problems in MS has long been a goal of scientists. It is thought that such information could lead to highly specific therapies aimed at those immune system components involved in the disease, while leaving the rest of the immune system intact and functioning.

This search has been an important focus of research in recent years. This includes exploring what makes an immune system that is normally directed against outside invaders become misdirected against normal body tissues. Why the body mistakes "self" tissue for "foreign" invaders, and searching for the actual target of immune responses in the brain and spinal cord. Scientists are trying to determine the nature of T cells and antibodies that are primed to attack this target.

Another promising avenue of immunological research is directed at understanding how and why immune system cells move from the bloodstream into the central nervous system. This phenomenon, called "trafficking," may be one of the most important aspects of immune system problems in MS. Ordinarily, activated immune cells that could cause damage in the central nervous system are prevented from moving from the blood to the nervous system. In MS, the blood-brain barrier that keeps activated immune cells in the blood is breached and the potentially damaging cells enter the nervous system. Why is the blood-brain barrier breached in MS? How can the resulting movement of cells into the nervous system be stopped? Within recent years, a sufficient body of information has accumulated that points to the development of therapies that can block the blood-brain barrier breach and reduce or prevent immune cells from trafficking into the brain. Continuing work is needed to develop drugs that more effectively and safely reduce trafficking of immune cells into the central nervous system.

A difficulty in the MS research is the uncertainty about what specific antigens in myelin are being targeted in the immune reaction. One difficulty may be that there could be multiple myelin antigens involved. It is possible that different people may have different antigenic responses. To complicate things further, there tends to be a shifting in the immune responses. This means that specific T-cell treatments aimed at taking advantage of the originally proposed "restricted" immune responses in MS would not likely to be effective for a wide spectrum of patients with MS, and treatments effective at one time in the disease may not continue to be effective.

One relatively new focus in immunological research in MS has been on chemical messengers of the immune system called *cytokines* and *chemokines*. Cytokines and chemokines are produced by immune and other cells that regulate immune system activity. Many scientists believe that cytokines may be important "final pathways" involved in all immune responses—some cytokines encourage inflammation, which can be damaging in MS, and others suppress inflammation, which may be protective in MS. By manipulating cytokine activity so that pro-inflammatory responses are suppressed and anti-inflammatory responses are encouraged, it may not be necessary to understand specific immune cell responses in MS to combat the disease. And a second group of immune messengers, chemokines, sends important information signals throughout the body, helping to direct immune responses where they need to be most active. Controlling these chemical messengers may provide a kind of relatively non-specific treatment for MS.

Interferons, which are one type of cytokine, are an example of this dichotomy: Interferon beta has been shown to be anti-inflammatory and has been beneficial for treating MS, while there is evidence that interferon gamma may make the disease worse, at least at certain stages of the disease. Enhancing the activity of interferon beta might be an effective treatment; suppressing gamma interferons at certain states of the disease might be successful as well. A number of approved therapies for MS provide interferon beta by injection.

Research is giving us a better understanding of the cytokine "networks" and chemokine signaling pathways that are involved in MS and we hope to learn how to block "bad" cytokines and chemokines and enhance the effects of "good" ones.

Much of what we know about immunology and autoimmunity, including the actions of cytokines and chemokines, is shared among different autoimmune diseases. However, even if such complex immune networks are understood in a different disease, the outcomes are not always predictable in MS. For example, an important cytokine called tumor necrosis factor alpha (TNFα) was found to be involved in nervous system tissue damage in animal models of MS and believed to be functioning abnormally in MS itself. Blocking the action of TNFα in animal studies prevented or improved disease. A similar phenomenon was seen in animal models of rheumatoid arthritis that resulted in successful clinical trials for an agent that blocks TNFα in that disease, which is now available to treat arthritis patients. It was disappointing to find in clinical trials in MS that such TNFα blockers actually worsened MS. As before, as informative as animal and other disease research may be for MS, it is not always possible to predict MS-specific results. This is why careful, stepwise research needs to be conducted. Controlling cytokine activity in MS, such as interleukin-2 (IL-2), which can foster harmful inflammatory activity in the brain in animal models and in MS, is a fruitful area for the development of monoclonal antibody that can block the activity of IL-2.

While most work in MS immunology has focused on the T-cell response, cytokines, and chemokines, antibodies produced by B cells are increasingly believed to be important in MS pathology as well, and some of the newest effective treatments are directed at reducing B cells. The recent focus on antibodies as an important part of the MS pathology has led to attempts to control antibody responses using agents that specifically block the immune B cells that produce them.

*Hormones*

Also important is research on the role of hormones in MS. It is well known that MS is three times as common in women as in men. And it is well known that pregnant women with MS tend to have stabilization or improvement of their disease in the second and third trimesters of pregnancy, when estrogen levels are high, only to experience a higher risk for a disease exacerbation in the first several months after delivery, when estrogen levels drop. Changes in estrogen levels during pregnancy are thought to help regulate immune function: The immune system is suppressed in pregnancy to prevent a "rejection" of the fetus, which is recognized as being foreign by the mother's immune system. Therefore, hormone regulation of immune responses in MS has been an important area of MS research in recent years. Estrogen can actually improve EAE, the animal model of MS; testosterone, a male sex hormone, can make the disease worse. Would hormone levels also help control MS in humans by regulating immune function? This is under study.

### Genetic Research—Links to Susceptibility, Course, and Causation

Research on the genetic basis of MS has clarified some of the patterns of MS in families and populations. Population studies tell us that specific groups of people may be protected from MS and others may be more susceptible, with different rates of MS in different parts of the world (see Chapter 2). Moving beyond population studies, genetics research has become highly "molecular" in nature as scientists race to uncover genetic factors that underlie the disease and may help determine who is susceptible. The worldwide effort that led to the understanding of the human genome has helped us understand the genetic code that defines humans and was a major step in unraveling the complexities of diseases with genetic components. Whole genomic screens in MS have supported hypotheses about its autoimmune nature. They still have not explained the exact genetic basis of the disease. Genomic screen studies have now led to a focus on analysis of genetic haplotypes—blocks of genes that tend to be inherited together and that may be used for easier analysis of genetic factors in diseases like MS.

The possibility of specific gene therapies is no longer the stuff of science fiction, even though its application to human disease is in the early stages. The first attempts unfortunately were unsuccessful in disorders such as metabolic diseases and muscular dystrophy. There are very strict ethical and governmental restraints on gene therapy studies in humans. For gene therapy to become a potential treatment in a disease like MS, we need to understand completely the genetic factors that underlie the disease and devise ways to "correct" any defects that may be present. We are a long way from this goal and, given the nature of the disease, it may not be possible to achieve it at all.

A more immediate consequence of genetic research in MS may be the development of techniques to more readily determine susceptibility to MS in the general population and in families in which the disease already occurs. Genetic factors may even one day provide some clues to the prognosis for any individual with the disease, helping to predict the type of MS that a person will have and even its severity.

The genetic research has supported the belief that MS is autoimmune in nature. Immune function is under strict genetic control, and the genes of people with MS that control immune function are in some ways different from the immune system genes of healthy individuals. Among these are genes involved in helping the immune system determine which body tissues are its own and which substances are foreign—a bacterium or virus or even a transplanted liver or kidney from a genetically different donor. This ability to distinguish between self and foreign allows the immune system to mount an effective response against foreign substances but not against tissues or cells that are part of its own body. Genes controlling this recognition process are called human leukocyte antigens (HLA genes), histocompatibility genes, or major histocompatibility genes (MHC genes). Based on both early population studies in which HLA typing was done on blood samples and more recent results from highly molecular state-of-the-art whole genome screens of individuals with MS in the United States, Canada, and the United Kingdom, the HLA genes are, to date, the strongest link that we have to an MS genetic factor.

Genetic studies are helping us to know more about the immune nature of the disease, how much of the disease susceptibility may be related to genetic problems in immune system function, and how much of it may be related to other non-immunological factors or even to environmental or infectious factors.

An interesting recent genetic observation is a link between MS and vitamin D. It was shown that proteins activated by vitamin D in the body bind to a particular DNA sequence lying next to the DRB1-1501 variant associated with MS risk.

## Microbiome – How Bacteria in the Gut Affect the Immune System

The microbiome is the population of bacteria in the small and large intestine of the digestive system, which has more cells than in the rest of the body. There is increasing information on how the balance of the bacteria in the gut is important to health, and how alteration can affect many diseases and affect the immune system. There is evidence that the microbiome is involved in cardiovascular disease, obesity, and inflammatory bowel disease. Early research suggests the microbiome in MS patients may be different from other people and further research will try to find out the details and what factors might alter it back to normal. We also know that factors of interest in MS such as vitamin D deficiency, smoking, and alcohol can affect the microbiome. There are promising studies in laboratory animals to show that demyelinating disease (EAE) similar to MS can be worsened or improved by altering the microbiome in various ways. There are studies underway to see how the microbiome may be involved in the disease and how therapeutic trials could be designed.

## Infectious Disease Research—Clues to Triggers, Causes, and Possibly Treatments

Genes and the immune system are clearly involved with MS, but what event actually triggers the development of MS in people who are susceptible? For over a century it was suspected that an infection might be the trigger for MS, but it has been hard to prove and the evidence is incomplete.

Viral infections can cause human diseases with characteristics similar to those of MS, and these are usually one-time acute events. Certain viral diseases in laboratory animals also result in myelin damage like that seen in MS. For decades there has been very clear evidence that some viral infections, particularly upper respiratory tract viral infections, may set off acute exacerbations of MS in individuals who already have the disease. These observations, along with the knowledge that MS is more common in temperate regions and rare in tropical regions, have generated years of scientific hypotheses about infectious agents and MS. Some infectious diseases have a geographic pattern, as MS does, and it was noted many years ago that polio, when it was widespread, had a pattern not dissimilar to MS. There are many other infections common in temperate zones, but less common at the Equator, and vice versa.

Researchers have hunted for a specific identifiable virus related to MS, with the hope that this will result in a relatively simple explanation for the disease, and also with the hope that combating such a virus with a specific vaccination will result in a safe and effective preventive treatment or a specific virus-focused disease treatment. However, the search for *the* MS virus has been unfruitful. Several dozen common and uncommon viruses have been postulated to be related to MS based on either epidemiologic studies, the presence of higher levels of antibodies against a given virus in individuals with MS, or, more recently, evidence from very sophisticated polymerase chain reaction (PCR) analysis that can detect the "footprint" of a viral protein in body fluids and tissues even if the virus has been long eliminated by the immune system.

In most cases follow-up studies confirming the relationship of MS to a specific virus have not been convincing. Most such claims have been a result of inadequate experimental sampling or laboratory contamination. Nonetheless, there remains the possibility that infections may be related to MS.

In recent years, most of the focus has been on viruses that are very common in the general population—not necessarily isolated only in individuals with MS—such as human herpesvirus 6, which causes roseola in infants, and Epstein-Barr virus (EBV), which is known as the cause of infectious mononucleosis. Virtually everyone in the population has been exposed to these viruses, making it hard to assess a connection to MS.

A common bacterial infection has similarly been linked to MS. *Chlamydia pneumoniae*, the cause of "walking pneumonia," is an infectious agent to which most humans have been exposed. Reports have claimed an association with this bacterium in individuals with MS and have shown its presence in MS tissues. But many years of follow-up research have raised skepticism about the original reports, and a causal relationship between this bacterium and MS has not been proven.

How can common infectious agents be involved with MS when relatively few humans have the disease? Are these false leads and not really causes of MS? Are such agents simply associated with MS or are they "cofactors" that are required, but not in themselves sufficient, to cause the disease? If so, what else might be required for the disease to appear? This is where *genetic susceptibility* may have its impact: While a common infectious agent may be a trigger for MS, perhaps the disease will only occur in people who carry a genetic susceptibility to it. It is probable that both—a triggering agent and the "right" genetic background—are required and neither alone is sufficient for MS to develop.

This may be the case, but many investigators believe it is likely that no specific virus, bacterium, or other infectious agent will be found to be a cause of MS. Instead they are concentrating on research that explores how a susceptible person's immune system reacts to a variety of viral or other infections, or how immune function is tied to hormonal and other factors that might explain the initiation of the MS process. Studies from the mid-1990s to now, largely in laboratory animals, have helped to explain how an immune system that has lost its ability to distinguish self from non-self-tissue can be tricked by certain infectious agents into mounting an attack against its own myelin. The "trick" might be a very close similarity of molecular structure among some viruses, bacteria, and myelin itself—called *molecular mimicry* to reflect the similarity of molecular structure between some parts of myelin and some infectious agents. An effective and natural immune response mounted against a common infectious agent might result in a damaging cross-reaction with myelin itself if the molecular structure of the infectious agent mimics part of the molecular structure of myelin. This scenario of "mistaken identity" may explain much of the origin of MS and help to determine how the disease can be prevented from occurring in susceptible people.

## Glial Cell Research—What Is Damaged? What Can Be Repaired?

The symptoms of MS are directly due to inflammation and breakdown of myelin and the cells that make myelin called *oligodendrocytes*. Most likely as a secondary (but still early) process, nerve fibers that are wrapped and insulated by myelin also are often damaged in MS. The biology of oligodendrocytes and other glial cells in the central nervous system is a vital and expanding area of research. This includes study of how oligodendrocytes develop and form myelin in early stages of life, how they are affected by immune system responses, how the nervous system responds when myelin is lost, how scars are formed when myelin is lost, and what the potential is for myelin regeneration and recovery.

Basic biochemical studies of myelin using increasingly sophisticated techniques have closely analyzed nervous system tissue in people with MS, and such studies are used to determine if there are any abnormalities in the myelin or oligodendrocytes that might make these tissues and cells vulnerable to immune system attack. Historically, biochemical and anatomic research have repeatedly demonstrated that myelin, or white matter, is "normal" in individuals with MS, suggesting that the autoimmune attack in MS is truly a question of immune cells not recognizing normal self-tissue.

However, by the mid-1990s, a new technology stemming from magnetic resonance imaging (MRI), called *magnetic resonance spectroscopy* (MRS), began to show that normal-appearing white matter (myelin) in the brains of people with MS may actually have subtle abnormalities. It is not clear if these subtle imaging signals truly reveal myelin tissues or oligodendrocytic cells that are potentially vulnerable to immune attack or whether such signals are a result of a very early, previously undetected disease process. Cause and effect here, as elsewhere in biomedical research, is difficult to sort out. But such studies show not only the power of newer technologies but also the need to constantly reassess scientific beliefs and facts. Subsequently there have been pathological studies that also show that there is evidence of abnormal change in the areas that initially looked normal. We still need to consider, therefore, that there may be inherent abnormalities in white matter and myelin in individuals who develop MS and that the immune response is directed against this abnormal tissue. Or the disease is more widespread than suspected from clinical findings and MRI.

## Regeneration and Repair

Early on it was not recognized that myelin in the central nervous system could be regenerated after it was damaged. In the 1980s it was found that there was a degree of new myelin development in individuals whose brains showed extensive immune system damage and scarring due to MS. This myelin regeneration was insufficient to overcome the devastation caused by the disease, but it provided new hope that myelin could be more effectively repaired. It is likely that regeneration is very active early in the disease but repeated damage over time makes it harder to repair the myelin.

Knowing that damaged central nervous system oligodendrocytes can regenerate and form new myelin, many laboratories have focused on ways to enhance myelin growth and development in animals and in humans. In most cases of MS, particularly early cases, when myelin insulation around nerve fibers is damaged or lost, the central axon remains intact and can continue to function when myelin is restored, even though the new myelin is thinner than before. This is why we see recovery after an attack of MS.

Scientists are pursuing many experimental approaches to meet this challenge. These include identifying the early-stage myelin-making cells in the nervous system, called *oligodendrocyte progenitors*, that are capable, even in adults, of forming new tissue after immune system damage; using "growth factors" to stimulate myelin regeneration; taking advantage of chemical and physical signals that flow between myelin and nerve fibers to stimulate more rapid and efficient myelin growth and nerve regeneration; modulating immune system functions by blocking special immunoglobulins and antibodies that may be inhibiting myelin growth; and transplanting myelin-making cells from healthy donors or from healthy parts of a person's own nervous system to diseased or damaged nervous system sites.

## Stem Cell Research

Concepts of transplantation of myelin-making cells or of nerve cells by necessity involve research related to stem cells. Many of the ethical and religious concerns were solved when it became possible to develop stem cells from the tissues of the person who would in turn receive the stem cells. A key problem in cell or tissue transplantation is the issue of immune system rejection of the transplanted cells and tissues, based on a lack of genetic compatibility of the donor with the recipient, so this is overcome by using the person's own stem cells. So, the potential of therapeutic cloning of cells from the patient is a major advance. This research is opening doors to future ways to treat MS.

There are a number of studies that use bone marrow depletion by drugs and then replacement with the patient's own stem cells. This a difficult and complex therapy for a patient, but most of the cases have been advancing MS that failed on other therapies. The results have been very dramatic and positive.

To date, studies focused on myelin and nerve regeneration and replacement in MS (not using bone marrow suppression) have been largely limited to laboratory experimentation. Studies using certain immunoglobulins to suppress a theorized immunologic inhibition of myelin growth have been done in humans with MS, with mixed results; more work is planned. One small study that attempted to show re-myelination by transplanting peripheral nervous system glial cells into the brains of individuals with MS did not meet with success. But these are the first steps, and over time, more such efforts will be made, and eventually one or more of the cutting-edge techniques may prove to be successful. All of this research provides hope that myelin regrowth and functional recovery for individuals with MS may be possible in the future.

However, no matter what the potential for myelin and nerve fiber regeneration and growth, it is vital to emphasize two key problems related to MS: (a) the continuing immunological reaction, if unchecked, will tend to overcome efforts for regeneration; and (b) for some individuals, especially those with advanced MS, long-standing nerve fiber damage is likely to be a major component of their disability. Even if myelin can be repaired for such individuals, if the nerve fiber, the axon, is damaged, it is unlikely that conduction can be restored. Thus, research focusing on myelin and nerve regeneration must move hand-in-hand with efforts to stop the underlying immune system process—both to prevent patients from becoming seriously disabled in the first place and to hold in check immune system activity that will simply continue to damage any repaired cells and tissues. It is also another reason to treat MS early to take advantage of current therapies to reduce the activity of the disease.

## *Clinical Research—Treating the Whole Patient*

*Clinical research* directly involves individuals who have MS—not test tubes, not laboratory animals, but individuals living with a chronic disabling disease who experience symptoms, impediments to activities of daily living, and who have to live with consequent impacts on employment, family life, and social interactions. All MS research, no matter how fundamental, is aimed at finding treatments and a cure and at improving the quality of life for people living with MS. Studies in basic immunology, virology, and glial biology, in laboratory test tubes or in animal models of MS, all become applied in the clinic to help us translate such fundamental disease information into studies of people with MS. Clinical trials (see Chapter 11) focus on testing the safety and efficacy of new drugs and agents developed to treat MS and its symptoms (Figure 1).

Also important is the refinement and development of new techniques for reaching a diagnosis. Such techniques can be used to follow disease progress, particularly the relatively new imaging techniques based on magnetic resonance technology that allow direct observation of lesions in the brain and spinal cord (MRI and related technologies). New developments in analysis of MRI, blood, and cerebrospinal fluid also have importance in diagnosis, in tracking disease change over time, and in monitoring the results of experimental clinical studies. These technologies played a role in recent refinements of criteria used to diagnosis MS. In particular, the value of imaging and how it should be used has been codified into new MS diagnostic criteria through the widely used McDonald MS Diagnostic Criteria first put forth in 2001 and since refined in 2005 and 2010 (see Chapter 1).

Figure 1.   The spectrum of MS research.

| Basic Research → | Clinical Research → | Patient Management, Care and Rehabilitation → Research | Health Care Delivery and Policy Research |
|---|---|---|---|
| aims to | aims to | aims to | aims to |
| Understand Biologic Mechanisms → | Apply Basic Understanding → to Treat, Prevent, Cure | Improve Symptoms and Quality of Life → | Optimize Delivery of Care and Guide Public Policy |

While new treatments are being developed to help reduce the symptoms and progression of MS, helping individuals and their families cope with the disease, obtain the best possible medical care, and function at the highest possible level in society are essential aspects of research in the areas of psychosocial studies as well as health care delivery and policy research.

Understanding the psychologic and emotional aspects of MS has become a major focus of research in recent years. We realize that the brain pathology of the disease creates problems in cognitive and emotional function. Increased information in these areas is leading to new techniques to help with coping and rehabilitation, as well as interventions that can be applied in a clinical setting.

Although not limited to MS, the problems of access to care and services for people with chronic disease are increasingly unwieldy and are becoming the focus of high-quality health care delivery and policy research. Data gathered from such studies have a direct impact on altering public perception of chronic disease and on changing for the better legislative policy, entitlement programs, and societal policy for all people with disabilities.

Current research in MS is broad based and comprehensive. Funding for this research traditionally has come from governmental agencies, MS societies in many countries around the world, and, more recently, pharmaceutical and biotechnology companies. The results have increased understanding of the disease, provided new and specific therapies, and significantly enhanced the quality of life for people with MS. Basic and applied research are needed more than ever before to close the gaps in our knowledge of MS and move us closer to full treatment, prevention, and cure.

# CHAPTER 11

# Searching for Treatments: The "Ins" and "Outs" of Clinical Trials

B iomedical research in MS is intended to better understand the underlying mechanism and cause of the disease, which will lead to safe and effective therapy. The process is to explore research areas of immunology, virology, genetics, and neurophysiology to develop more focused therapies to benefit people with MS. When the research develops a potentially helpful drug, device or other therapy, the way to assess the benefit and safety of the therapy is by a *randomized, double-blinded clinical trial (RCT)*.

## The Randomized Clinical Trial

The RCT is designed to avoid bias in the assessment of results of treatment. Many things may appear to work when the results are no better than chance, and are biased by the desire to see a positive result.

In a RCT the drug to be studied is given to a large group of patients who are from a randomized population of MS patients and compared to a matched group who are reasonably the same so the results can be compared. One group is given the drug and the other an identical appearing placebo (or a comparable drug to study one against the other). The physicians, nurses and patients don't know who has the active drug and the inactive drug (blinded to the therapy). The only group who knows and oversees the trial as it goes along is a safety committee that makes sure nothing untoward happens. The RCT is the gold standard for the study of a drug.

It may seem an easy task to test a promising new drug, but consider the steps. First there has to be some solid scientific basis for considering a clinical trial of a drug and this may have come only after years of basic research. Then it is a long process to design the study, and determine how many patients have to be studied, for how long, to obtain a convincing statistical result. Then it has to go through a rigorous ethical review by an ethics committee. Then, if the study is not funded by the company who developed the drug, it will have to be presented to a funding agency in hopes that it will receive support. The application process may take a year or more. When funded, the recruitment of hundreds of patients may take one or two years, and the duration each patient must be followed is usually many years. After the trial is ended and all patients have arrived at the end of their treatment phase, it would take a year to collect all the data, do the statistical analysis, submit the results to a major medical meeting, and submit the finished research paper to a journal.

It would be nice if this could be faster, and many efforts are being made, with assurance that the quality of the results would not be lessened, but it still is a long procedure in order to get it right. The interferons were discovered in the 1970s but approved for therapy of MS after trials in the 1990s. It was twenty-five years from the discovery of glatiramer acetate to having it approved by the Food and Drug Administration for MS therapy. New technologies such as MRI are allowing us to do some trials more quickly but it still takes time and costs are often in the $15 million to $30 million range. We should also recognize that all this time, patient involvement, expense, and hope could end in failure, because the drug was ineffective, or had too many risks, or good but no better than available therapies. Poorly done clinical trials that result in misleading conclusions are wasteful at best and potentially dangerous for the intended population needing the treatment if they provide erroneous conclusions.

## The Special Problems of MS Trials

### Placebo Effects

Almost every drug used in every disease has a placebo effect, a feeling or sense of improvement that is due to the mind's positive perception of a result, unrelated to the effect of the treatment. And in the case of a placebo, which has no effect, the placebo effect again is due to the mind's perception, and the feelings are real, not imaginary. For example, in a study patients were told the drug (actually an inert placebo) was a stimulant and the patients' had an increased heart rate, increased blood pressure, and more rapid reaction times, but when told it was a sleeping pill they had the opposite reaction. Some pain and headache studies have very high placebo effects. In all the trials of MS drugs that showed benefit, the placebo group had some positive results as well. What the study has to show is that the drug effect is greater than occurs with a placebo. Placebo effects are very complex, as a red pill has a greater effect as a stimulant, and a blue pill has a greater effect on sleep. Also taking two placebo pills has a greater effect than one. And being told the placebo pill is very expensive has a greater effect, as does putting it in a package that has a known trade name over a plain package.

People with MS generally are highly motivated to search for a treatment or cure for their disease and hope for benefit in any treatment. This positive motivation can actually interfere with the objective assessment of any drug or device. Working with a sympathetic physician who also strongly believes in the value of an experimental treatment can help to reinforce placebo effects and can give rise to false-positive outcomes in clinical trials.

Simply participating in a clinical trial can result in a person's sense of well-being and increased hope and excitement at the prospect that an experimental agent will have benefit. As we mentioned, the placebo effect is not imaginary. The positive psychologic factors can even affect immune system function, thus leading to a real change in immunology that could have a direct impact on this immune-mediated disease. The interaction between psychology, physiology, and disease outcomes in MS is not well understood, but when they occur, they can seem to cause disease improvement—usually temporary unfortunately, since the underlying disease process might be unaffected. Such placebo effects are particularly present when results of experimental treatment rely on self-reporting of symptoms or physical state by a treated patient rather than on the more rigorous objective assessment of performance by an examining physician or on objective laboratory findings. This was noted in clinical trials of CCSVI when a large number of patients said they felt improvement in symptoms, but there was no improvement and sometimes worsening in objective measurements of their MS.

While important and potentially useful, placebo effects must be carefully separated from a true therapeutic drug effect. Treatments are costly, often inconvenient, and usually have associated side effects. If the impact of a treatment is, in fact, no better than a placebo response, there is no reason to use the drug! So, any useful drug for MS must have an impact that is greater than the placebo effect.

### The Natural Disease Variability of MS

The high degree of variability in MS makes the design of clinical trials difficult. The patients have different involvement, different courses, and because it is a life-long disease, the changes are usually slight in any year. In any individual, the disease may go through seemingly spontaneous remission and worsening that are unpredictable in occurrence, severity, and duration; no two individuals experience the same problems in the same ways. Spontaneous stabilization in previously progressive disease or a spontaneous remission of symptoms could easily be confused with a drug effect even if the drug is having no impact whatsoever.

### Understanding the Predicted Drug Effect

New agents for MS are usually chosen for testing because their known or suspected mechanism of action bears some relation to what we know about the disease. For instance, because the disease is widely believed to have an immune system origin, most new agents being tested in MS work through modulating immune functions. However, drugs may have different effects on different MS disease types. Agents that may be predicted to alter the frequency or severity of acute attacks of MS may have no benefit on longer term progression of disease, which may be due more to tissue degeneration than to inflammation.

A trial is designed to study a defined outcome, so certain patients who fit that criteria are candidates, but not others. For instance, if the study is to see if a drug has an effect on acute attacks, only patients who are having a certain number of acute attacks each year would be included.

Finally, some drugs may seem to cause improvement but actually only have indirect effects on the MS disease process. This can be the case for agents aimed at treating symptoms of MS like spasticity, fatigue, or depression, in which improvement may be real, but only the symptom and not the underlying disease is affected. This does not make the intervention less valuable, but it is important to distinguish between symptom improvement and actual impact on the underlying disease pathology that might come from disease-modifying agents. Understanding the true effect of any drug on the disease process requires a detailed knowledge of the drug's action and careful clinical assessment of effects on the disease.

### Availability of Safe and Useful Therapies

Since 1993 a total of fifteen drugs have been approved for the treatment of MS by the Food and Drug Administration and by other drug regulatory authorities in countries around the world. The list of approved drugs in each country may vary as each country has its own process to approve new drugs. The approval process requires convincing clinical trial data, which are examined in great detail.

The availability of treatments for some forms of MS actually complicates the search for new therapies, as placebo trials are less accepted now that many effective therapies are available. Increasingly the new agent must be tested against a known therapy. This has been specifically addressed in recent revisions of the Declaration of Helsinki, an international agreement that sets out guidelines for all human research. The Declaration states that it is an ethical obligation to provide "best available therapy" to all patients involved in research. It would be unethical to withhold known effective therapy, so trials in the future will mostly compare the experimental therapy with an accepted therapy rather than a placebo.

Beyond ethics, there are other issues involved in conducting placebo-controlled studies. Many patients don't want to enter a trial where they may receive a placebo rather than the study drug. This makes recruitment of patients difficult.

## Comparison of New Treatments Against Available Therapies

New treatments that are being developed need to be at least as good as, but hopefully, better than those already available. One way to judge is to conduct a "head-to-head" clinical trial that can determine clinical superiority of one agent over the other. Superiority might be determined by showing increased efficacy of one agent compared to the other, but also by increased safety, increased ease of delivery or compliance, or all of these. For statistical reasons, and because trials are conducted differently, it is difficult to compare the results of two separate placebo-controlled trials of two different agents, each tested alone against placebo, and to say that one is better than the other. All studies have a different patient population, are done in different locations, and are done at different times, all of which make direct comparisons between outcomes of different trials done at different times impossible. Head-to-head studies are difficult and expensive but more and more trials will be by this method.

These and other problems associated with MS clinical trials can best be overcome by extremely rigorous experimental designs for the studies. The generally accepted methods of study are time consuming and expensive, and needed innovation is hard to come by, but such rigorous trial designs hold the best chance of obtaining a clearcut answer about the efficacy and safety of any agent in MS.

## Steps in MS Clinical Trials

### Scientific Rationale

Both scientific rigor and the rules of regulatory agencies such as the Food and Drug Administration, and related agencies in Canada and Europe dictate a set path for development and testing new treatments for human diseases. These include demonstration of biologic relevance, safety, and efficacy in a stepwise fashion that can take many years to accomplish.

There must be a strong scientific rationale for being tested in this disease. Based on our knowledge of the MS process and on prior experimental studies of the drug in the laboratory, in animal disease models for MS, or in human disorders with similarities to MS, scientists will conclude that a drug may have a potential role in the treatment or management of MS. The drug likely will have no impact on disease outcome and will be wasteful of the time and effort of participating individuals with MS and their physicians, as well as the financial resources required for the study. Many "alternative" therapies can be faulted on this first criterion: a lack of bona fide biologic rationale for even being considered in a disease such as MS.

If a scientific rationale has developed for a potential therapy, it goes through a detailed set of "preclinical" studies, either in laboratory Petri dishes and test tubes (in vitro) or in living animals (in vivo) to better understand the action of the agent, the pharmacologic dynamics of its use, and its safety in a setting in which humans are not yet exposed to the agent. Such preclinical testing usually continues even after an agent has been given to humans for evaluation.

### *"Preliminary" or Phase 1 Studies*

Given a strong scientific rationale and acceptable results from preclinical testing in laboratory and animal research, human trials almost always begin with toxicity or safety studies in a very small number of people with the disease. This is a "preliminary" or *phase 1* clinical trial. In such early experiments, physicians look for evidence that the agent is safe for use in humans—the most vital consideration in any medical intervention. If such studies demonstrate that the agent is safe, a physician may pursue further studies to get a sense of possible efficacy. Phase 1 studies will also often begin to explore different doses or routes of delivery (e.g., oral, injection) of the experimental agent, to help define the safety and tolerability spectrum of the agent.

### *"Pilot" or Phase 2 Clinical Trials*

These studies usually involve larger, statistically relevant numbers of patients (often twenty to 250 or more) to assess key factors such as:

1. Determining the effectiveness of the drug in halting progression, reducing relapse rate, or improving symptoms and function;
2. Obtaining additional information about toxicity and safety; and
3. Refining knowledge about the best possible dose and route of delivery.

Such pilot studies aim to be objective in obtaining the required answers. We need to compare patient performance while on these drugs with a person's pre-drug status or against the known performance of a similar group of individuals not receiving treatment. Even better, patients on the trial drug might be compared with an identical group of patients who are on a parallel "control" track but being given sham or placebo treatment when ethically and practically possible, or with patients who are being actively treated with the existing best available therapy for that form of disease.

True objectivity is enhanced in controlled studies if both the patients and the physicians are "blinded" or "masked" to the treatment status of individual subjects. In other words, neither knows which group of patients is receiving the experimental drug and which group is being given control treatment. Such "double-blinded" studies are hard to achieve, given the fact that many test agents have side effects that may be "unblinding" to the patient or examining physician. Also, some therapies are hard to hide if the patient gets injections on one schedule compared to a treatment that is oral or by a different injection route or schedule. But rigorous efforts at blinding are essential to reduce the likelihood of bias.

Increasingly, phase 1 and 2 studies are being combined into a "phase 1-2" study to speed the initial assessment of toxicity and efficacy. Magnetic resonance imaging (MRI) to detect the impact of treatment on lesion development in the central nervous system is now used as a key outcome in such studies in MS, and often is the primary outcome that is monitored. MRI is an effective marker of disease activity and disease pathology, and since MRI changes tend to occur relatively rapidly compared with more difficult-to-detect clinical changes they can shorten a trial if MRI change is taken as the outcome. If another outcome, such as reduction of disability, is measured, the studies are longer and MRI would be used for assessment of secondary outcomes.

Results from such phase 1-2 studies can often take several years to obtain. They may or may not show statistical benefit to people receiving the drug compared with people receiving control therapy, and may or may not show acceptable levels of side effects and tolerability. An experimental agent usually is abandoned as a possible therapy if there is no benefit, or if there are uncontrollable or dangerous side effects. On the other hand, if the possibility of benefit remains after the study, and side effects are acceptable, a further clinical trial, usually with a primary focus on change in clinical status, will be undertaken to confirm and expand the studies.

*"Definitive" or Phase 3 Clinical Trials*

These trials usually are the final step toward making a decision about the value of a proposed therapy. As in phase 2 studies, the key questions are efficacy and safety. Large, statistically determined numbers of participants are essential, and the study often is conducted at a number of different sites and often is international in scope to ensure that the drug can be used in an equivalent fashion by many physicians in many care settings. These studies require large numbers of patients over a long period and are very expensive.

Rigorous adherence to blinding of patients and examining physicians is essential. Randomization of patients to the study and the control group is essential so that the groups are as similar in all meaningful ways as possible. Investigators try to pick patients similar in age, sex distribution, type, duration and degree of disability. At the conclusion of the study period, when the blinding code is broken and the performance of drug-treated patients can be compared with that of the control group patients, there should be sufficient information to determine if the tested agent is truly safe and effective. Phase 3 studies in MS virtually always track the impact of an experimental agent on measurable change in the patient and additional studies might be added as "secondary outcomes" of interest. In order to achieve regulatory acceptance, it is required that the therapy has an impact on the clinical course of the disease.

Recent definitive clinical trials for MS have included as many as 1,500 individuals or more, have involved fifty to one hundred or more participating centers, often distributed around the world, and have taken multiple years to complete. These are the "gold standard" studies from which physicians and patients may have the best confidence that the results are sound.

There are variations in these study designs, often depending on the amount of information available about a new drug from the laboratory, from use in other diseases, or from prior use in MS. Not all new agents go through a test phase in animal models of MS. And in some cases, phase 2 and phase 3 studies are combined into a single large phase 2-3 study when there is sufficient information available from previous studies on dosing and route of delivery. These are also the elements and data required by the Food and Drug Administration and similar regulatory bodies in many countries, which closely monitor clinical trials at every step. It is ultimately the regulatory authority's assessment of the results of benefit and safety and the care with which a study is done that determines whether any agent may be marketed as a treatment for MS.

### *"Postmarketing" or Phase 4 Studies*

Once governmental regulatory approval has been granted and a new agent can be marketed and advertised as a treatment for MS, there often is a series of further studies, which are termed "post-marketing" or *phase 4* studies. These usually are designed to collect long-term information about safety and adverse reactions to the agent, to evaluate its continued efficacy over time, and to explore the use of the drug for different forms of disease.

In some cases, regulatory authorities mandate phase 4 studies to collect data that were missing or insufficient in the definitive analysis and that are important in understanding the use of the new medication. Sometimes the outcome of these mandated phase 4 studies can determine continued marketability of new agents. Should data become available that change the original understanding of the safety and efficacy of the new agent and compromise its use, regulatory authorities may remove the treatment from the market.

## *Financing Clinical Trials*

Drug studies are time consuming and expensive. Such studies most often are supported financially by pharmaceutical and biotechnology companies that invest significant "research and development" resources in these experiments. Grants from the federal government or voluntary health agencies, such as the National Multiple Sclerosis Society and its counterparts around the world, also may fund part or all of the cost of clinical trials. It is rare (and often considered unethical) to request that a patient who volunteers to participate as an experimental subject be asked to pay for that privilege.

## *Who Participates in Clinical Trials?*

The decision for any person with MS to participate in an experimental clinical trial is an intensely personal one and is highly subjective. Since there is always the potential for risk of any untested agent, a potential study participant must be fully informed by the treating physician with a clear assessment of the potential risk factors in the study. Informed consent, including close personal discussion with the physician and nurse as well as required written permission from the study participant, is a legal requirement that protects the rights of all participants.

A true sense of altruism, coupled with a sense of adventure, often characterize those who volunteer to participate in such studies, since participation in either an active treatment or sham group ultimately may help tens of thousands of people with MS. The clinical trial volunteer is a true hero.

## *Why Can't Some Patients Participate in Clinical Trials?*

Disappointed patients will ask, "Doctor, why can't I be in your clinical trial?"

Clinical trials generally are limited to a fixed number of individuals, who must be located geographically close to one of the clinical centers where the study is undertaken. Since most studies require intense and frequent clinic visits at specific predetermined times throughout several years, difficulties in travel from home to the clinic may be considered in determining whether someone will be accepted into a study.

The design of trials is such that generally only one type of MS— for instance, relapsing-remitting disease—is involved in the study. This excludes people with any other form of MS. Even within the group of interest, further restrictions, called inclusion and exclusion criteria, will be enforced in virtually all studies: disease limited to a certain duration or a certain level of disability; restricted age of participants; exclusions based on prior medications or participation in previous trials of agents for which there might be dangerous or confusing effects with the new experimental treatment.

For any particular test drug, other restrictions also may apply, depending on the known characteristics of the test medication. There are often prohibitions against pregnancy as new drugs don't yet have safety information about the mother or fetus. Some medical conditions cause confusion with MS symptoms or add medications that would confuse the record of side effects from the new drug. If a patient is disappointed by not being entered in a trial, they may take some solace from the realization that positive findings eventually are available to all patients

## *Where Can I Learn About Ongoing Clinical Trials?*

Finding out about clinical trials in MS should be a joint project of the patient and the physician. The network of physicians who organize and participate in MS clinical trials is ever growing, and in consultation with a personal physician, an interested patient usually can learn of any pending studies locally or in nearby communities, often with the assistance of the local branch or chapter of the National Multiple Sclerosis Society, Multiple Sclerosis Society of Canada, or their over thirty affiliated member organizations around the world. The U.S. National Multiple Sclerosis Society (www.nationalmssociety.org) has an extensive listing of ongoing and newly recruiting MS clinical trials in the United States and elsewhere, as does the Consortium of Multiple Sclerosis Centers (www.mscare.org) through its NARCOMS affiliate group; the Multiple Sclerosis International Federation (www.msif.org) carries similar information about trials around the world. Other sources, which might include information about MS clinical trials but are not specific or restricted to MS, include Centerwatch (www .centerwatch.com) and the U.S. Department of Health and Human Services (www.clincaltrials.gov).

# CHAPTER 12

# How Multiple Sclerosis Organizations Can Help

People with MS have many needs and concerns related to their diagnosis and struggles with MS, and some of these are shared by family members and close friends. The issues are different at different stages of the disease, the nature of the symptoms or disability, and the family and work situation. The needs will also vary due to the different personality characteristics, previous life events, and learning and coping styles of the individuals.

The family physician or neurologist is a frequent source of information. While this is certainly appropriate for issues related to the disease symptoms and treatment, a medical practice is not an adequate resource to accommodate the extensive nonmedical needs of those with MS, their families, friends, and other concerned persons such as employers, teachers, and health professionals. In North America, the primary resources for addressing nonmedical MS-related needs are the National Multiple Sclerosis Society in the United States and the Multiple Sclerosis Society of Canada, the

Multiple Sclerosis Association of America, the Multiple Sclerosis Foundation, the Consortium of Multiple Sclerosis Centers, the International Organization of Multiple Sclerosis Nurses, Can Do MS, and the Multiple Sclerosis Coalition. This chapter provides general information about these organizations, as well as the specific ways these organizations can help you.

## The National Multiple Sclerosis Society

The National Multiple Sclerosis Society (NMSS) was the first non-profit organization in the United States to support national and international research on the prevention, cure, and treatment of MS. Equally important, the Society's goals include the provision of nationwide programs to assist people with MS and their families and the provision of information about MS to those with the disease, family members, professionals, and the public. Programs are designed to help people with MS to maintain their independence and lifestyle. The Society's mission—to end the devastating effects of MS—addresses the negative impact of the disease in the present through education and services to support a positive quality of life and into the future through research and advocacy.

The NMSS was founded in 1946 by Sylvia Lawry, whose brother had MS. In her search to learn more about the disease, she found that very few people in the country professed any interest in the disease. Ms. Lawry placed an advertisement in *The New York Times* seeking any information about successful treatments for MS. A number of people who were also touched by MS responded. They had no news of a cure, but asked that Ms. Lawry share whatever helpful information she received. And so the National Multiple Sclerosis Society was born.

The NMSS continues to grow. A fifty-state network of chapters provides assistance and education. The home offices in New York City, Denver, and Washington, DC, direct MS-related research and advocacy, provide some specific services, and provide support, structure, and guidance for chapters. Policies and national priorities are established by a National Board of Directors, composed of business and professional leaders with a special interest in MS. The Board is assisted by a nationally representative group of individuals with MS, the National Programs Advisory Council. Each local chapter is governed by a Board of Trustees. Staff at both national and chapter levels work in partnership with volunteers and the community to implement the necessary and desired programs. There is an ongoing process of identifying needs and eliciting feedback regarding the value of programs. This involves people with MS, their families, and the professionals who serve them, and provides direction for Society activities.

## Philosophy of NMSS Programs

The NMSS and its chapters are committed to empowering people with MS to live as independently as possible within the limits of their disabilities and to the maximum of their capabilities within the least restrictive environment. This goal is achieved through programs, services, and activities that:

- Promote and support knowledge, health, and independence
- Inform and educate people with MS and their families, professionals, public officials, and the general public about MS
- Provide support programs that help people with MS and their families cope with the changes and challenges that MS presents
- Help people gain access to community resources and quality specialty health care
- Stimulate changes and developments in the community and public policy beneficial to people affected by MS
- Fill gaps in community resources

The Society believes that all people with MS and their families in the United States should have access to certain basic programs and ensures this through its chapter certification process.

All people with MS are offered services without discrimination. Access is not affected by a person's race, color, religion, age, disability, sexual orientation, or the individual's relationship with a chapter. Chapters do hold "targeted" programs to meet the needs of specific groups; for example, education programs for those newly diagnosed, young professionals' groups, and the gay/lesbian community.

The confidentiality of members with MS and their family members ("clients") is strictly maintained.

## Who Does the NMSS Serve?

The Society's mission reflects a dedication to "end the devastating effects of multiple sclerosis." At the center of chapter programs are people who have MS. Since the disease affects others as well, NMSS clients are all who come to the Society for information and/or professional assistance. The secondary focus of its programs is the MS "family circle"—spouses, children, parents, relatives, and significant others. Coworkers and close friends are included in this circle as well. Family members and significant others can also utilize chapter programs.

The NMSS is a leading source of information on MS for the general public. It also provides education to health professionals, service providers, and community agencies. This information and education can have significant impact on quality of life, increasing access to quality health care and community resources, and promoting understanding from others.

## Quality of Life Goals

The NMSS organizes services under three main Quality of Life Goals: MS Knowledge, Health, and Independence. Specific services are addressed within this framework.

### Knowledge

The NMSS facilitates the acquisition of essential knowledge about MS by providing information and education to clients, families, professionals, and the public. Information is the first and most frequent request the NMSS receives from people with MS. Client surveys consistently request more information about MS: symptoms, diagnosis, programs, treatment, research, and related issues such as employment, health insurance, disability rights, and family issues.

Seeking information about MS is usually a first step in the coping process. Getting accurate up-to-date information can assist you to make informed decisions, become aware of needs and resources, and take some control over this unpredictable and complex disease. One of the main functions of the NMSS is to serve as the repository of the most current and accurate information on MS. This includes:

- Information can be obtained by calling 1-800-FIGHT-MS (1-800-344-4867)

- Website with updated information about treatments, current research, and programs (http://www.nationalmssociety.org)

- *Knowledge Is Power* educational program (serial mailings) for people newly diagnosed with MS and their families, available through all chapters or on the website

- *Moving Forward* group educational program for people newly diagnosed with MS and their families

- Educational programs on various topics throughout the year

- Annual national education program

- Booklets, articles, and information sheets on MS-related topics (see Resources)

- Lending library of books, audio- and/or videotapes, with mail access

- *Inside* MS national bimonthly magazine plus chapter newsletter issued quarterly or more often

*Health*

The NMSS helps people with MS to achieve optimal health physically, emotionally, and in their relationships.

### PHYSICAL HEALTH

People with MS must deal with concerns about physical impairments related to the disease and their impact on general physical health. NMSS programs and services address physical health needs by:

- Promoting state-of-the-art MS health care and facilitating access for people with MS through formal affiliations with MS clinical facilities and professional education programs

- Providing referrals to neurologists, physical therapists, and other medical/rehabilitation professionals knowledgeable about MS

- Swimming and other exercise programs sponsored or co-sponsored by some chapters or referral to existing programs in the community

- Wellness programs

- Affiliation with local MS clinical facilities to facilitate access to, and coordination of, health services

- Participation in local and national advocacy issues related to physical health, for example, health insurance reform, through Action Alert Network. (Call your local chapter to join or sign up on the Society's website.)

### EMOTIONAL HEALTH

Emotional health is a state of psychological well-being, including an individual's adaptive capacities. It is demonstrated by successful interactions with others and with the social environment. Difficulties with adaptation to a chronic illness are normal and respond favorably to a variety of interventions.

Although NMSS chapters are not primarily mental health agencies, they can help individuals and their significant others in their adaptation to chronic illness. Chapters provide short-term counseling: defined as "reflective listening and problem solving." The social isolation that often results from having a chronic illness can be reduced through peer relationships and group programs that bring people together.

NMSS chapters offer assistance with problem solving, including:

- *"Someone to Listen"* peer support program, which meets the second most requested service—to speak with another person who has MS. "Peers" are specially trained to provide information and support to the person with MS.

- Local counselor/therapist referrals.

- Self-help groups—leaders have often received group leadership training through the Society.

- Peer support programs.

**FAMILY SUPPORT**

Families of people with MS are important to the NMSS, which has formally adopted the Family Service America, Inc. definition of family: "A family consists of two or more people, whether living together or apart, related by blood, marriage, adoption, or commitment to care for one another."

This definition highlights the inclusion of all varieties of family configurations. The NMSS recognizes the enormous, ongoing stress that the entire family experiences, as well as the critical support provided by the family to the person with MS. Programs emphasize the strengths of the family and bolster these strengths by offering education and other means of support and assistance.

The NMSS sponsors a variety of family programs that combine education, counseling, and social activities. Some chapters have family counseling programs, referrals to experienced community counselors in others. The *Children with MS* program provides support, networking, education, and counseling for children/teens with MS and their parents (call the Denver home office: 303-813-6623).

*Independence*

The NMSS is committed to promoting the highest possible level of independence for people with MS.

### INDEPENDENT LIVING AND ACCESSIBILITY

The NMSS can provide referrals to centers for independent living, equipment vendors, accessible housing, and others.

All chapter offices and program locations are accessible to people with disabilities.

### EMPLOYMENT

Referrals and consultations are available to help people continue employment despite MS-related obstacles.

### LONG-TERM CARE SERVICES

Programs are available to help people who are moderately to severely limited by MS-related disability receive necessary personal services and other assistance.

## The Multiple Sclerosis Society of Canada

Founded in 1948, the Multiple Sclerosis Society of Canada has a growing membership with seven regional divisions and more than 120 chapters. The head office is located in Toronto, Ontario, and division offices are located in Halifax, Montreal, Toronto, Winnipeg, Regina, Edmonton, and Vancouver. The mission is "to be a leader in finding a cure for MS and enabling people affected by MS to enhance their quality of life." The Multiple Sclerosis Society of Canada funds a research program totaling about $6 million annually. It also has a $20 million endMS program to encourage young trainees to have their careers dedicated to MS research.

### Client Services

The Multiple Sclerosis Society of Canada provides a wide variety of programs and services for those affected by MS. These include the following.

### INFORMATION AND REFERRAL

- Multiple Sclerosis Society of Canada publications
- ASK MS and National Information Resource Centre

- Lending libraries
- Information and referrals over the phone or by email

**EDUCATION**

- Conferences and workshops

**SUPPORT**

- Individual advocacy
- Support and self-help groups
- Recreation and social programs

**ADVOCACY**

- Helping individuals with MS obtain needed services

**FUNDING**

- Equipment purchase or loan programs
- Special assistance programs

Services vary across the country depending on the kind of provincial government and community programs available, since the Society does not duplicate services available through other sources. The Society currently spends nearly $9 million annually on services and education programs for people who have MS, their family members, and all others affected by MS.

### Awareness Activities

The Multiple Sclerosis Society of Canada is firmly committed to informing Canadians about MS and how they can join the fight against MS. The national office coordinates an overall public awareness campaign that is complemented by division and chapter activities.

### Government Relations/Social Action

The Multiple Sclerosis Society of Canada works with people who have MS to ensure that they have the opportunity to participate fully in all aspects of life. Volunteers across the country endeavor to change government policies at all levels, private industry practices, and public attitudes in ways that will positively benefit people with MS.

### Fund Raising

The Multiple Sclerosis Society of Canada has growing total revenues annually. The funds are used to support research, client services, public education, social action, and volunteer resources. Most of this income comes from public donations, bequests, and special fund-raising programs conducted by the Society. The major fund-raising programs are the MS Carnation Campaign, the RONA MS Bike Tour, the MS Read-A-Thon, the Super Cities WALK for MS, the direct marketing program, and major gifts/planned giving.

### History

A small group of dedicated volunteers in Montreal founded the Multiple Sclerosis Society of Canada in 1948 after contact with the newly established National Multiple Sclerosis Society in the United States. Support of MS research began in 1949.

Headquarters for the Society remained in Montreal until the mid-1960s, when the offices were moved to Toronto. Other advances came with the establishment of regional divisions; there are now seven divisions across Canada from coast to coast. The Multiple Sclerosis International Federation, of which the Canadian Society is a charter member, was established in 1967.

### MS Clinics

The Multiple Sclerosis Society of Canada is proud to work with a network of specialized MS clinics across the country. Clinic services vary, but most offer a wide range of services, delivered by a multidisciplinary health care team. These services usually include:

- Expert diagnostic and treatment services for people with MS

- Clinical research, especially in the area of MS treatment options

- Educational and support programs for people with MS and their families and caregivers

To learn more about the clinic in your area and the services it provides, contact the Multiple Sclerosis Society of Canada for contact information on the clinic in your area by calling toll-free in Canada at 1-800-268-7582.

### *The Multiple Sclerosis Association of America*

The Multiple Sclerosis Association of America (MSAA) is a national nonprofit organization founded in 1970 dedicated to enriching the quality of life for everyone affected by MS. The MSAA provides ongoing support and direct services to individuals with MS and people close to them. It also serves to promote greater understanding of the needs and challenges of those who face physical obstacles. Its philosophy and effort have focused on enriching the quality of day-to-day living for everyone affected by MS. It helps each individual on a personal level and relies on volunteers and support from the general public. The MSAA's national office in Cherry Hill, New Jersey, serves clients throughout the United States. Its regional offices, the Midwest Regional Office, Northwest Regional Office, Southeast Regional Office, Northeast Regional Office, South—Central Regional Office and Western Regional Office, provide additional assistance on a more local basis, facilitating outreach and awareness. Regional offices conduct awareness and educational conferences and workshops and bring people together through networking and events and conduct fundraising activities. Overseeing MSAA's activities is a national Board of Directors comprised of accomplished professionals from across the country, volunteering their time. Providing medical consultation is MSAA's Chief Medical Officer, who reviews all of MSAA's medical information and chairs its Healthcare Advisory Council, which brings significant leadership, knowledge, and expertise in the fields of neurology, nursing, and physical therapy and provides strategic support and guidance on health-related issues.

*Vital Programs and Services*

MSAA's website (http://www.msassociation.org) is an excellent resource for anyone interested in learning more about MS featuring topics such as "What is MS," "Types of MS," and "Treatments of MS." There is a "Newly Diagnosed" section offering answers and support. MSAA publications provide a great deal of helpful and important information and cover a wide range of subjects such as medical research and treatments, symptom management, complementary and alternative therapies, as well as general information. Its national magazine, *The Motivator*, includes articles on vital issues such as new research, treatments, and personal stories. All publications are available free of charge and may be viewed, downloaded, or ordered at www.msassociation.org or by calling toll-free 1-800-532-7667. The Lending Library offers a collection of nearly 300 MS resources on diagnosis, symptoms, treatments, general health, along with books that inspire through personal experiences and life stories. MSAA loans and mails the books and DVDs free of charge, along with instructions for returning them free of charge.

MSAA provides people with MS with equipment ranging from grab bars to wheelchairs; cooling accessories for heat-sensitive individuals; a mobile phone app, *My MS Manager*, for use free of charge on an iPhone, iPad or iPod touch. Visit http://www.msassociation .org/mobile to download *My MS Manager*. A new program called S.E.A.R.C.H has been introduced to assist the MS community about different treatment choices. It is designed as a memory aid, the acronym representing the key areas that need to be discussed with one's health care team when "searching" for the most appropriate MS treatment. S.E.A.R.C.H. stands for safety, effectiveness, affordability, risks, convenience, and health outcomes. Written materials about the program can be downloaded at http://www.msassociation.org/ search or requested at 1-800-532-7667.

MSAA provides assistance in acquiring magnetic resonance imaging (MRI) scans for patients without insurance or who have been denied coverage for an MRI. The *Staying Connected* program is a networking program that facilitates peer support. It is an online community of individuals with MS and their care partners who are interested in corresponding via email with others who are affected by MS. Email correspondence through this program is especially helpful for those who are unable to attend traditional support group meetings but want to stay connected to the MS community. The *Staying Connected* network program's online directory is password protected and available through MSAA's website.

### The Multiple Sclerosis Foundation

The Multiple Sclerosis Foundation (MSF) provides a comprehensive approach to helping people with MS maintain their health and well-being by offering programming and support to keep them self-sufficient and their homes safe, and by conduction educational programs to heighten public awareness and promote understanding about the disease. MSF is a service-based, non-profit organization with national headquarters in Fort Lauderdale, Florida. It serves the nation from one central location eliminating the need for branch offices in order to maintain a more cost-effective and efficient operation while maintaining the highest quality service. It networks with independent, grassroots organizations to give it a local presence in communities around the nation.

The MSF was established in 1986. It is a publicly funded 501 organization and the funds it raises go directly into services designed to improve the quality of life for people with MS. All of its services including information, literature, and subscriptions to its publications are provided free of charge. Some programs are needs-based and dependent on income and other factors while other programs are available to all individuals affected by MS. The MSF sponsors Home Care Grant Programs, Support Groups, Peer Counseling, and a yearly Cruise for the Cause where people with MS and their families cruise together to interact with MS health care professionals to gain knowledge about MS and support. It has a Lending Library and excellent publications on the different aspects of MS for patients and their families. Information about MSF programs can be obtained by calling 1-888-MSFOCUS or on its website, http://www.msfocus.org.

### The Consortium of MS Centers

The Consortium of MS Centers (CMSC) is an organization of MS health care providers intent on improving the lives of those affected by MS. Its members are neurologists, nurses, physical therapists, neuropsychologists, and social workers who work with MS patients. It was organized in 1986 under the direction of neurologists interested in the clinical care of MS. It has grown to become a multidisciplinary organization providing a team approach to MS care and a network for all health care professionals and others specializing in the care of persons with MS. It has over 200 member centers in the United States, Canada, and Europe, representing over 4,000 health care professionals worldwide who provide care for more than 150,000 individuals with MS.

CMSC provides leadership in clinical research and education; develops vehicles to share information and knowledge among members; disseminates information to the health care community and to persons affected by MS.. Through its CMSC North American Research Committee on Multiple Sclerosis (NARCOMS) based at the University of Alabama at Birmingham, it maintains a patient registry, website, expert forum and research registry to promote MS research. It has an online journal, the *International Journal of Multiple Sclerosis Care*, to promote multi-disciplinary approaches to treating persons with MS. While this is an organization for health care professionals rather than patients, patients will find articles of interest to them on its website (http://www.mscare.org).

### The International Organization of Multiple Sclerosis Nurses

The International Organization of Multiple Sclerosis Nurses (IOMSN) was founded on May 30, 1997 and is the first and only international organization focusing solely on the needs and goals of professional nurses, anywhere in the world, who care for people with MS. By mentoring, educating, networking, sharing—the IOMSN supports nurses in their continuing effort to offer hope. The IOMSN establishes standards of nursing care in MS, supports research, and educates the health care community about MS.

Out of this group came the development of an examination to certify nurses who provide MS care. This is a group that those of you with MS will want your nurses to join. While it is only for MS nurses, its website will provide information helpful to patients and connect you to other sites that will be of interest. The website is http://www.iomsn.org.

### Can Do MS

Can Do MS is a leading provider of innovative lifestyle empowerment programs for people with MS and their support partners. Leveraging the powerful legacy and principles of former Olympian and organizational founder, Jimmie Heuga, Can Do MS has helped thousands of people living with MS reclaim a sense of dignity, control, and freedom by empowering them with the knowledge, skills, tools and confidence to transform challenges into possibilities.

Can Do MS does programs all over the United States but it also has events and webinars listed on their website at http://www .mscando.org.

## The MS Coalition

The MS Coalition (MSC) is another organization that benefits people who have MS. It was founded in 2005 by three independent MS organizations, the MSAA, the MSF and the NMSS, in an effort to work together to benefit individuals with MS. Since that time it has grown to a nine-member organization, all of whom provide critical MS programs and services. Its members are the Multiple Sclerosis Association of America (MSAA), the Multiple Sclerosis

Foundation (MSF), the National Multiple Sclerosis Society (NMSS), the United Spinal Association, Accelerated Cure Project for Multiple Sclerosis, The Consortium of Multiple Sclerosis Centers (CMSC), Can Do MS, and the International Organization of Multiple Sclerosis Nurses (IOMSN). It is important for you to know about this organization because its vision is to improve the quality of life for those affected by MS through a collaborative network of independent MS organizations. Its mission is to increase opportunities for cooperation and provide greater opportunity to leverage the effective use of resources for the benefit of the MS community.

The first chapter of this book began by making you aware of the history of MS. Hopefully you will realize from its other chapters how far we have come. In the coming years you will note that we continue to have rapid improvements in the treatment of the disease as we move forward to work for better treatments and a cure.

# Glossary

**ACTIVITIES OF DAILY LIVING (ADLs)**

ADLs include any daily activity a person performs for self-care (feeding, grooming, bathing, dressing), work, homemaking, and leisure. The ability to perform ADLs is often used as a measure of ability/disability in MS.

**ACUTE**

Having a rapid or sudden onset.

**ACUTE DISSEMINATED ENCEPHALOMYELITIS (ADEM)**

A demyelinating disorder, usually in children, usually following a viral infection and rarely vaccination. The clinical features and MRI may resemble MS, but the disorder usually happens in one acute event. Oligoclonal bans are usually absent in the cerebral spinal fluid, which is helpful in separating this from MS, and if there are bans, they are only in the acute phase and then disappear, whereas they persist in MS.

## ADRENOCORTICOTROPIC HORMONE (ACTH)

A naturally occurring pituitary hormone that stimulates the adrenal gland to produce corticosteroids. It was uses to treat acute attacks of MS in the past but has mostly been replaced by methylprednisolone, and is not easily available now.

## ANTIBODIES (Ab)

Immunoglobulins or large Y-shaped proteins of the immune system that are primarily produced by plasma cells and used by the immune system to identify and neutralize pathogens such as viruses and bacteria, and also proteins recognized as "foreign" antigens. *See* Antigen.

## ANTICHOLINERGIC

Refers to the action of certain medications commonly used in the management of neurogenic bladder dysfunction. These medications inhibit the transmission of parasympathetic nerve impulses and thereby reduce spasms of smooth muscle in the bladder.

## ANTIGEN

Any substance that triggers the immune system to produce an antibody; generally refers to infectious organisms, toxic substances, or proteins the immune system identifies as being "foreign". *See* Antibodies.

## ASSISTIVE DEVICES

Any tools that are designed, fabricated, and/or adapted to assist a person in performing a particular task (e.g., cane, walker, shower chair, adapted kitchen utensils).

## ATAXIA

The incoordination and unsteadiness that result from the brain's failure to regulate the body's posture and the strength and direction of limb movements. Ataxia is most often caused by disease activity in the cerebellum.

## AUTOIMMUNE DISEASE

An immune system malfunction in which the body's immune system causes illness by attacking its own cells, organs, or tissues. Multiple sclerosis is believed to be an autoimmune disease, along with systemic lupus erythematosus, rheumatoid arthritis, scleroderma, and many others.

## AUTONOMIC NERVOUS SYSTEM

The part of the nervous system that regulates "involuntary" vital functions, including the activity of the cardiac (heart) muscle, blood vessels, smooth muscles (e.g., of the bladder and bowel), and glands.

## AXON

The extension of a nerve cell that conducts impulses to other nerve cells or muscles.

## B CELL

A type of lymphocyte (white blood cell) manufactured in the bone marrow that makes antibodies.

## BABINSKI REFLEX

A neurologic sign in MS in which stroking the outside sole of the foot with a pointed object causes an upward (extensor) movement of the big toe rather than the normal (flexor) downward movement of the toes. It indicates an abnormality in the motor tracks of the central nervous system. *See* Sign.

## BLOOD-BRAIN BARRIER

A semipermeable cell layer around blood vessels in the brain and spinal cord that prevents large molecules, immune cells, and potentially damaging substances and disease-causing organisms (e.g., viruses) from passing out of the bloodstream into the central nervous system (brain and spinal cord). A break in the blood-brain barrier may underlie the disease process in MS by allowing immune cells to enter.

## BRAIN ATROPHY

Shrinkage of the brain that seems to be due, at least in part, to the loss of myelin and axons. Evidence of atrophy is present in most patients when they have their initial symptoms of MS, indicating the disease has been going on long before. It continues during the disease but therapies can slow this process.

### BRAINSTEM

The part of the central nervous system that houses the nerve centers of the head as well as the centers for respiration and heart control. It is the area between the base of the brain and the spinal cord.

### CATHETER, URINARY

A hollow, flexible tube, made of plastic or rubber, which can be inserted through the urinary opening into the bladder to drain urine.

### CENTRAL NERVOUS SYSTEM

The part of the nervous system that includes the brain, brainstem, spinal cord, and optic nerves.

### CEREBELLUM

A part of the brain situated in the brain stem that controls balance and coordination of movement.

### CEREBROSPINAL FLUID (CSF)

A watery, colorless, clear fluid that bathes and protects the brain and spinal cord. The composition of this fluid can be altered by a variety of diseases. Certain changes in the CSF that are characteristic of MS can be detected with a lumbar puncture (spinal tap), a test sometimes used to help make the MS diagnosis.

### CEREBRUM

The large, upper part of the brain, with two halves (hemispheres) responsible for thought, memory, sensation, and motor movements.

### CLINICAL FINDING

An observation made during a medical examination indicating change or impairment in a physical or mental function.

### CLINICALLY ISOLATED SYNDROME (CIS)

A first neurological event (e.g., an episode of optic neuritis) that suggests demyelination in the central nervous system, and is accompanied by several "silent" or asymptomatic lesions on MRI that are typical of MS. Individuals with CIS are at high risk for developing clinically definite MS.

## CLONUS
A sign of spasticity in which a repetitive reflex jerking happens in the lower leg when the foot is forcibly pushed from under the forefoot. The stretching evokes a repetitive reflex indicating there is spasticity in the lower leg muscles.

## COGNITION
High-level functions carried out by the human brain, including comprehension and formation of speech, visual perception and construction, calculation ability, attention (information processing), memory, and executive functions such as planning, problem-solving, and self-monitoring.

## COGNITIVE IMPAIRMENT
Changes in cognitive function caused by trauma or disease process. Some degree of cognitive impairment occurs in approximately 50 to 60 percent of people with MS, with some memory, information processing, and executive functions being the most commonly affected functions.

## COGNITIVE REHABILITATION
Techniques designed to improve the functioning of individuals whose cognition is impaired because of physical trauma or disease. Rehabilitation strategies are designed to improve the impaired function via repetitive drills or practice, or to compensate impaired functions that are not likely to improve. Cognitive rehabilitation is provided by psychologists and neuropsychologists, speech/language therapists, and occupational therapists. While these three types of specialists use different assessment tools and treatment strategies, they share the common goal of attempting to improve the individual's ability to function as independently and safely as possible in the home and work environment.

## COMPUTED TOMOGRAPHY (CT SCAN)
A noninvasive diagnostic radiology technique. A computer integrates x-ray scanned "slices" of the organ being examined into a cross-sectional picture.

## CONTRACTION, MUSCLE

A shortening of muscle fibers and muscle that produces movement around a joint.

## COORDINATION

An organized working together of muscles and groups of muscles aimed at bringing about an accurate and coordinated purposeful movement such as walking or standing or reaching for an object.

## CORTICOSTEROIDS

*See* Glucocorticoid hormones.

## CORTISONE

A glucocorticoid steroid hormone, produced by the adrenal glands or synthetically, that has anti-inflammatory and immune-system suppressing properties. Prednisone, prednisolone, and methylprednisolone also belong to this group of substances used in MS to decrease the duration of attacks.

## CRANIAL NERVES

Twelve nerves that carry sensory or motor fibers to the face and neck. Included among this group of twelve nerves are the optic nerves (vision), auditory nerves (hearing), trigeminal nerves (sensation along the face and tongue), olfactory nerves (smell), and vagus nerves (pharynx and vocal cords). Evaluation of cranial nerve function is part of the standard neurological exam.

## DEEP TENDON REFLEXES

The involuntary jerks that are normally produced at certain spots on a limb when the tendons are tapped in a way that stretches them, usually with a reflex hammer. Reflexes are tested as part of the standard neurological exam.

## DEMYELINATION

A loss of myelin in the white matter of the nervous system.

## DIPLOPIA

Double vision, or the simultaneous awareness of two images of the same object that results from a failure of the two eyes to work in a coordinated fashion. Covering one eye will erase one of the images.

## DISABILITY
As defined by the World Health Organization, a disability (resulting from an impairment) is a restriction or lack of ability to perform an activity in the manner or within the range considered normal for a human being.

## DOUBLE-BLIND CLINICAL STUDY
A study in which none of the participants, including experimental subjects, examining doctors, attending nurses, or any other research staff, know who is taking the test drug and who is taking a control or placebo agent. The purpose of this research design is to avoid bias of the test results. In all studies, safety procedures are designed to "break the blind" if medical circumstances require it.

## DYSESTHESIA
Distorted or unpleasant sensations experienced by a person when the skin is touched.

## ELECTROENCEPHALOGRAPHY (EEG)
A diagnostic procedure that records, via electrodes attached to various areas of the person's head, electrical activity generated by brain cells. It is particularly important to detect evidence of seizure activity.

## ELECTROMYOGRAPHY (EMG)
A diagnostic procedure that records muscle electrical potentials through electrodes. It is often combined with tests of the conduction in the sensory and motor nerves.

## ETIOLOGY
The study of all factors that may be involved in the cause of a disease, including the patient's susceptibility, the nature of the disease-causing agent, and the way in which the person's body is invaded by the agent.

## EVOKED POTENTIALS (EPs)
Recordings of the nervous system's electrical response to the stimulation of specific sensory pathways (e.g., visual, auditory, general sensory). EPs can demonstrate lesions along specific nerve pathways

whether or not the lesions are producing symptoms, thus making this test useful in confirming the diagnosis of MS.

### EXACERBATION

The appearance of new symptoms or the aggravation of old ones (synonymous with attack, relapse, flare-up, or worsening); usually associated with inflammation and demyelination in the brain or spinal cord.

### EXPERIMENTAL ALLERGIC ENCEPHALOMYELITIS (EAE)

An autoimmune disease resembling MS that is induced in genetically susceptible research animals. Before testing on humans, a potential treatment for MS may first be tested on laboratory animals with EAE in order to suggest the treatment's efficacy and safety in humans. EAE is not MS but resembles it enough to be used as a model for many aspects of MS.

### EXTENSOR SPASM

A symptom of spasticity in which the legs straighten suddenly into a stiff, extended position. These spasms, which typically last for several minutes, occur most commonly in bed at night or on rising from bed.

### FLACCID

A decrease in muscle tone resulting in loose, "floppy" limbs.

### FLEXOR SPASM

Involuntary, sometimes painful contractions of the flexor muscles, which pull the legs upward into a clenched position. They often occur during sleep, but can also occur when the person is in a seated position.

### FOOD AND DRUG ADMINISTRATION (FDA)

The U.S. federal agency that is responsible for establishing and enforcing governmental regulations pertaining to the manufacture and sale of food, drugs, and cosmetics. Its role is to certify benefits of medication and prevent the sale of impure or dangerous substances. Any new drug that is proposed for the treatment of MS must be approved by the FDA.

## FOOT DROP

A condition of weakness in the muscles of the foot and ankle, caused by poor nerve conduction, which interferes with a person's ability to elevate the forefoot, producing a dragging of the foot when walking. The toes touch the ground before the heel, and may cause the person to trip or lose balance.

## FRONTAL LOBES

The anterior (front) part of each of the cerebral hemispheres that make up the cerebrum. The back part of the frontal lobe is the motor cortex, which controls voluntary movement; the area of the frontal lobe that is further forward is concerned with learning, behavior, judgment, and personality.

## GLUCOCORTICOID HORMONES

Steroid hormones that are produced by the adrenal glands in response to stimulation by adrenocorticotropic hormone (ACTH) from the pituitary. These hormones, which can also be manufactured synthetically (prednisone, prednisolone, methylprednisolone, betamethasone, dexamethasone), serve both an immunosuppressive and an anti-inflammatory role in the treatment of MS exacerbations: They help control overactive immune response and interfere with the release of certain inflammation-producing enzymes.

## HANDICAP

As defined by the World Health Organization, a handicap is a disadvantage, resulting from an impairment and disability, that interferes with a person's efforts to fulfill a role that is normal for that person. Handicap is therefore a social concept, representing the social and environmental consequences of a person's impairments and disabilities.

## HELPER T-LYMPHOCYTES

White blood cells that are a major contributor to the immune system's inflammatory response against myelin.

## IMMUNE SYSTEM

A complex system of cells and dissolvable proteins that protect the body against disease-producing organisms and other foreign invaders.

**IMMUNOCOMPETENT CELLS**
White blood cells (B and T lymphocytes and others) that defend against invading agents in the body.

**IMMUNOSUPPRESSION**
In MS, a form of treatment that slows or inhibits the body's natural immune responses, including those directed against the body's own tissues. Examples of immunosuppressive treatments in MS include cyclophosphamide, cyclosporine, methotrexate, and azathioprine.

**IMPAIRMENT**
As defined by the World Health Organization, an impairment is any loss of function directly resulting from injury or disease.

**INCIDENCE**
The number of new cases of a disease in a specified population over a defined period of time. It is often used in a form of the number of cases in a defined population (such as 100,000) in a year.

**INCONTINENCE**
The inability to control passage of urine or feces.

**INFLAMMATION**
A tissue's immunologic response to injury, characterized by mobilization of white blood cells and antibodies, swelling, and fluid accumulation.

**INTENTION TREMOR**
Rhythmic shaking that occurs in the course of a purposeful movement, such as reaching to pick something up or bringing an outstretched finger in to touch one's nose.

**INTERFERON**
A group of immune system proteins, produced and released in the presence of a virus, bacteria, parasite or tumor cells. They modify the body's immune response by activating nearby cells to inhibit the multiplication of viruses. The tendency to interfere with viruses gave rise to the name. The benefits of interferons in therapy relates to its

immune effects, not just to the anti-viral effects. Several interferons have been approved by the Food and Drug Administration for treatment of relapsing-remitting MS.

## LUMBAR PUNCTURE
A diagnostic procedure to sample cerebrospinal fluid (CSF) by inserting a hollow needle into the spinal canal in the lumbar area of the lower back. It is often called a spinal tap. The CSF can be tested for various features such as cells, sugar, proteins infectious agents, and in MS, for oligoclonal banding patterns of proteins.

## LYMPHOCYTE
A subtype of white blood cells that is part of the immune system. Lymphocytes can be subdivided into B lymphocytes, which originate in the bone marrow and produce antibodies; T lymphocytes, which are produced in the bone marrow and mature in the thymus; and natural killer cells, which can bind to certain tumor and virus infected cells and kill them by inserting granules containing a substance called perforin. Helper T lymphocytes heighten immune responses; suppressor T lymphocytes suppress them.

## MACROPHAGE
A white blood cell with scavenger characteristics that ingests and destroys foreign substances, such as bacteria and cell debris.

## MAGNETIC RESONANCE IMAGING (MRI)
A diagnostic procedure that produces computer-generated visual images of body parts by using strong magnetic fields. An important diagnostic tool in MS, MRI makes it possible to visualize and count lesions in the white matter of the brain and spinal cord.

## MINIMAL RECORD OF DISABILITY (MRD)
A standardized method for quantifying the clinical status of a person with MS. The MRD is made up of five parts: demographic information; the Neurological Functional Systems, which assign scores to clinical findings for each of the various neurological systems in the brain and spinal cord (pyramidal, cerebellar, brainstem, sensory,

visual, mental, bowel and bladder); the Disability Status Scale, which gives a single composite score for the person's disease; the Incapacity Status Scale, which is an inventory of functional disabilities relating to activities of daily living; the Environmental Status Scale, which provides an assessment of social handicap resulting from chronic illness. The MRD assist doctors and other professionals in assessing the impact of MS and in planning and coordinating the care of people with MS.

### MONOCLONAL ANTIBODIES
Laboratory-produced antibodies, which can be designed to react against a specific antigen in order to alter the immune response.

### MOTOR NEURONS
Nerve cells of the brain and spinal cord that enable movement of muscles in various parts of the body.

### MUSCLE TONE
A characteristic of a muscle tension brought about by the constant flow of nerve stimuli to that muscle. Abnormal muscle tone can be defined as: hypertonus (increased muscle tone, as in spasticity); hypotonus (reduced muscle tone or flaccid paralysis); or atony (loss of muscle tone). Muscle tone is evaluated as part of the standard neurological exam in MS.

### MYELIN
A fatty white coating of nerve fibers in the central nervous system, composed of lipids (fats) and protein. Myelin serves as insulation and as an aid to rapid nerve fiber conduction. When myelin is damaged in MS, nerve fiber conduction is faulty or absent.

### MYELIN BASIC PROTEIN
A protein comprising about 30 percent of all myelin of the central nervous system that may be found in higher than normal concentrations in the cerebrospinal fluid of individuals with MS and other diseases that damage myelin. Some believe myelin basic protein is an antigen against which autoimmune responses are triggered in MS.

## MYELITIS

An inflammatory disease of the spinal cord. In transverse myelitis, the inflammation spreads across the tissue of the spinal cord, resulting in a loss of its normal function to transmit nerve impulses up and down.

## MYELOPATHY

A lesion of the spinal cord that may be partial or complete. It is not uncommon as a presenting feature of MS, and the clinician needs to look for other evidence of lesions elsewhere, clinically, on the MRI and with oligoclonal banding, to confirm MS. (Other terms used are acute or subacute, and transverse myelopathy.)

## NERVE

A bundle of nerve fibers (axons). Fibers are either afferent (leading toward the brain and serving in the perception of sensory stimuli of the skin, joints, muscles, and inner organs) or efferent (leading away from the brain and mediating contractions of muscles or organs).

## NERVOUS SYSTEM

Includes all of the neural structures in the body: The central nervous system consists of the brain, spinal cord, and optic nerves; the peripheral nervous system consists of the nerve roots and nerves throughout the body.

## NEUROGENIC BLADDER

Bladder dysfunction associated with neurological malfunction in the nervous system and characterized by a failure to empty, failure to store, or a combination of the two. Symptoms that result from these three types of dysfunction include urinary urgency, frequency, hesitancy, nocturia, and incontinence.

## NEUROLOGIST

Physician who specializes in the diagnosis and treatment of conditions related to the nervous system.

## NEURON

The basic nerve cell of the nervous system. A neuron consists of a nucleus within a cell body and one or more processes (extensions) called dendrites and axons.

### OCCUPATIONAL THERAPIST (OT)

OTs assess functioning in activities of everyday living that are essential for independent living, including dressing, bathing, grooming, meal preparation, writing, and driving. They design treatment to develop, recover, or maintain daily living or working skills.

### OLIGOCLONAL BANDS

A diagnostic sign indicating abnormal levels of certain antibodies in the cerebrospinal fluid; seen in approximately 90 percent of people with MS, but not specific to MS. There are a number of procedures that can show the protein patterns in the CSF and blood and it is important to observe when the bands are seen in the CSF and are not just a reflection of the same pattern in the blood.

### OLIGODENDROCYTE

A cell in the central nervous system that is responsible for making and supporting myelin.

### OPTIC NEURITIS

Inflammation or demyelination of the optic (visual) nerve. It usually recovers but can leave some permanent visual change. Visual evoked potential studies can show slowed conduction in the optic nerve even when the person now feels the visual symptoms have fully recovered.

### ORTHOSIS

A mechanical appliance (such as a leg brace or splint) that is specially designed to control, correct, or compensate for impaired limb function.

### PARESTHESIA

A sensation of burning, prickling, or tingling on the skin that is often seen in MS.

### PAROXYSMAL SYMPTOMS

Symptoms that have sudden onset, apparently in response to some kind of movement or sensory stimulation, last for a few moments, and then subside. Paroxysmal symptoms tend to occur frequently in those individuals who have them, and follow a similar pattern from one episode to the next. Examples of paroxysmal symptoms include acute episodes of trigeminal neuralgia (sharp facial pain), tonic seizures (intense spasm of limb or limbs on one side of the body), dysarthria (slurred speech often accompanied by loss of balance and coordination), and various paresthesias (sensory disturbances ranging from tingling to severe pain).

## PHYSIATRIST
Physicians who specialize in the rehabilitation of physical impairments.

## PHYSICAL THERAPIST, PHYSIOTHERAPIST (PT)
PTs evaluate and improve movement and function of the body, with particular attention to physical mobility, balance, posture, fatigue, and pain.

## PLACEBO
An inactive compound. It is a term applied to a medicine with little or no effect but might have a positive result because of anticipation of benefit in the patient. In a clinical trial, the placebo is made to look similar to the test drug to be able to assess its benefit, safety, and limitations.

## PLACEBO EFFECT
An apparently beneficial result of therapy that occurs because of the patient's expectation that the therapy will help. The placebo, which is inert, does not have the effect; it is an effect produced by the mind of the receiver.

## PLAQUE
An area of inflamed or demyelinated central nervous system tissue.

## POSTURAL TREMOR
Rhythmic shaking that occurs when the muscles are tensed to hold an object or stay in a given position.

## PREVALENCE
The number of all new and old cases of a disease in a defined population at a particular point in time.

### PRIMARY PROGRESSIVE MS
A clinical course of MS characterized from the beginning by a progressive disease.

### PROGNOSIS
Prediction of the future course of the disease.

### PROGRESSIVE-RELAPSING MS
A clinical course of MS that shows disease progression from the beginning, but with clear, acute relapses along the way.

### PSEUDO-EXACERBATION
A temporary aggravation of disease symptoms, sometimes resulting from an elevation in body temperature or other stressor (e.g., an infection, severe fatigue, constipation), that disappears once the stressor is removed. A pseudo-exacerbation involves temporary flare-ups of prior or existing symptoms rather than new disease activity or progression.

### PYRAMIDAL TRACTS
Motor nerve pathways in the brain and spinal cord that connect nerve cells in the brain to the motor cells located in the cranial, thoracic, and lumbar parts of the spinal cord. Damage to these tracts causes spastic paralysis or weakness.

### REFLEX
An involuntary response of the nervous system to a stimulus, such as the stretch reflex, which is elicited by tapping a tendon with a reflex hammer, resulting in a contraction. Increased, diminished, or absent reflexes can be indicative of neurological damage, including MS, and are therefore tested as part of the standard neurological exam.

### RELAPSE
Also known as an attack, flare-up, or exacerbation. The appearance of new symptoms or the aggravation of old ones, lasting at least 24 hours; usually associated with inflammation and demyelination in the brain or spinal cord.

### RELAPSING-REMITTING MS
A clinical course of MS that is characterized by clearly defined, acute attacks (relapses) with full or partial recovery and no disease progression between attacks.

### REMISSION
A lessening in the severity of symptoms or their temporary disappearance during the course of the illness.

### REMYELINATION
The repair of damaged myelin. Myelin repair occurs spontaneously in MS but the new myelin is thinner and conducts a little more slowly.

### SCLEROSIS
Hardening or scarring of tissue. In MS, sclerosis is the replacement of lost myelin around central nervous system nerve cells with scar tissue.

### SECONDARY PROGRESSIVE MS
A clinical course of MS that initially is relapsing-remitting and then becomes progressive at a variable rate, with or without occasional relapses along the way. The disease-modifying medications are thought to provide benefit for those who continue to have relapses.

### SENSORY
Related to bodily sensations such as pain, smell, taste, temperature, vision, hearing, and position in space.

### SIGN
An objective physical problem or abnormality identified by the physician during the neurological examination, including altered eye movements and other changes in the appearance or function of the visual system; altered reflexes; weakness; spasticity; and sensory changes.

### SPASTICITY
Abnormal increase in muscle tone, manifested as a springlike resistance of an extremity to moving or being moved.

**SPHINCTER**
A circular band of muscle fibers that tightens or closes a natural opening of the body, such as the external anal sphincter, which closes the anus, and the internal and external urinary sphincters, which close the urinary canal.

**SPINAL TAP**
*See* Lumbar puncture

**STEROIDS**
*See* Glucocorticoid hormones.

**SYMPTOM**
A subjectively perceived problem or complaint reported by the patient. In MS, common symptoms include visual problems, fatigue, sensory changes, weakness or paralysis of the limbs, tremor, lack of coordination, poor balance, bladder or bowel changes, and psychological changes. *See* Sign.

**TONIC SEIZURE**
An intense spasm that lasts for a few minutes and affects one or both limbs on one side of the body. Like other types of paroxysmal symptoms in MS, these spasms occur abruptly and fairly frequently in those individuals who have them, and are similar from one brief episode to the next. The attacks may be triggered by movement or occur spontaneously. *See* Paroxysmal symptom.

**TRIGEMINAL NEURALGIA**
Lightning-like, stabbing acute pain in the face caused by demyelination of nerve fibers at the site where the sensory (trigeminal) nerve root for that part of the face enters the brainstem.

**URINARY FREQUENCY**
Need or urge to urinate more frequently than normal due to small hyperactive bladder.

**URINARY HESITANCY**
The inability to void urine spontaneously even though the urge to do so is present.

## URINARY URGENCY

The inability to postpone urination once the need to void has been felt.

## VERTIGO

A dizzying sensation of the environment spinning, often accompanied by nausea and vomiting.

# *Additional Readings*

There are many books with information about MS. Some are scientific, some educational, some give advice about management of various symptoms and some of therapies people are putting forward, and others are personal experiences of people with MS. It can be bewildering—Amazon has over 75 books on MS currently for sale. This is a brief list of helpful books:

**Books from Demos Medical Publishing on MS**

Rae-Grant A. et al. 2013. *Multiple Sclerosis and Related Disorders (Second Edition forthcoming in 2018)*.

Bowling, A. 2014. *Optimal Health with Multiple Sclerosis: A Guide to Integrating Lifestyle, Alternative, and Conventional Medicine*

Bowling, A. 2007. *Complementary and Alternative Medicine and Multiple Sclerosis.*

Kalb, R. 2012. *Multiple Sclerosis: The Questions You Have, the Answers You Need, Fifth Edition.*

Murray, T. J. 2005. *Multiple Sclerosis: The History of a Disease.*

Saunders, C. 2011. *What Nurses Know ... Multiple Sclerosis.*

Schwartz, S. 2017. *Multiple Sclerosis: Tips and Strategies for Making Life Easier, Third Edition.*

Shenkman, M. 2009. *Estate Planning for People With Chronic Disease.*


**Other References**

Marcia Finlayson. 2012. *Multiple Sclerosis Rehabilitation: From Impairment to Participation.* CRC Press.

Barbara Giesser. 2016. *Primer on Multiple Sclerosis, Second Edition.* Oxford University Press.

Dennis Greenberger and Christine Padesky. Mind over mood. 2015. *Change How You Feel by Changing the Way You Think, Second Edition.* Guilford Press.

Alirenza Minagar. 2015. *Multiple Sclerosis: A Mechanistic View,* Academic Press.

Catherine Edward. 2008. *The Brow of Dawn: One Woman's Journey With MS.* Bunim and Berigan.

# Resources

There are many resources available to help you meet the challenges of multiple sclerosis. This list is by no means complete; it is designed as a starting point in your efforts to identify the resources you need. Each resource will lead to others.

## Information Sources

**National Health Information Center** (P.O. Box 1133, Washington, DC 20013; Tel: 800-336-4797; Internet: www.health.gov/nhic). The Center maintains a library and a database of health-related organizations. It also provides referrals related to health issues for consumers and professionals.

## Agencies and Organizations

**National Multiple Sclerosis Society (NMSS)** (733 Third Avenue, New York, NY 10017; Tel: 800-FIGHT-MS; Internet: www.nationalmsssociety.org). The NMSS is a nonprofit organization that supports national and international research into the prevention, cure, and treatment of MS. The Society's goals include provision of nationwide services to assist people with MS and their families, and provision of information to those with MS, their families, professionals, and the public. The programs and services of the Society promote knowledge, health, and independence while providing education and emotional support:

- Toll-free access by calling 800-FIGHT-MS (800-344-4867).

- Website with updated information about treatments, current research, and programs (http://www.-nationalmssociety. org); local home page in many areas.

- Knowledge Is Power—an eight-segment, learn-at-home program (serial mailings) for people newly diagnosed with MS and their families.

- MS Learn Online—online, interactive web casts on a wide variety of topics.

- Printed materials on a variety of topics available by calling 800-FIGHT-MS (800-344-4867) or in the Library section of the National Multiple Sclerosis Society website at http:// www.-nationalmssociety.org/library.asp.

- Educational programs on various topics throughout the year, provided through individual chapters.

- Annual national education conference, provided through individual chapters.

- Swimming and other exercise programs sponsored or cosponsored by some chapters, or referral to existing programs in the community.

- Wellness programs in some chapters.

**Multiple Sclerosis Society of Canada** (250 Bloor Street East, Suite 100, Toronto, ON, M4W 3P9 Canada; Tel 416-922-6065; in

Canada: 800-268-7582; Internet: www.mssociety.ca). A national organization that funds research, promotes public education, and produces publications in both English and French. They provide an "ASK MS Information System" database of articles on a wide variety of topics including treatment, research, and social services. Regional divisions and chapters are located throughout Canada.

**Consortium of Multiple Sclerosis Centers** (CMSC) (c/o 59 Main Street, Suite A, Hackensack, NJ 07601; Tel: 201-487-1050, Internet: www.mscare.org). The CMSC is made up of numerous MS centers throughout the United States and Canada. The Consortium's mission is to disseminate information to clinicians, increase resources and opportunities for research, and advance the standard of care for MS. The CMSC is a multidisciplinary organization, bringing together health care professionals from many fields involved in MS patient care.

**Department of Veterans Affairs** (VA) (810 Vermont Avenue, N.W., Washington, DC 20420; Tel: 202-273-5400; Internet: www.va.gov). The VA provides a wide range of benefits and services to those who have served in the armed forces, their dependents, beneficiaries of deceased veterans, and dependent children of veterans with severe disabilities.

**Equal Employment Opportunity Commission** (EEOC) (Office of Communication and Legislative Affairs, 1801 L Street, N.W., 10th Floor, Washington, DC 20507; Tel: 800-669-3362 (to order publications); 800-669-4000 (to speak to an investigator); 202-663-4900; Internet: www.eeoc.gov). The EEOC is responsible for monitoring the section of the Americans with Disabilities Act (ADA) on employment regulations. Copies of the regulations are available.

**Can Do MS** (27 Main St., Suite 303, Edwards, CO 81632; Tel; 1-800-367-3101; Internet: http://www.mscando.org). Can Do MS is a non-profit organization dedicated to improving the lives of people and families living with MS through interactive, educational programs unique to any in the world. With an interdisciplinary team of MS experts in fields such as neurology; psychology; occupational, physical, and speech therapy; and nutrition, the CAN DO,

JUMPSTART, and other Can Do MS programs offer a supportive, nurturing environment in which participants learn to take control of their lives and their health by focusing on what they "can do" instead of what they cannot. The Center's programs, offered throughout North America, help participants set realistic personal goals, construct an individualized lifestyle plan, and gain the strategies and skills necessary to be successful in improving their lives. Can Do MS programs also address the needs and education of support partners and family members.

**United Spinal Association (USA)** (75-20 Astoria Boulevard, Jackson Heights, NY 11370; Tel: 718-803-3782; Internet: www .unitedspinal.org). USA is a private, nonprofit organization dedicated to serving the needs of its members as well as other people with spinal cord injury or disorder. While offering a wide range of benefits to members with spinal cord dysfunction (including hospital liaison, sports and recreation, wheelchair repair, adaptive architectural consultations, research and educational services, communications, and information services), they will also provide brochures and information on a variety of subjects, free of charge to the general public.

**Well Spouse Foundation** (610 Lexington Avenue, New York, NY 10022-6005; Tel: 212-644-1241; 800-838-0879; Internet: www. wellspouse.org). An emotional support network for people married to or living with a chronically ill partner. Advocacy for home health and long-term care and a newsletter are among the services offered.

## Electronic Information Sources

There are many sources of information available free through the Internet on the world wide web. If you are an experienced "net surfer," switch to your favorite search facility and enter the keywords "MS" or "multiple sclerosis." This will generally give you a listing of dozens of websites that pertain to MS. Keep in mind, however, that the world wide web is a free and open medium; while many of the websites have excellent and useful information, others may contain highly unusual and inaccurate information. A good place to start ...

***Complete Drug Reference*** (Compiled by United States Pharmacopoeia, published by Consumer Report Books, A division of Consumers Union, Yonkers, NY.) This comprehensive, readable, and easy-to-use drug reference includes almost every prescription and non-prescription medication available in the United States and Canada. A new edition is published yearly.

# Index

# *About the Author*

**T. Jock Murray, OC, ONS, MD, FRCPC, MACP, FAAN, FRCP, MCFP, FCAHS (Honorary LLD, DSc, DFA, D.Litt, LLD)**

Dr. T. Jock Murray is professor emeritus of Medicine and Neurology and former Dean of Medicine at Dalhousie University in Halifax, Nova Scotia, Canada. He served as president of the Canadian Neurological Society, vice president of the American Academy of Neurology and two terms as chairman of the American College of Physicians. Although he has international awards for his contributions to medical education, medical history, and medical administration, his clinical and research devotion was always to patients with multiple sclerosis. He has published over three hundred medical papers, held ninety-one funded research grants and authored eight books and forty-eight book chapters. He was a founder of the Consortium of MS Centers and the Canadian Network of MS Centers, and was awarded the Dr. Labe Scheinberg Award for contributions to MS research. His publication of *Multiple Sclerosis: The History of a Disease*, was awarded the ForeWord Silver Medal as the best book on history in 2005. He has been awarded five honorary degrees, the Order of Nova Scotia and is an Officer of the Order of Canada. In 2014 he was elected to the Canadian Medical Hall of Fame. He is proudest of his wife, Janet, who contributed in a huge way to all of the above, and his four children and seven grandchildren.

# The Dangerous Legacy

## A Pirate's Calling
## Book One

Darren Simon

The Dangerous Legacy
©2016 Darren Simon

Swartz Creek, MI 48473
Cover design by Clarissa Yeo

Tell-Tale Publishing Group

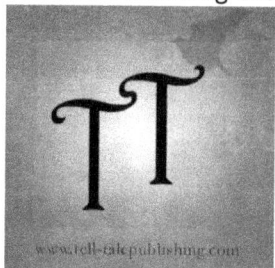

Tell-Tale Imprint

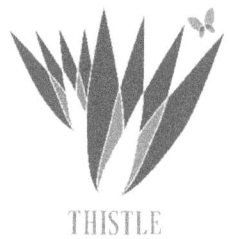

THISTLE

A Young Adult Novel

.

I wish to dedicate this book to my loving wife and two sons who inspire me every day to continue to pursue this dream of writing. I also want to thank my parents – my father who shared his love for reading with me and my mother who every week took me on outings to the library. Finally, I'd like to thank my editors, including Cindy Vallar, for the knowledge of the pirate world she shared, and the team at Tell-Tale Publishing for all the support.

# Prologue
## 1715 – Middle of the Caribbean

Jonathan Every stormed into the captain's cabin and banged his fist on the thick wooden desk. His thin frame trembled under a torn white shirt. Bony knees shook inside a pair of tattered calf-length breeches. A tingling sensation stretched across his back, shoulder blade to shoulder blade. He felt it whenever danger approached.

Captain Trayvon Bishop sat quietly behind the desk, rum-filled tankard in one hand, a pistol in the other. He took a long swig; the amber liquid dripped from his chin onto his dirty brown waistcoat. "Aye, Mr. Every, what is troubling you now?"

"You must set a new course or everyone on this ship is going to die! Heed my warning. He knows of my existence. He shall come for me, and when he does, no one aboard shall be safe." Jonathan paced as he rubbed his hands together.

"You should speak more pleasant words to me," Captain Bishop chuckled. "It is ill-advised to trouble me while enjoying a good rum. Let me fill a tankard for you, and we shall drink to the King's health. Our course is steady and you shall be back in London soon enough." Bishop turned to the shelf behind him and reached for a mug.

*I must make him understand.* Jonathan charged around the desk and grabbed Bishop by the edges of his waistcoat. The tankard fell to the ground and splashed rum onto Jonathan's already-stained breeches. "You are a fool, Captain Bishop. You condemn your ship, all these men, to Davy Jones's locker."

Thud. The butt of the captain's pistol crashed down on Jonathan's head. He tumbled to the floor, dazed. Hands pressed against his head, he fought off queasiness. Clarity slowly returned, and when it did, his head throbbed. He tried to stand, but the captain kicked him back down with a heavy boot.

"How dare you, sir." Bishop flipped the pistol around and aimed the nine-inch barrel at Jonathan's head. "I should kill you now and be done with it. I took you aboard *Chalice* as a kindness. And look at you, Mr. Every. I provide you the clothing of a sailor over that skeleton of a frame, as though you have ever done a day's honest labor aboard a ship. Who are you to challenge me? You best get those blue eyes off me, sir. My kindness may not last."

*What kindness? I paid a heavy price for safe passage to London.* "My apologies, Captain. I mean no disrespect. I only wish you to understand the risk you take."

Bishop leaned in closer and pressed the barrel harder against Jonathan's skull. "What is it you mean to declare? Who do you fear so much? What have you not shared? Tell me now."

Jonathan shivered under the pistol's icy chill. "Jem Slayer is the one!"

Bishop's large hazel eyes widened. His dark-bearded face turned white. He stumbled against his desk and lowered the pistol to his side with a shaky hand. "What have you done? What curse have you brought aboard my ship? You made me swear an oath to guide you home and now you would have me honor that to my own death?"

"For that I am truly sorry. There was no other way." Jonathan stood on wobbly legs and staggered toward the captain.

"I should spill your blood now, but Slayer would gut me with his sword if your life belongs to him." Bishop took a deep breath, perhaps to steady himself. "I shall get you to London, but if that wretched pirate finds us, I hand you over to him. Clear?"

"Yes."

"By God, I would sooner face a kraken—"

*Chalice* abruptly stopped. Jonathan and the captain lost balance and crashed into a cabin wall. "What the blazes?" Bishop uttered as he recovered, grabbed his pistol, and rushed from the cabin onto his ship's deck.

Jonathan's heart pounded. He clutched his chest to steady his pulse and started to follow Bishop. He got as far as the cabin door when a scalding pain, as if phantom flames charred his back, knocked him to his knees and signaled the inevitable. *He has come for me!* With teeth clenched, he stood and continued through the cabin doorway onto the deck. He stopped at Bishop's side.

"Navigator, what the devil has happened?" Captain Bishop gazed at his ship's three masts and massive squared sails, which had lost contact with the wind. They hung limply from *Chalice's* masts.

"I have never seen the like, Captain." The navigator, his deeply lined face surrounded by a long gray beard, stood on the quarterdeck. His hands gripped the wheel that steered *Chalice*. "The wind just died. My old bones tell me something is quite wrong, Captain. The sea is sending something evil our way."

"You must ready the canons." Jonathan winced as the pain in his back worsened.

"This is a merchant ship, not a warship. We are not prepared for battle." Bishop stared at the sea. The calm waters reflected the mid-afternoon Caribbean sun. The sea revealed no sign of Slayer, no sign of any danger.

Jonathan leaned against the captain. "You must have guns."

Bishop rubbed his forehead. "Mr. Jones," he ordered a scruffy man in a blue unbuttoned waistcoat, "take some men below deck and ready our 6-pounders."

"Captain—" Jones began, but Bishop cut him off.

"Just do it!" he ordered as he turned to the rest of the men on deck. "The rest of you, grab the oars. We need to get *Chalice* underway toward a new wind. Haste, men! And keep watch for any approaching ships."

"Captain, two points fine on the starboard side! See it?" One of the sailors pointed off the right bow.

A wall of mist slithered along the sea and moved toward them silently. Jonathan gulped. "It is him. He has found me. I have doomed you all."

"It is fog—nothing more." Captain Bishop shrugged off Jonathan's warning. "Mr. Jones, are the guns ready?"

"Three are ready," Jones answered.

"Avast! That shall have to do." Bishop reached for a spyglass in his belt and aimed it in the direction of the mist. "Bloody rot," he cursed as he handed the spyglass to Jonathan. Like an impenetrable barrier, the mist hid whatever awful thing might be inside.

Jonathan shook his head. "The guns shall not matter now."

Every man aboard stood still and quiet as the mist came within fifty yards of their ship and stopped. The mist hovered there, its contents cloaked. Nothing happened. The sea remained quiet. Too quiet. Captain Bishop released a lungful of air. "Mr. Jones, fire a round into the center of that mist."

"Aye, Captain." A thunderous eruption followed as one of *Chalice's* guns unleashed a round. Jonathan waited for an explosion to indicate their shot had found a target, but silence followed. The shot disappeared into the mist. If the shot struck water, the round made no splash. Nothing, until…

The mist lit up like fire. A chorus of explosions followed as if a storm rose from the sea. Projectiles screamed through the air. They signaled *Chalice's* fate.

Jonathan managed a quick glance at Bishop before two black iron cannonballs slammed into the hull. The vessel shook as timbers split. Splinters and larger wood fragments tore through the crew's flesh and dropped several men. Their shrieks echoed in his ears. A third cannonball struck the ship's tallest mast and toppled the main sail. That strike rendered any chance of escape impossible. Not that the vile pirate Slayer would allow any escape. *Chalice* was dead, along with several of its crew.

"Captain, you are hurt!" Jonathan wrapped an arm around Bishop. Blood dripped from Bishop's forehead down his cheek and onto a deck already drenched in blood. He didn't respond. His eyes seemed drawn to the body of the old navigator, who lay dead on the quarterdeck, *Chalice's* wheel on top of him. "Captain!"

Bishop's head snapped up, as if suddenly alert. "Every able-bodied man, to arms!"

"I think that is an unwise order." The words hovered over the deck as if spoken by an apparition.

Jonathan scanned in every direction. Black smoke from smoldering timber lingered over the deck and clouded his view until a pair of glowing red eyes cut through the darkness. The eyes burned brighter as they heralded a man who emerged from the chaos. Dressed in black, his head topped by a black three-cornered hat with a raven's feather attached, the man held a handkerchief to his nose. His blazing eyes were the only visible feature to his face, but they were enough. It was him—the pirate *Slayer!*

Other pirates flanked him, including a large bald-headed, bare-chested beast who seemed more giant than man.

"Oh how I hate the stench of death." The glow in Slayer's eyes vanished, replaced by deep-set black orbs that surveyed *Chalice.*

Captain Bishop cleared his throat. "Who are you, sir, and why have you attacked my ship? Surely no pirate would destroy his prize."

"I guess that makes me special, for you see I am a pirate and so much more than your little mind can fathom." Slayer approached Bishop. "I believe you know my name, sir. Speak it."

"I would assume you are the pirate Jem Slayer." Bishop blinked rapidly, the only indication of his fear.

"Very good, Captain." Slayer removed the handkerchief from his nose and placed it against Bishop's bleeding forehead. "It is a nasty wound you have. I am sorry to have caused it, but then, in a way, you brought this on yourself and these men."

"You foul—"

"Now, now, Captain, you know of that which I speak." Slayer circled Bishop. "There is one among you, my dear Captain, who is no sailor, but rather a paid guest to whom you have granted safe passage to escape me."

Jonathan waited for Bishop to turn him over to Slayer. For whatever reason, though, the captain didn't. Bishop didn't even turn his eyes toward him. *Why? For what reason does he persist in protecting me?*

"Your silence guarantees every man aboard this ship a painful death." Slayer slapped Bishop with the back of his hand. Still Bishop refused to speak. "All right then, brave Captain." Slayer unsheathed his sword and pointed the long curved blade at Bishop's chest.

"Wait!" Jonathan stepped forward. "No need to kill him. I am here."

"Oh, well spoken. And I see you wear a disguise, like a real sailor." Slayer laughed then still plunged his blade into Bishop's chest. His eyes wide as if he knew death was upon him, Bishop gasped as Slayer slowly twisted the blade. A cough of blood, a final gurgled breath, and Bishop's head slumped. His body crumbled to the deck as Slayer kicked him away from the blade.

"No!" Jonathan dropped to his knees. He shivered from the searing pain in his back.

Slayer pointed his bloodied blade toward Jonathan. "Mr. Black, please remove this one's shirt."

The giant pirate, armed with a long sword attached to a red sash across his hairy chest, followed orders. He reached for Jonathan with arms as big as cannon barrels. A wide smile revealed a mouth filled with yellow, broken teeth. "Come now, little man. Do not fight 'ol Maximilian Black, or I'll crush your tiny neck." With one massive hand he grasped Jonathan's neck and, with his other, ripped off the shirt. Black twirled him around to reveal his bare back.

"Astonishing," Slayer quipped. "You carry the mark of the sword. You, in fact, are the one I have sought."

"Enough!" Jonathan broke free of Black's grip, stumbled to the deck, and screamed. His back sizzled as a line of fire rose from his skin and traced the mark Slayer spoke of, a birthmark in the shape of a sword. Jonathan slowly stood. "You are right about me. I am the one you seek, Slayer. I know why you have come. I should never have fled. It is my destiny to face you." He reached to his back as if to claw at the flames. Instead, his hand plunged into the fire-covered birthmark, penetrated skin and found the handle of a sword magically hidden in his body.

As if his skin split in two, he pulled the burning blade from his back. Bone formed the handle. In place of steel, a long narrow flame crackled and danced as it formed the blade.

Slayer's eyes glowed red again. He wiped the blood from his own blade and sheathed the weapon. "Must we go through this exercise? Accept that my magic is superior, you bilge rat, and save yourself much pain."

Jonathan raised the burning blade. "My name is Jonathan Every. I shall do now what I should have done long ago." He rushed at Slayer, his sword's fiery blade pointed at the pirate's heart.

Slayer stood motionless, his arms crossed at his chest. A snicker escaped his lips. A red energy beam flashed from his glowing eyes and struck Jonathan in the chest. The blast threw him backward ten feet. He smashed against a barrel and fell to the deck.

As smoke rose from the wound, Jonathan clumsily climbed to his feet. He still held onto his burning sword with shaky hands. Once more, a bit slower, he swung the blade at Slayer. The pirate side stepped the blow. Jonathan swung wide as Slayer fired another red beam that sliced into Jonathan's back and knocked him to his knees. *Have to get back up. Have to fight on.* He took a deep breath and stood once again.

"Must we continue?" Slayer gripped his sword's handle.

Jonathan shouted and lunged. The pirate deflected the fire blade and slashed with his own sword across the length of Jonathan's chest. The blade tore deep through skin and muscle. Jonathan's blood spilled onto the deck as he stumbled against a wooden crate and fought to remain on his feet.

He tried to breathe, but could only manage shallow breaths. Slayer's blow had emptied his lungs. The end neared, but Jonathan had enough strength for one more action. "If I cannot defeat you I may still thwart your plans." He drove the burning blade into his own stomach. A smile crossed his face as he fell to the deck. Through labored breaths, he stuttered, "P-p-perhaps S-S-Slayer, another of my kind—one stronger than I-I—shall k-k-kill…"

Jonathan fell silent. Death came.

# The Dangerous Legacy

# Chapter 1
## Present Day—The Bet

"Here's the bet." Zack stared at his shorter cousin. "We jump from the pier. The first one back to shore wins. The loser leaves the pier forever. Agreed?"

"Agreed." Sam Every swallowed hard. He gazed first at his cousin and then at the gathered crowd of teenagers.

One thought filled his mind over and over. *Stupid, stupid, stupid. I can't beat Zack. He's fifteen, two years older than me. Plus, he's a muscled-up surfer. I'm a skinny violin-playing orchestra nerd.* He forced that thought away and tried to steady his nerves as an icy sweat fell from his forehead. *But I'm a good swimmer. Maybe today could be my day. Besides, it's a stupid bet. No one could hold someone to a lifetime ban of the pier.* Either way, there was no going back. "Let's do this." Sam took a step toward Zack.

"All right, cuz." Zack brushed his long blond hair away from his steel blue eyes and smiled from ear to ear. Sam nodded. A slight quiver ran through his body as he followed Zack to the railing. "Still time to call it, cuz," Zack offered. "Say the word. We can end this and you and your geek friends can leave the pier for good right now."

"Let's dive already, *cuz*." Sam's voice was shaky. His statement brought nods of approval and laughter from the crowd. Zack silenced the onlookers with a menacing stare.

"You had your chance." Zack swung his legs over the railing and leaned toward the water.

With a deep sigh, Sam cautiously joined his cousin on the railing. He peered toward the glassy, dark water. It was a long way down. *How did I get myself into this?* he wondered as his heart danced wildly. The answer quickly played through his mind. The day had started with a phone call.

"Hey, what's up?" The voice on the line belonged to his best friend, Greg.

"Not much."

"Let's hang. Be ready. I'm on my way." The line went dead before Sam could answer. He quickly showered and brushed his teeth. He stopped mid-brush to gaze at his image in the mirror. *Man, I need to work out and grow about two more feet.* He studied his thin, short frame and soft stomach. Even his face was too bony. *Oh well.* His eyes focused on his brown hair that fell in disarray to his shoulders. He never combed it. He liked it messy. It separated him from the rest of the more clean-cut orchestra nerds at school, like he was a rebel.

Twenty minutes later, Greg's mountain bike skidded to a halt in front of the house. He wore a Hawaiian shirt dotted with palm trees and calf-length shorts. Sam laughed at his best friend. What an outfit. Greg was the tallest in the group. With his tan skin and ponytail, the basic looks of a surfer jock--except for a slightly rounded stomach--he had the best chance of someday becoming popular.

Greg was not alone. John and Dean, two other members of their pack, had decided to join them. "John, Dean, how's it going?" Sam jumped on his own bike.

"Where we headed, dudes?" John asked. He huffed loudly from the bike ride. Built thick with no neck and arms and legs the size of small tree trunks, he tired easily.

"The beach, man—where else are we going to check out some girls?" Greg winked and pointed both forefingers west toward the ocean.

Dean, a Hawaiian native and the smallest of their group, rolled his eyes. "Greg's all about the girls. If only he could talk to them."

"Not funny." Greg punched Dean in the arm.

"Beach sounds good; pier sounds better." Sam started to ride. "I'm craving a hotdog, and we can see just as many girls on the boardwalk."

"Fine," Greg nodded. "On our way, guys."

The day held great promise. The pier was one of Sam's favorite places with food, music, fair-like gaming attractions and plenty of girls. Whether they gave you the time of day or not, there was an excitement that came when near girls with the hope one might offer a smile.

Fifteen minutes later, they passed through the shadows of the pier's covered parking structure onto the sun-soaked boardwalk. The late morning air warmed Sam's face. The comforting odor of hot dogs and musty sea filled the air. Crowds of locals and tourists gathered together in the harmony of the pier. He and his friends made their way along the cobblestone walkway and soon spotted their destination—an area along the railings where an older wooden section of the pier gave way to a newer concrete structure.

As they parked themselves along the railing, Sam focused on the sea and a group of seals about a hundred yards out to sea on top of a buoy.

"Man, check out who's coming," Greg warned. "What do they want?"

Sam shifted his attention from the water to the pier and bowed his head. Carlos, Freddy, TJ and their leader, Zack—Sam's cousin—approached, each with a gleaming surfboard in tow and dressed in expensive black bodysuits.

"Hey, losers, what brings you to the pier?" An evil smile crossed Zack's face. His perfectly white teeth reflected the sun. "The beach is for surfers, not dweebs."

"The beach is for everyone, Zack. Back off." Sam swallowed hard.

"Oh. My ghost cousin feels tough today."

Sam's skin heated as he blushed.

"Hey, cuz, why don't you take off that shirt of yours and show everybody that cool birthmark?" Zack reached for Sam's shirt. "Have you seen that thing? It's shaped like a giant sword across his back."

Sam backed away from his cousin. He shivered as a tingling sensation spread along the outline of his birthmark. *What is that?*

"Shut up, Zack," John stepped forward.

"Relax, guys, I'm just playing with you." Zack glowered at John but still smiled. He handed his surfboard to TJ and placed his arms around Dean and Greg. "It's a great day isn't it, guys? The kind of day meant for a swim." He peered over the railing to the water about fifty feet below. "How about it, guys, feel like a swim?" Zack motioned to Carlos and Freddy and before Sam could react, Carlos grabbed him by the arms and pushed him against the railing. Freddy did the same to John. "Throw them over," Zack ordered.

Sam struggled against Carlos as the tingling in his back intensified, like someone pricked him with hundreds of needles. A lucky elbow jab against Carlos' side, and Sam freed himself. His friends were not so lucky. Like pro wrestlers in a grudge match, Zack's stronger bunch locked them in submission holds. He couldn't let his friends face the brunt of Zack's bullying. It wasn't fair. *This is between me and Zack. I have to stop him. But how? Say something—anything—to save your friends.* "Zack, if you're so big and strong, dive from the pier yourself and swim back to shore. Show everyone just how great you really are—or are you scared?"

Zack glared silently at Sam. His smile disappeared while he seemed to weigh the challenge, but his upper lip quickly rose in a sneer. "Sure, cuz, I'll jump. But you have to do it, too."

That's how the bet had started.

Sam tensed his muscles. A million thoughts raced through his mind. What could have possessed him to make a bet that involved a dive off the pier? He could have chosen so many other challenges. It was as if a will stronger than his own spoke for him and chose a water dare. Then there was his back. What was that strange tingling? With so many questions, he was sure of only one thought, *I could die doing this!*

"All right, we jump on the count of three." Zack leaned farther over the water and started the countdown "Three." Sam held his breath. "Two." He willed himself to ease his grip on the railing. "One."

Sam jumped.

# Chapter 2
## The Leap

His body twisted and his arms flailed as Sam fell toward the water. He tightened his stomach to prepare for the impact. *This is going to hurt.* He slammed into the sea in a belly-flop position. The salty, icy water stung his face and burned his nose. Lost in a maze of bubbles, he couldn't find the surface and sank fast. When he finally spotted light, he rushed toward it. *Air. I need to breathe.* Moments later he broke the surface and gulped oxygen; then whirled to find the shore.

He expected to see his cousin already on shore in a victory dance. Instead, laughter greeted him from above. Zack nearly doubled over as he cackled like a hyena from atop the pier. Others snorted and hooted just as loud. "Cuz, you're such a loser." Zack formed an "L" with this thumb and forefinger. "I can't believe you fell for that!"

The laughter from above continued as Sam floated in the water. *He never jumped. Zack is such a jerk,* he fumed, but he couldn't think of a clever comeback. Embarrassed, he began the long swim back to shore. *I should just punch Zack in the face.*

He took a few strokes but stopped when something tugged at his feet. Confused, Sam glanced down but saw nothing in the water around him. He pushed forward but immediately felt another tug. *Weird.* He checked for seaweed around his ankles but found nothing. A more violent tug pulled him under the water. *Sharks! It must be sharks!* Sam resurfaced briefly. He thrashed wildly as his hands and feet clawed at the water. Whatever it was dragged him beneath the water again—deeper and deeper. It would not let go. *What's happening?*

He screamed silently underwater as his mind fogged and lungs burned. He stopped kicking long enough to stare into the abyss. As the water calmed, it revealed what held him. A bony hand! Skeletal fingers wrapped around his right ankle! Sam's eyes followed the hand up a seaweed-covered arm that belonged to the ghostly figure of a girl! *What the...?* He thrashed and kicked again, but she would not let go. He gulped water and started to choke. *I don't want to die. Please.* His vision grayed and his chest constricted.

A jerk on his leg brought his gaze to her eyes, black orbs surrounded by a sea of white and full of determination. Her long, ash-colored hair floated like seaweed against a green bone-thin face. Her tattered dress reminded him of clothes worn centuries ago.

Then darkness enveloped him.

# Chapter 3
## Was It a Brain Fart?

Sam coughed and vomited a bit of water until pinpricks of light dotted the darkness. A shadowy, gray world came into focus. He coughed up a bit more seawater as shadows formed into shapes and colors. He squinted against the warm sun. Silhouettes of maybe a dozen people stood over him and voices murmured.

"Leave it to my band geek cousin to almost drown on a bet." Zack, the first person Sam recognized, knelt over him. Water dripped off his gleaming surfer hair.

"What? What happened?" Sam asked.

"I'll tell you what happened." Zack stood. "I just saved your sorry butt."

As Sam became fully conscious, he lifted himself into a sitting position and twisted in every direction. He had reached the shore somehow. Many of the same people who had watched from the pier stood around him. They smiled, whispered and pointed. *Perfect.* Dean, John and Greg stood just to the right of Zack. They, too, were wet, as if they had jumped into the water after him.

The one person Sam didn't see was… "Hey, what about that girl who was in the water?"

"Who?" Zack ran his hands through his hair and flexed his muscles.

"That girl—the one who grabbed me—pulled me down." Sam ran to the water. "She's the reason I almost drowned."

"Man, you must have hit your heard or something? You're talking crazy," Zack chuckled along with the rest of the crowd.

"No, I'm telling you there is a girl out there." Sam waded through the water only to be pulled back by Greg and John. "She might still be in trouble!"

"Cuz, either you're making up some lame excuse for almost drowning or that water did you some damage. Either way, you owe me your life, so you have to do what I say. I don't want to see you on my beach again." Zack backed away, turned and walked off, his buddies and followers not far behind.

*Maybe Zack's right. Maybe I am crazy.* Sam glanced at his friends, who stayed. "Something tells me Zack doesn't deserve all the credit for rescuing me."

"Zack was the first one into the water," Greg answered, "but we weren't about to let him take all the glory. If there was some saving to do, and possibly girls to look really cool in front of, we had to jump in, too. It had nothing to do with saving you."

They all laughed "Thanks, guys," Sam placed a hand on Greg's shoulder. "You risked your lives for me."

"Don't mention it," John said. "Just buy us some hot dogs for lunch and we'll call it even."

Sam gazed at the ocean. "It sounds crazy, but I really did see something, or someone, out there in the water just under the pier—a girl probably no older than us."

"We didn't see anyone else when we went in after you." Dean raised an eyebrow. "Your mind could be messing with you. I mean there couldn't be anyone else out there. She would have to come up for air, right? I mean, you know, she'd have to."

"Unless …," Greg suggested, nudging John in the ribs with an elbow.

"Unless what?" Sam asked.

"Unless you saw a mermaid."

John laughed as he pushed Greg's elbow away. "That would be so hot."

"You know it." Greg blew a kiss toward the water.

"If only," Dean giggled. "But since we live in reality—except for Greg who lives in a fantasy world most of the time—mermaids aren't real. Sam, man, most likely your mind's playing games."

"Yeah, you're right." Sam kept his eyes fixed on the sea and slowly backed out of the water. "Since I'm no longer allowed on the beach, let's head to the mall and I'll buy us those hot dogs. We can play a few games of air hockey at the arcade."

As he and his friends walked from the beach, Sam shot one more glance toward the water. *I did see a girl out there.* His stomach churned and his mind spun. Those dark eyes of hers, so determined, had called out to him, like she needed him. It was almost like she had pleaded with him to stay with her. *But why? Does she want to drown me? Is she a zombie wanting a zombie boyfriend?* He shivered but laughed inside. *No, she wants something else, but what? I'm going to have to investigate this further even if no one believes me—even if this is nothing more than a brain fart.*

# Chapter 4
## The Sea Beckons

"They need you. You must save them. We all need you."

"What? Who needs me?" A dense fog surrounded Sam. He couldn't see who spoke.

There was no response, but the ghostly voice repeated the words as if from far away. "They need you! They need you! They need you!"

"Who needs me? I don't understand." A small wave of salty water lifted Sam's body and splashed him in the face. The water stung his eyes. *Wait a second, where am I?* Another wave pushed him up and slapped him. *I'm in the water!* He whirled his body in every direction and splashed to stay afloat. The gray fog was an impenetrable barrier that blocked his view of everything but the murky, choppy seawater that immediately surrounded him.

The voice returned. "Why have you not come? Why do you leave them to suffer? Save them! Save them! Save them!"

Sam shivered. "Hold on, man. Don't lose it."

The voice sounded female. Might it belong to the girl underneath the pier? But is she real? By the time he'd gone to sleep last night, he just wasn't sure. Sleep! *That's right. I went to sleep. I must still be sleeping. This is just a dream. I'm still safe in my room. But it feels real. Whether a dream or not, I should make contact.* "Look, I don't know what you're talking about. Who needs to be saved? Why am I the only one who can save them?"

Still no response, but a soft breeze drifted over the water and tickled his face. Fingertips seemed to caress his cheeks and run through his brown hair until the breeze grew into a gust. Waves, formed by the rushing wind, tossed him like a ragdoll. He kicked and splashed as one wave after another bombarded him and threatened to drag him under the sea. Then, as suddenly as the assault began, it ended. The fog broke, the wind silenced, and the sea became still. Sam pushed his hair away from his eyes and with a gasp spun in every direction. He floated alone in a vast blue ocean that stretched for miles in any direction. "Oh my God!" He again spun in search of signs of life—a boat, an island, a plane, something!

At least the fog had given him a sense of a finite space, like the inside of a box. That was better than being adrift in an endless sea. *How did I get out here? This can't be real!* He swam wildly; his heart raced. He panted and choked as salt water spilled into his mouth. "Stay calm," he mumbled as he willed each breath, each heartbeat to match the rhythm of the swells that rolled upon him.

"Uh, I'd like to return to my room," he pleaded. His answer was an unexpected wave that smacked his face and temporarily blinded him. When his vision cleared, he was no longer alone. She floated next to him—the ghostly girl with dark eyes and long wild hair dampened against her head.

"Ahhh!" Sam swam away, but for some reason he stopped and turned to look at the girl. Soft freckles dotted shallow green cheeks. Her eyes were rimmed with the blackness of death. Wrinkles puckered her lips as if she'd been in the water a long time. Actually, she would be beautiful if she didn't look like she had drowned and the frosty water had preserved her body. Her face was expressionless until she cocked her head and a tear fell from her right eye.

"Help them," she whispered and reached for him with her ghostly pale right arm.

Despite himself, Sam screamed. "Noooooooo!"

He fell out of bed onto his floor. His scream still echoed through his room. The salty taste of seawater clung to his tongue. *Was it real? Was it a dream? It had to be a dream. It just had to be.*

With labored movements, Sam stood and flipped the switch on the wall; comforting light shed throughout the room. He glanced at the clock on his dresser. Only three in the morning. Several hours remained until first light. "All right, let's listen to some music." He jammed his iPod into his ears. The calming melody of a Bach violin concerto replaced his troubled thoughts. He turned up the volume, reached for his own violin, and paced the room, his violin hugged tightly against his chest. He stayed far away from the bed, but sleep eventually beckoned.

Sam awoke in a chair, head on his desktop, a sheet of paper glued to his mouth from dried drool. He tugged the paper from his lips and checked the clock. It read six in the morning. With a yawn, he stood and stretched. While he shook off the stiffness of an uncomfortable sleep, one thought filled his mind. *Head back to the pier.*

The ride was quick and the brisk morning air relieved any remaining sluggishness from the night. Once at the pier, he rode to the exact spot where he had jumped into the water just a day earlier. A mist hovered over the ocean and gray clouds blanketed the sun. A cargo ship's low, mournful cry signaled its passage along the coastal waters. Seagulls launched into the morning sky to begin their daylong dance for food. Pelicans kept watch on a nearby outcropping of rocks. They stretched their wings but otherwise showed little movement.

Sam balanced on his mountain bike as he peered over the railing at the water. His eyes strained to pierce the dark glassy surface to the world beneath the sea where he had nearly drowned.

*Should I jump in again?* He knew he shouldn't, but he wanted to prove to himself that he had just imagined things yesterday.

He scanned the pier. A few people strolled along the boardwalk, but otherwise it was quiet. If he jumped in, no one would notice. "Do it. It's the only way you'll forget about this." He was prepared for the jump dressed in swim trunks and a lightweight T-shirt. One more look around to ensure no one watched, and he climbed over the railing.

"You can do this," he repeated over and over to himself, but his hands trembled and would not release the railing. His feet refused to leap. More than once he made the motion to jump, but his limbs would not obey. "Come on, man!" He closed his eyes and counted down to one in one last attempt to leap. When that failed, he opened his eyes and saw something rise from the water. A hand! Long, thin fingers stretched from the shadowy sea beneath the pier and reached toward him.

Sam shook his head. His stomach knotted. *It can't be. I'm not seeing that. But I am seeing it. I know I'm seeing it. I just wish I wasn't.* He closed his eyes again and when he reopened them, the hand had disappeared. He laughed. *You're going crazy. You're letting this stupid thing get to you.* "What are you thinking?" he scolded himself. He swung his legs back over the railing onto the pier. He wasn't about to jump into the water. *I mean for what? Because I'm seeing things? Let it go.*

Sam sat on his bike and looked toward the horizon. The clouds had already started to part and the morning sun split the mist. In the distance, he spotted something out of the corner of his eyes—a sailing vessel, only not one like those modern sailboats nestled by the pier's harbor. *It's a pirate ship!* He wasn't sure why that was his first thought, but the craft in the distance looked like a ship from a time long ago, like those he had studied about from the early eighteenth century. His history teacher had called it the golden age of piracy. Three masts with squared sails rose high above the vessel. Another thought came to him. *The dress the girl is wearing is probably from that same time. What's going on? Why am I seeing this stuff?* "Go away!"

When he uttered the words, the ship vanished, like the hand in the water. Sam scooted away from the railing in silence. The little hairs at the base of his neck tickled him. *This is all very weird.*

# Chapter 5
## Scrawled In Blood

Sam eyed the clock on the wall just above as he pushed the cart through the narrow aisle. Only four in the afternoon! *Ugh*! He wanted to go home, but his shift as a volunteer at the library didn't end until five.

He shook his head and stared at the front counter where his mom, the head librarian of the small city branch, helped a woman and little girl check out a book. *This is not how I should be spending my summer days. I never should have volunteered. Dude! What were you thinking? I know. You thought cute, brainy girls come to the library. No! Haven't seen anyone but moms and kids! This bites.*

He lifted a book from his cart and placed it in the exact spot on a shelf based on its reference number. What a waste of time. Some dorky kid would pick it up again and put it back in the wrong place. It happened every day; and every day for three hours he walked this stupid cart around the library and placed books back where they belonged. *Totally useless.*

With the book back on the shelf he moved farther down the aisle, until—clump—something struck his head. "Ouch!" Sam rubbed his head and looked over his shoulder to search for anything that might have hit him. A book lay on the floor at his feet. It must have fallen from a top shelf.

He picked it up and checked for a reference number but found none. *Strange.* He studied it more carefully. The black cover, soft and dusty, had no title. Inside, hand written scribbles filled ragged, stained pages. The first page had a date at the top. *1718.* "It's a diary?" he asked. "There is no way this is really that old!"

Sam turned the stiff pages and carefully pried apart the ones that stuck together. Much of the writing had smeared and faded but one entry was as clear as if it had been written that day. He read it aloud. "Beware the pirate Jem Slayer, for he is most evil. All who face his wrath are doomed to a painful death until the Chosen One rises."

*Cool.* Sam's thoughts turned to his vision of a ship—maybe a pirate ship—in the morning while at the pier. He laughed at himself and shook his head. He hadn't really seen a pirate ship off coast, just like no hand had risen from the water. This book or diary had to be a coincidence.

Sam closed the book and peered at the higher shelves to see where it might have fallen from, but none of the books in this section dealt with pirates. It must have been misplaced, as usual. "Mom, I don't know where to put this. It has no reference number." Sam approached his mom at the front desk. "It fell from a shelf and hit me in the head. Can I sue? Just kidding. But it shouldn't be in that section, so what should I do with it? I think it's pretty old. It's like a diary or something."

"Let me see that." His mom put on her reading glasses. "I don't recognize it either. But look at the date. If this is authentic, it could be a real treasure. But I imagine it's just a copy. Maybe someone just recently submitted this for our book collection drive, and we just haven't assigned it a reference number yet. I'll contact some local historians and have them take a look at it. For now, let's keep it safe in the vault downstairs. Can you take it down for me?"

"Come on, Mom. You know I hate the basement."

"Honey, do this for me and you can cut out early."

Sam sighed, grabbed the book and crossed the library to an employee-only door that led to the basement. That's where books not yet assigned reference numbers rested in piles on tables and shelves. His mom locked the special books in the vault, a closet in the basement filled with books sealed in air-tight plastic envelopes.

On a normal day the basement, a cramped space no bigger than his own bedroom with boxes and stacks of books to the ceiling, gave him the creeps. Given all that had happened, even if only his imagination, the feeling amplified. Moisture dripped from his forehead. His heart boomed in his chest as he stepped lightly down the staircase to the basement.

Alone, he headed toward the vault. A crunch from the stairway caught his attention. "Who's there?" He expected to see another volunteer or staff member on the steps, but no one stood in the stairway. He remained by himself in the room. *Uh, let's hurry and get out of here.* Sam unlocked the vault's door, opened it a crack and peeked inside. Nothing but books filled the shelves. With a deep breath, he dashed inside, snatched an empty envelope, placed the book inside and sealed it.

A bump sounded from somewhere in the basement. Sam glanced through the vault's doorway, but he was still alone. *I don't like this.* Footsteps followed; they clip-clopped toward the vault. "Okay, enough jokes! Come on, guys, I mean it!" One of the other volunteers had to be responsible. They often played tricks on each other. He still didn't like it. The steps moved closer to the vault door, then stopped.

"That's it! I'm out of here!" Before he could take a step, the vault door slammed and the latch clicked; he was locked inside. "What's happening?" He pounded on the door. "Let me out!"

No one responded. Sam stopped his attack on the door as his back tingled, like it did a day earlier at the beach. The sensation rose along the large sword-shaped birthmark from his lower back to his shoulder blades. *What's happening to me! Forget your back.*

*Just figure out a way out of here.* He slowed his breathing and quieted his thoughts. *Think, dude. Call your mom on your cell.*

He grasped the cell phone from a pant pocket and dialed until he realized the phone was dead. "What? No! That can't be! It had enough juice to last the day!" Sam shook his phone, and it started to ring. *Great! Someone's calling! Maybe Mom's wondering why I'm taking so long.* Sam checked the caller ID, but the message read *Unknown Caller*. "Hello?" he whispered into the phone. No one answered—at first. "Hello!" This time he shouted into the phone.

"Why have you not come?" The caller spoke in a hushed voice. "The children need you."

"What? Who's this? This isn't funny." Sam waited for an answer, but none came. The phone went silent. The signal disappeared. He was about to pound on the door again when something moved in the vault. The diary! On its own, it slid out of the envelope and unseen hands flipped through the pages. Sam whimpered and backed against the door. "This can't be real! It's my imagination. That's all. None of this is real!"

The diary opened to two dusty white empty pages. With shallow breaths, Sam leaned toward the diary until—plop—a red drop splashed onto a page. A second drop followed, then a third and fourth. He peered at the ceiling. *It can't be!* A circle of crimson liquid had formed on a ceiling panel and drops spilled onto the pages. *Is it blood?* He followed the red drops with his eyes down to the diary. At first, the droplets splashed randomly onto a page, but the red sticky liquid pooled and words formed— handwritten words that became a sentence. He read it aloud. "Samuel Every. Face your destiny. Return to the water."

"No!" Sam reached for the diary and slammed it shut.

At that moment, the vault door swung open and there stood his mom. "Honey, what are you doing? Why have you been down here so long?"

"Mom, the door was locked... the diary... and the blood." Sam rushed from the vault.

"Sam Every, what are you talking about?" His mom frowned. "The door wasn't locked. But are you hurt? Are you bleeding?"

"No, the blood! Don't you see?" Sam pointed to the ceiling. The blood had disappeared. He laughed. "I don't believe it. Mom, blood fell from the ceiling onto the pages of the diary. Look for yourself."

His mom picked up the diary and turned through the pages. No blood. "Honey, are you feeling all right? Maybe I shouldn't send you to the basement anymore. Your imagination gets the best of you. I think you've worked enough today. Do you want to wait and I'll drive you home after I close up the library?"

Sam shook his head. His heart slowed, his breathing calmed. "No, I'm fine. It's just a short ride home. I'll take my bike." As he walked from the basement, Sam glared at the diary one more time. *Why am I going crazy?*

# Chapter 6
## Not You Too, Computer

Sam reached home without any further strange happenings. As night fell, his parents and two younger brothers watched television while he hid in his room. *There's nothing wrong with me,* he reasoned, as music spilled into his ears from his iPod. *It's just my imagination. That explains everything. I'm not being haunted. I just need to relax and enjoy my summer. It's all good.*

Seated at his desk, he placed his violin to his chin, took up the bow and tried to mirror the Bach concerto that streamed through his earphones. When tired of Bach, he fiddled a heavy metal tune he had started to write. Through the third chorus, his eyes grew heavy. Sleep called, but he slapped his face to stay awake.

By midnight, his family was fast asleep. Sam slunk from his room to the kitchen. He devoured a peanut butter and jelly sandwich, downed a glass of milk and with a full stomach returned to his room. After another hour on the Internet, his head drooped. He snapped back awake but the images on the computer blurred. His head drooped for a second time. "Enough of this! I can't live in fear. I'm going to sleep. You hear me, ghost?" Sam shut down the computer, switched off the bedroom light and fell into bed. Sleep came quickly.

Light sliced through his closed eyelids. His computer hummed to life. Sam's eyes shot open to a room bathed in the soft blue glow generated by the computer screen. He froze; his eyes scanned the room. "Not again." *Am I still asleep? Am I dreaming? A computer just doesn't turn itself on, does it? Maybe there was a power surge. Yeah, that would explain it—a power surge.* He forced down a load of saliva, lifted himself from his bed and crept to his computer.

With shaky legs, he sat at the desk and peered at the monitor. Words formed, only not in any font his computer could produce. They appeared in ghostly white letters, like cursive handwriting, against a sea of blue. He mouthed the words as they filled the screen. *Chosen One, return to the water. The young ones are in danger. They shall all die.*

"What? This is crazy! I must be dreaming again. Wake up, fool!" More words etched into the screen. *Why have you not come?* "What do you mean?"

The words on the screen faded and the screen grew dark. He glanced away until the monitor blazed to life once again. This time one word flashed at the top of the screen. *Why?* As if an invisible hand typed the word over and over again, that single word filled the screen. *Why? Why? Why? Why—?*

His body trembled as he leaned closer to the screen. The words suddenly stopped, then disappeared. Like an explosion, a face appeared on the screen. Hers! The girl in the water. The girl who invaded his dreams. She stared at him with deep-set eyes cast within an ashen face. Sam fell backward out of his chair and crashed onto the floor.

He glared at the computer screen, but the girl's face had vanished. The screen was off, as if it had never been on. *I'm losing it. That's the only explanation. How could I be some Chosen One?*

# Chapter 7
## Heeding The Call

*Oh my back.* Sam opened his eyes and stared sideways at a pile of dirty clothes on his bedroom floor. He had fallen asleep on the floor, curled up like a baby. Slowly, painfully he lifted himself until he could see the clock on his dresser. *5:30 in the morning. Too early. Need more sleep.*

He glanced at his computer. The screen was dark. With rubbery arms, he climbed to his feet and took heavy steps to his bedroom window. A misty trail floated by—a normal occurrence from the morning fog that blowed inland off the ocean. He opened the window and a chill drifted into the room. The dank odor of seawater quickly spread.

He looked at his computer again. *Did anything really happen last night? Is some girl, whose body lies in the ocean, haunting me? I have to go back to the pier where this all began.* It was the only way to find the truth. If an apparition wanted to reach out from the beyond to deliver a message, he should allow her to accomplish that mission.

Sam entered his attached bathroom and stared into the mirror. "Are you telling me you believe someone is trying to reach out to you from a watery grave? Come on, man. How stupid can you be?" He splashed cool water over his face. "Look, I'll just ride down to the pier and see what happens. I mean it can't hurt anything—right?"

He brushed his teeth and continued his conversation. "Let's just say someone is trying to make contact. Why with me? I'm nobody. And what was written on the computer last night… *'the Chosen One?'* That makes no sense."

Sam, still sleepy, staggered back into his room and shed his pajamas. He drew on his swimming trunks and a T-shirt. He slid a pair of jeans over the swimming trunks. "This is stupid. I'm not going. Besides what if my jerk cousin is there? He'll chase me off."

He slid into a pair of sandals and went downstairs to the kitchen where he grabbed a cold bagel and took a swig from the carton of orange juice. His mom protested every time he drank straight from the carton, but she was off to work, so what she didn't know wouldn't hurt. He carried on the conversation with himself between bites of bagel. "If I don't go, I'm a wuss. It means I really think some ghost is haunting me, and I'm scared. Don't be so lame. Just go. I should just ride down to the beach, stop at the pier and get it out of my system."

After he finished half of the bagel and took a few more gulps of orange juice, he grabbed his house keys and quietly snuck out the back door—careful not to awake his dad, who had the day off from work, or his brothers.

"No, screw it. Let's go inside, get back in bed and later call the guys. Maybe they'll want to hit the mall." He didn't listen; instead he climbed on his bike and rolled down the driveway to the front of the house.

"Go back. Go back," Sam urged himself as he rode down his street and soon reached Pacific Coast Highway. "I guess I'm going to do this." He continued to wrestle with the idea until he reached the pier's entrance. *Still time to turn back,* he thought as he teetered on the edge of the pavement and the pier's cobblestone entryway.

"What are you doing here?" he asked himself. "What do you think will happen?" *Maybe you are the Chosen One.* He laughed at that idea, took a deep breath, and crossed onto the walkway.

Shops wouldn't open for an hour, but the pier was abuzz with morning activity. Surfers made their way down to the nearby beach. People gathered with their fishing poles along the old wooden section. Seagulls and pelicans stood guard. A few people strolled along the pier where he headed. A mist covered the ocean and the arctic-like morning air lingered as he rode to the spot from which he had leaped two days ago. A fog horn sounded in the distance, a tanker's mournful call just like the one that called out yesterday and so many times before.

At the section where he had jumped, Sam climbed off his bike and leaned against the railing. The water flowed calmly; it rolled against the pier's pylons and reflected the gray overcast sky, as if the sea mourned for the return of the shimmering sun.

"All right, what now?" He watched the water for signs of something strange, but nothing seemed out of the ordinary. "Look, I'm here. What do you want?" He wasn't sure he wanted an answer—none came.

Sam shook his head. "This is so dumb. I'm out of here. I mean I don't know if you're real. Even if you are, I don't know what you want from me. So go haunt someone else."

He turned to his bike, where Zack waited for him. "Hey, cuz, didn't I tell you to stay away from my beach." Zack grinned and shrugged. "And after I saved your life, this is the thanks I get—you disobey me?"

Sam bit his lip. A run-in with his cousin was the last thing he needed, especially when Zack was with his surfing cronies who blocked all possible escape routes. "Look, Zack, thanks for what you did. I mean it. I'm leaving."

"I don't think so." Zack laughed and turned to each of his friends. "No, you broke the rules and now I have no choice. You have to pay."

"Just back off, Zack." Sam retreated against the railing and winced as the skin on his back heated, as if sunburned. Why did his back react to these situations—to threats? *It's never happened to me before these last few days. Why now?*

"What do you say we strip him down to his tighty whities, take his bike and let him find his way home?" Zack eyed his buddies.

Sam's hands formed into fists. "That's very original, Zackary."

"No one calls me Zackary." It was the final push for Zack. "Let's do this, guys. Get him!"

Before his cousin reacted, Sam did the one thing Zack never expected. He threw a hard punch that caught Zack on the nose and knocked him backward. Sam acted on that moment of surprise; he wildly threw himself against Zack's friend TJ and steamrolled over him. With an escape route clear, he scrambled toward the parking garage. If he could enter into that shadowy layer, he could duck behind a car and hide. *Have to make it!*

Taunts sounded from behind him. "No way you can get away from us," Zack threatened.

*Come on, get to the garage!* His lungs burned as he reached the garage and entered into the parking structure's darkened first level. Since it was still so early in the morning, only a few vehicles were scattered through the garage—not much to choose from to hide. He selected an old delivery van parked off to the right and slid underneath the vehicle. Sweat dripped from his brow as he held his breath and waited. From the hiding place, he saw the legs of his cousin and the others enter the garage.

"Cuz, we're coming for you," Zack warned. "There's nowhere you can hide. Why don't you make this easy on yourself. I was just kidding before, but now I can't let this go."

Sam quivered. Maybe he had overreacted when he hit his cousin. It felt good and was long overdue, but he was in a real fix now. *Please don't see me.* His cousin and the others slithered closer as they searched the garage. They were almost upon him. Sam held his breath. His body froze. He waited for Zack to bend down with an evil smile and crazy eyes, but his cousin and the others walked right past the van.

"Yes!" Sam whispered. He slid farther under the van and listened carefully as Zack commanded his friends.

"He's got to be in here. Split up," Zack ordered. The others ran in different directions. When they were out of sight, Sam quietly crawled from under the van and stealthily sprinted to the opening of the parking structure.

"Hey, cuz, where you going?"

Sam stopped and glanced back. Zack and his surfing friends were perched atop nearby cars. "That's right, cuz, you're not going to escape that easily." Zack jumped down from a car hood. "Since you sucker punched me, be a man and fight me now."

*Yeah, maybe I should fight him, but it won't be a fair fight. No matter what, Zack's buddies will jump me.* In a last desperate attempt to escape, he dashed from the dark parking structure onto the pier toward his bike. He ran fast, but not fast enough. Zack closed the gap. A quick glance back showed his cousin was just a few feet behind him. Sam eyed the railing ahead. He had only one choice—jump from the pier and hope Zack didn't follow.

"I got you, cuz!" Zack shouted from just an arm's distance away. "You have nowhere else to run."

If Zack expected Sam to stop, he was mistaken. A step from the railing, with one last burst of energy, Sam leaped. He landed both of his feet on the top railing and pushed off into a swan dive, arms extended to the water. He tensed his body for a frigid, wet smack in the face. In the half second before he hit the water, Sam contemplated his next move. He hadn't really thought that far ahead. *Too late now,* he thought as he struck the water in a near belly flop. The icy water stung, like a thousand snowballs had hit him at once. Bubbles from the splash surrounded him as he sank deeper into the murky water.

Sam thrashed about; his arms flailed in all directions, but he had no control over his movements. He continued to slip farther down below the surface. *Relax! Find the light. It has to be there. Stop and think.* He twisted around until he spotted the light. *There!* His composure regained, he swam toward the air. As he broke the surface, he coughed out the chilly water and forced in air. Laughter filtered down from above—his cousin's.

"Glad I don't have to save your life again." Zack and his friends applauded. Sam didn't bother to respond. "Listen, cuz, I got some surfing to do, so I can't hang with you anymore. It's been fun. Oh, and just to make sure no one steals your bike, maybe we should give it to you. Dudes …" Zack's friends picked up Sam's bike and lifted it over their heads.

"No!" Sam shouted as he treaded water.

"Oh, yes." Zack laughed and walked away. With one mighty heave, his friends threw Sam's bike into the water and the two-wheeler quickly sank. Rather than let the sea claim his bike, Sam took a deep breath and dove under the water to try to save it. Deeper and deeper he traveled until he grabbed his right front tire. He tugged and strained to bring the bike to the surface. *Come on, lift! Swim up!* His lungs ached for air, but he and the bike started to rise. *I'm going to make it. Zack won't win today.*

A tug on his foot stopped him. *No!* A second tug followed and Sam peered down. The water swallowed his scream.

# Chapter 8
## Follow That Ghost

The ghostly girl he had seen two days ago, the girl in his dreams, clung to his sandal-covered right foot. Her other hand grabbed his calf. Like a snake, she wrapped her right arm around his torso. *She's going to drown me!* Sam fought to free himself. His lungs screamed, throat tightened, head grew numb. His vision tunneled in on itself. Still she climbed until her face was even with his; her dark eyes never blinked as she stared at him.

*Let me go!* Sam spoke with his thoughts. His head grew heavy; unconsciousness beckoned. He was about to die—there was nothing he could do about it.

Unable to hold his breath any longer, he opened his mouth and instead of salty water, warm air gushed into his lungs. His heart beat again, his mind cleared. He still lived—because of a kiss.

The apparition had placed her lips over his and the warmest kiss he had ever experienced brought him back to life. Slowly, she removed her lips from his. Her eyes, still rimmed by shadows, were determined, but soft and concerned. "Chosen One, are you all right?" Her lips never moved. A gentle but commanding voice echoed in his thoughts. He detected a British accent.

Sam whirled in each direction. He hadn't drowned; somehow he breathed underwater. The sea had become warm, energizing, even comforting as if it was the most natural thing for him to be under water. "Chosen One," the girl repeated.

"What have you done to me? Who are you?" He thought his response just as the girl seemed to speak with her mind. "This is all freaking me out."

He tried to swim away, but the ghost girl gripped his hands and held him in place. "Let me go! Please! I don't want to be your zombie boyfriend! I don't want to die!"

"Chosen One, you don't need to fear me." She released him. "You are free to go if you wish it."

Sam eyed the streaks of light that signaled the water surface. He reached up as if to swim toward the world above, but stopped and searched her face, still shallow and green, for answers. Was she a ghost? Was she something else? Had he hit his head on a pylon and this was his imagination? Getting no answers to these questions, he asked, "How am I breathing underwater?"

"Because of me," she answered, still through thoughts.

"How are we talking this way—I mean without words?"

"Again, because I have made it so." She smiled and Sam thought the bones in her cheeks might burst through what little skin she had.

"Are you a mermaid?"

The girl laughed and looked at her feet, which were shoeless and barely exposed under her long dress. She had no fin. "I'm no mermaid, but I've sometimes wished to be one." Her accent was definitely British. Not proper and formal, like he heard spoken at Buckingham Palace during his family's visit to England. She spoke fast, words mixed together, like many spoke on the streets of London.

"Are you a ghost? Is your body at the bottom of the ocean?"

"I'm no ghost." This time the girl did not laugh. Her words flowed as if she had chanted them, but her tone darkened.

"Are you sure you're not a ghost because you kind of look like death."

"Chosen One, you must trust me."

"Why are you calling me the Chosen One?" Sam asked as a school of fish swam close.

"Because that is who you are." Sarah moved closer, her face inches from his. "Please trust me."

*This isn't really happening*, he told himself. *This is a dream. That's all. I'm not really talking to a dead girl? I'm not breathing underwater. I'm back home in my bed fast asleep. So let's see where this dream takes me.* "All right—I trust you."

The ghost girl gripped his hand and kissed him again on the lips. It only lasted a second or two, but the effect was the same as the first kiss. It warmed him. Did she kiss him to sustain his ability to breathe or because she was happy with his answer? "Now, take my hand. We've a journey to undertake." The girl clasped his hand tightly.

"Wait! You haven't told me who you are." Sam glanced at her bony fingers interlocked in his. The touch tingled.

"In time. Now we must go."

"Can you at least tell me your name?"

"Sarah." She drew out the 'S', as if she sang a musical note, and let the 'H' hover.

Sam nodded. "Sarah, where are we going? Why is it so important?"

She was silent for a moment. Her face grew rigid, her eyes narrowed. "I've come to take you to the past so you can face your destiny."

"What destiny?" Sam's stomach tightened as if he prepared for a punch.

"You must stop the pirate Jem Slayer, that bloody dog, and save the children he's kidnapped!"

"I don't under—" He cut himself off as he remembered the diary in the library that mentioned the evil Jem Slayer. Had this girl left diary for him? It had to be her. But had the events in the library happened or was that part of the dream, too?

"Chosen One, we must hurry! Come with me before it's too late. The past, the present and the future are all at stake."

# Chapter 9
## The Portal to His Fate

Sam blew out an air bubble and watched it rise toward the beams of sunlight that pricked holes in the water's darkness. He didn't understand anything Sarah said and still doubted any of this was real, but he followed her anyway.

"Hold my hand and come with me." Sarah's telepathic words sounded like both a request and a command. "Don't be afraid."

"I'm not afraid." He tried to sound brave.

"Good, then let's go." In one fluid motion, she swam farther toward the sea floor and zipped by fish and discarded junk as if she might really be a mermaid.

*This is all just so freaky. What am I doing? I should be running from her.* Sam resisted the urge to flee. This had to be a dream and an inner force nudged him to discover where it led. The farther out to sea they glided, the more the ocean bottom came alive with clarity and color. Sam rubbed his eyes, which functioned as well as they did out of water—maybe even better. *Amazing!*

Schools of golden and silver fish swam in all directions. Rock formations rose up from the ocean floor while crabs jutted in and out of their hiding places. Starfish clung to the rocks. Soda bottles, tires, even a couch, littered the ocean floor, and sea creatures of all shapes and sizes dwelt in them.

Still, Sarah led him deeper into the ocean. The underwater pylons from the pier became specs in the distance. *Where is she taking me? Who does she think I am? Why does she think I'm this Chosen One?* He quieted all the questions. *Don't show fear. Look cool.*

In spite of his desire to learn what this was all about, he hesitated when Sarah pointed to an underwater cave up ahead.

While the world around him was brightly illuminated, that cave was bleak. Sam shuttered. Is that where she meant him to go? *I can't. If I go in there, I might never return home. Never see Mom and Dad and my little brothers. But, it's just a dream, isn't it? Anytime now I'll wake up and laugh about this.* "I'm not so sure about this." Sam ripped his hand out of Sarah's.

"Don't fear, Chosen One… at least not yet." She reached for his hand.

"What do you mean, not yet? And stop calling me Chosen One."

"Bloody hell, are you not Samuel Every?" Impatience marked her words as she rolled her eyes.

"Uh, yeah, I am." Sam swam a few feet away from her. "How do you know my name?"

"Your name and your face have appeared to me. You are the Chosen One, and you have abilities that can save us all."

"What abilities? I don't understand. Enough games." Sam thrashed at the water to escape Sarah, but she moved too fast.

She dashed in front of him and placed a hand on his shoulder. "You've nothing to fear from me."

"Yeah, then let me go."

She removed her hand from his shoulder. "I'll understand if you choose not to come. I don't want to mislead you. Slayer is a dangerous rat. If you come with me, your life shall be in danger. But if you don't face Slayer, the world you know shall end."

Sarah paused. Her black-rimmed eyes zeroed in on his. "I don't lightly ask you to take such risk, but you must. You're the only one who can save the children and save us all. It's your destiny."

*What does that mean?* His head spun, and he turned from Sarah to glance back toward the pier. The pylons had disappeared. How far had they come? How could he just leave his family? They would worry, maybe even think him dead. How could he do that to them? "I can't leave my family."

Sarah swam around to face him. "If you don't come with me, this world you know and everyone you love shall disappear because of that pig, Slayer. The only way to prevent that is to come with me. It's your choice."

*What is she saying? I should just go home… or wake up. But if this is a dream, what do I have to lose? Come on, man. You can't be a wuss, especially in your own dream. And this has to be a dream. It just has to be.* "You said my destiny awaits me?"

"Yes, I believe it does." Her greenish face came to life as she smiled.

"You said there are children in danger."

"Yes."

"And the way to save them and everyone else is through this cave."

"It is."

Sam gazed back one more time; he squinted as he tried to find the pier's pylons, but they were too far away. He was already far from home and he gulped. *If this is a dream I have nothing to fear. If this is real, how can I say no? I have to save my family—jeez the whole world. The Chosen One can't prove to be a coward.* He closed his eyes. *Goodbye, Mom, Dad, little bros.* He reopened them and grasped Sarah's hand. "All right, I'll come with you."

Sarah squeezed his hand tightly and in a couple of strokes, they reached the cave entrance. Its rounded mouth, the size of a manhole, revealed nothing about what might be inside. Before they entered, Sam studied the entrance, a light-swallowing black hole. *I can't see anything!* Sarah was the first to enter and with a slight tug on his hand, Sam followed. He half expected an explosion of light or for some universal doorway to open, but they simply swam through darkness so thick he couldn't even see Sarah next to him.

*Where is she leading me?*

# Chapter 10
## A Time of Pirates

They swam deeper into the cave. Sam glanced back once toward the entrance, and the ocean he knew slipped from sight. Walled in by the darkness of the cave, there was no way to tell how much farther they had to swim. The water grew icy in the bleakness of the cavern. Each breath came tougher, as if something heavy constricted his chest. *I need out. I need real air. This has to end sometime.* Sam shivered. He swam faster as his heart thumped like a hammer in his chest.

A pinprick of light appeared up ahead. *Yes!* The farther they swam, the more pronounced the brightness became. Beads of sunlight pierced the water's depth and illuminated an opening up ahead. *An exit! Thank God*! But that made no sense. The cave led him deeper underground. He never had the sensation that they had swam up toward an exit. *Just go with it,* Sam thought.

Five more strokes, another kick of his legs, and he and Sarah burst from the cave. Sam breathed a sigh of relief. The cold disappeared. The water grew warm—warmer than the waters back home.

*Where has this girl brought me?* He stared at the cave they had just exited. The way home was inside that narrow passage, but he turned away from the cave and followed Sarah as she led him farther into this new watery world. Schools of fish—all the colors of a rainbow—darted in and out of pink reefs. Two shipwrecks lined this ocean floor. The sunken vessels resembled the pirate-looking ship he'd seen off the pier.

Sam stopped. He couldn't take his eyes off the shipwrecks. *This can't be real. I'm not really seeing this.* The wrecks gently swayed as they rested on the ocean floor. One wooden carcass still had a large white sail attached to a mast. The sail floated in a ghostly dance over the torn-up deck. He studied the sail closely until his vision blurred and the sail transformed. A massive forehead jutted out with two black holes underneath—eyes—and a gaping mouth formed under sharply-edged cheeks. The sail became a skull, and the skull spoke. *"The Chosen One must die."*

"No!" Sam shouted. The undersea world around him slipped away as darkness overtook him.

"Chosen One, wake up." Sam heard the words in the distance. "Breathe. You're alive." The voice was familiar. That street-wise British accent mixed with concern and determination. *Sarah!*

Sam blinked several times and opened his eyes to a blue sky filled with bands of orange and purple clouds. He was on his back in wet sand. Water rushed up on shore and covered his feet. He slowly lifted himself onto his elbows. The motion made him sick, and he leaned over as vomit—a mix of salt water and phlegm—spilled from his mouth. His head pounded. A cold sweat covered his brow. When his stomach no longer heaved, he lifted himself onto his elbows one more time. "Where am I?"

"You'd do better to ask—when am I?"

Sarah's voice no longer filled his thoughts. He had actually heard her words.

He turned toward her and his eyes found a very different girl. Sunbeams danced across her face and broke through her ghostly appearance. Her face was no longer green, just pale and thin. The black rims around her eyes faded. Sparkles of red shimmered throughout her gray hair. The sun's energy seemed to soak into her. Death still seemed to linger around her, but she was a little less like a zombie. *And she's beautiful.* "What's happening to you? You look different—really different."

"Chosen One, we can't stay here, else we become shark bait." Sarah didn't answer his question as though she purposely chose to ignore him. "It's too dangerous here."

"What? Why?" Sam started to remember. Sarah had told him she would take him back in time to fight some dreaded pirate and to face his destiny. But that was impossible! How could they have traveled back in time? Was the cave actually a portal? *Do things like that actually exist? Or is this still a crazy dream?* If so, Sam hoped he would wake up soon. "You haven't told me where, or when, we are."

"This place is New Providence—a scurvy infested port filled with poxy-faced scoundrels," she answered, her voice lowered to a hush.

Sam studied their surroundings. They had surfaced inside a massive harbor crowded with anchored ships of different sizes. The wooden vessels rocked and creaked in the water as men shouted orders at each other and lowered crates and barrels into rowboats. Some of the ships had been run up on shore where a sandbar served as a natural dock. A small island, just beyond the harbor entrance, permitted ships to enter from one side of the island and depart from the other. Larger ships that probably required deeper water lay just beyond the island; their massive masts rose like a forest of trees over the sea. Most flew the British flag. Sam brought his attention to the shore where men, some in three-cornered hats and long coats that reached down to their legs and others shirtless in pants that extended down to their calves, loaded and unloaded cargo from small boats along the beach. The cargo was placed onto horse-drawn carriages and with a crack of a whip men in the carriages led the horses up the beach to a town of wooden shacks and tents.

A strange scene unfolded on the beach. Candles lined the water's edge, while men and women stared out to sea. The women, who wore long, drab-colored dresses and bonnets that mostly covered their faces, cried. The men, most in three-cornered hats with swords at their sides, sobbed and bowed their heads. They all seemed to pray.

Farther up on the beach, beyond the group, a stone fortress was under construction. *Or maybe it is being rebuilt because it looks really old.* Canons protruded from sections of unfinished walls, the rounded mouths of the barrels aimed toward the sea. Just like the anchored ships, a British flag flew high over the fortress. Gaping holes and burn marks spotted the walls. Beyond the fort was a sparse town made up of shacks and tents. Smoke rose from inside the town and a handful of tents were shredded.

"What's going on?" Sam rose to his knees. "What happened here?"

"Look out there." Sarah pointed toward the ocean.

A fleet of ships—Sam expected they might be warships— headed out to sea. "What is it? What am I seeing?"

"Two days prior, Slayer attacked the harbor and kidnapped twenty children. The British fleet, those royal fools, have been ordered after him, but they shall not reach him, and even if they do, the lot of them cannot defeat him." Sarah shook her head. "They underestimate his power. You are the only one who can bring him to justice." She eyed Sam, but quickly turned away.

"What?" he asked.

"Chosen One, this shall not be easy."

"Look, this is all a little weird, and, well, if this is a dream, I'd really like to wake up now."

Sarah's eyes flared with anger. "This is no dream. You must accept this is real. You must accept your destiny." She squeezed his hand. Sam winced and she quickly eased her grip. "Come with me. Let's make our way to safer ground and I'll explain all, so you can understand."

Sam held his head. It still hurt, as if someone tightened a vice grip against his forehead. If he moved, he would be sick again. "I don't feel too good. Can't we rest here a bit longer?"

"Your insides are feeling that bloody rot that I felt when I first went through the portal," she explained. "It'll pass. You must come with me now before we are discovered."

"By who?"

Sarah hesitated. "By anyone."

"Wait, Sarah, how did I get on shore? All I remember is being under the water, seeing those shipwrecks and then... a skull. I think I blacked out after that. What happened to me?"

"I brought you ashore." Sarah climbed to her feet, scampered to a nearby crate where she found a damp blanket. She then scurried back to Sam. "I think you had a vision, maybe from the sickness you suffered from the portal. We cannot worry about that now. Please, come." With more strength than Sam would have expected from a girl who still appeared half dead, Sarah lifted him to his feet. "Here," she ordered, "wrap this around yourself to hide your clothing. We don't want to draw attention to ourselves."

Before he could protest, she threw the damp blanket around him, grabbed his hand and led him toward the small town. He kept his eyes down, but still watched the sailors as they moved their cargo. They roughly lifted crates from boats and threw them onto the shore. One sailor who stood in a boat dropped a crate onto the beach too close to another's foot. An argument began.

"You scallywag—you best watch yourself or I'll gut you like a pig," said the sailor whose foot was almost crushed.

The sailor who dropped the crate jumped from the boat and stood before the sailor who threatened him. "You should hold your tongue or I'll bloody you with my bare hands, you scurvy dog." A third sailor threw water on both of them as others gathered around and laughed.

Meanwhile, clad in long red coats with muskets over their shoulders, British soldiers patrolled the beach. They took no notice of the argument between the sailors—or, at least, they didn't react to it.

Sarah didn't either. She walked bent over with a limp, her hair draped over her face, a clear effort to disguise herself. The only question was… from who? The sailors? The soldiers? Could no on here be trusted? She even held out her hand to individuals along the beach and asked for money like a poor beggar. Sam did the same, though his questions remained. *How bad are things if you can't even trust the soldiers?*

Two soldiers blocked their path with their muskets in hand. One soldier, tall, scarred and blue-eyed, placed a hand on Sarah's shoulder. "There now, this is no place for the likes of you, unless you want to be hauled out to sea like those other poor young souls."

Sam guessed he referred to the kidnapped children.

"No, sir," Sarah spoke in barely a whisper and avoided eye contact with the soldiers.

The second soldier laughed. "Look at these two; hardly worth anything. They are nothing more than mere scraps by the looks of them. Not even strong enough for work. No, these two have nothing to fear from any pirate."

"That may be," the scarred soldier said, "but Governor Rogers wants all children out of sight for their own protection."

"Are you blind?" the second soldier joked. "These two are no children. They are of age. Let them take their own risks. If pirates nab them, the lad shall toil away in a life of labor swabbing a deck and the girl shall find herself a galley slave, cooking away her life. How does that sound, young ones?"

"Just be off with you, and be quick about it," the scarred soldier ordered.

Sarah nodded and moved on quickly. Sam, head bowed, followed. They eventually passed the fort and moved onto a sandy roadway that led into the town—a small stretch of narrow dirt pathways and streets lined with shacks and tents. Some appeared to be businesses where merchants sold fruits, ship supplies and fabric.

Men, some with heads covered with bandanas, others with those three-cornered hats, staggered out of other shacks that reminded Sam of sports bars near the beach back home. They laughed and cursed. Some spilled liquid from mugs onto already-stained vests and long coats, clothing he had seen before in the Colonial display back home at the history museum. A group of men argued and shoved each other. All of them were armed with swords or wooden clubs. None seemed to care about the kidnapped children. Signs of battle littered the path. Windows were smashed, doorways blasted through and the charred remains of buildings smoldered.

Sam held his nose against the stench of burnt wood and spent gunpowder. Those smells, mixed with the reek of rum and urine, made him want to vomit again. Not even the ocean could wash away the collage of disgusting odors.

Sarah hastened her pace. "Hurry, we're almost there."

"Where?" Sam asked, but she didn't answer. They walked onto a side road overgrown with tropical greenery. Here there were small, modest residences, but not even those homes had been spared from the attack.

A mid-afternoon sun heated the air and made it even more difficult to breathe. Sam's clothes stuck to his skin and sweat dripped down his face. "I thought you said we're almost there," he huffed.

"Here." Sarah pointed to a hut. "We'll be safe here."

Sam wasn't so sure. The hut, not much bigger than an outhouse, tilted as though it could fall at any moment. A wooden door, barely attached by one hinge, covered the entrance.

"Before we enter, there's something you must know, Chosen One. Don't be frightened by what you see." Sarah opened the door and Sam glimpsed inside. *What? It can't be!* But it was. On the floor of the hut, on a bed of torn, stained sheets, was Sarah. Her eyes were closed and her hands were folded over her chest. She wore the same tattered dress as the Sarah who stood in the doorway, but the Sarah on the floor had turned blue, as though she had been dead for some time.

Sam fell to the ground outside the hut. "You are a ghost!"

# Chapter 11
## Two Become One

"Please, Chosen One! Allow me to explain." Sarah knelt toward him, her face still thin and pale, though no longer green, her gray hair marked by cinnamon streaks. "As I said before, I'm no ghost. Not exactly, anyway."

Sam slid away as she reached for him. "What is that supposed to mean?"

"Follow me into the hut and watch." She rose and walked through the doorway. Sam gritted his teeth and his body trembled. *Why do I keep following this girl? I should just run right now. Head back to the water. Find that portal.* Instead he scrambled to his feet, stepped cautiously to the doorway and peered into the hut.

Sarah stared at her corpse. "Watch."

She titled her head back, joined her hands as if in prayer, and chanted strange words in a language Sam didn't understand. Her chanting grew louder and she began to fade as if her body became more phantom than solid, like she really was a ghost. With one last nod and weak smile to Sam, she lowered herself to her corpse. As Sam stared wide-eyed, she disappeared into the body and the two became one.

Sam fought the urge to run. *What did I just see? What just happened?* He inched forward and knelt to the one remaining Sarah, who lay unmoving, eyes still closed, hands still crossed over her chest. "Sarah! Sarah!"

As she lay still, her face turned a deep brown while flesh and muscle filled in shallow, bony cheeks. Any remnants of black around her eyes vanished, and the streaks of cinnamon in her hair spread into long reddish locks that fell over her shoulders and vanquished any signs of gray. Even the flesh around her hands expanded and took on the same tanned hue as her face. "Woah!" Sam mouthed a little louder than he would have liked.

"Strange word," she mumbled weakly.

"Sarah!"

"I'm here, Chosen One." Her eyes fluttered and, after a few blinks, opened to reveal the same deep black spheres he had seen before. They still showed determination, but they were tired.

"Are you all right?" Sam started to reach for her hand, but recoiled. "I don't understand."

Sarah lifted herself into a sitting position. "I'm quite all right, although I'm bloody hungry and weak."

"What just happened?"

"I told you I was no ghost. I simply used my magic to separate my essence from my body as I searched for you through a time portal. That's why I appeared like a ghost to you."

Sam sat beside her. "But you didn't make me separate my essence—or whatever—to come back to this place. So why did you have to do it?"

Sarah grasped his hand and her grip felt warmer than ever. "I could've sought you out in my body, but I wasn't sure I could find you and since I'd never tried to enter a time portal. I wasn't sure I would survive the journey to the future. If I was to die, I didn't wish to die in your time. My place is here among the swine who dwell in New Providence, and since this hut has been my home, this was a fitting place for my body to rest."

"I still don't—"

"Chosen One. I've much to explain and so very little time." Urgency spilled into her words. She lowered her head before she spoke again. "Promise me you'll hear my words with an open mind. That's the only way you'll truly be able to understand."

"After all I've seen, yeah, I'll listen." He still wasn't sure any of this was real. He quietly prayed to wake up, but he remained stuck in this dream, if that's what it was.

"Be prepared, for it's a tale of darkness. It's a story that could foretell even darker times to come if we fail. I've brought you through a portal back to the Year of our Lord 1718." Sarah grabbed both of Sam's hands. "Your unique qualities make you the only soul throughout time who can stop Slayer."

Sam peered deeply into her dark eyes. *Is this girl for real? Is any of this for real? This has to be a dream, and I'd really like to wake up now.*

Sarah's hands tightened around his. "This place I've brought you—New Providence—is in the Caribbean where Slayer commands his army of pirates and his fleet of ships."

"So he's a big-time pirate." Sam half smiled.

"He's more than that. He's dangerous for reasons few understand. Jem Slayer is a practitioner of dark magic."

"What?"

"He's of a race of magic conjurers, and he's an evil dog. He has the gift, one he chooses to use for greed. Piracy provides him the perfect way to seek out wealth and power while disguising his magic and his true desire, at least until he's ready to unleash his full power to conquer the world, and maybe other worlds."

"Wait a second! Magic? Come on!" Sam pulled his hands free. He wiped sweat from his forehead, and pulled his sticky shirt away from his neck.

"Magic is real." Sarah moved a bit closer. "How else could I have sought you out and brought you to this time?"

"I'm not sure any of this is real. I could be dreaming. I could have hit my head in the water and be drowning even now."

"This is all real. Accept it."

"Let's say it is. How do you know so much about this pirate?" Sam slid over a few feet to the other end of the hut.

"I know because all those whose blood is filled with magic know each other. We're a race. Slayer, me, you—we're the same." Sarah reached over and placed a hand against Sam's chest. "You have magic, like me. It's in your blood."

Sam's mind spun. *Race. Blood. Magic. This just can't be true.*

Sarah brushed her hair from her face. "Chosen One, you know I'm right about Slayer and the reality of magic because you're one of us."

"No. It's not true." Sam peered at the door, his way out of all of this. Maybe if he crossed through, he would be back in his own bed, safe in his room.

Sarah closed her eyes as if to rest. "My abilities granted me the power to find you in time because you're one of us." She slowly opened her eyes. "You have great magic in you, more powerful even than my own."

"You're crazy. I'm just a normal teenager with enough problems of my own."

"You're more than you know. Soon you'll discover your magic. You'll need your abilities to face the challenge ahead of you."

"And Slayer's that challenge?"

"I had to bring you here because Slayer has discovered the hiding place of a mythical magic weapon called the Sword of Zel-Kar. If it's real, it'll allow him to rule the world."

"Nothing you are saying makes sense." Sam's head ached. "What's a Sword of Zel-Kar?"

"Zel-Kar was an ancient conjurer. He was so powerful that some say he discovered the secret to crafting a weapon—a sword—that could grant its user immortality. It was meant as a gift to the world to be used for good, but Zel-Kar's followers believed it could be used for evil. Stories passed down through time tell that they tried to convince him to destroy it, but Zel-Kar refused. A battle followed for control of the sword. Many died. When it was over, a repentant Zel-Kar hid the weapon from the world.

"To most of us, it is just myth, but not to Slayer. He has always believed in the existence of the sword, and has spent years searching for it." Sarah paused as her words echoed through the hut.

Sam remained silent, his hands clasped tightly together. "But the dude—Slayer—hasn't found it?"

"No, but he has found a legendary scroll from the ancient wizard he believes can lead him to it. The scroll is said to not only show where the sword is hidden but also commands that twenty innocent lives be sacrificed to claim the magic blade."

All of a sudden it dawned on Sam. "You mean the kidnapped children."

"Yes. As I told you, two days prior Slayer attacked New Providence from his ship, *The Reaper*. He inflicted the damage you saw. He and his men kidnapped twenty children of British soldiers, landowners, and some of the wealthier reformed pirates who signed the King's Pardon for acts of piracy, and recanted their pirating ways."

"The King's Pardon?"

"Yes, you heard the soldier mention Governor Rogers. Before Woodes Rogers got to New Providence, this was a haven for pirates. But when he arrived, he brought change. He reclaimed New Providence in the name of King George I from the pirates. He brought with him the King's Pardon. Any pirate who recanted his ways would be granted clemency as long as they turned themselves in to the colonial governors—not just in New Providence but throughout the British territories."

"But why would Slayer kidnap rich kids—I mean these wealthy children? Why not kidnap the poor or beggars or orphans? He's not going to ransom them. You said he plans to kill them. The British fleet might not be after him if he took the poor ones."

"Slayer is a powerful conjurer, but that bloody rat is still a crazy pirate. Slayer hates Rogers and all the pirates who accept the King's Pardon, so this is his way of making the governor look like a fool and laughing in the face of the Crown. Slayer sees any pirate who signs the pardon as an enemy."

Sam blew out some air. "So somehow we have to save the children and at the same time stop him from reaching the sword?"

"Yes. You're the only one who can save those children and ultimately keep Slayer from the sword."

"Why me?"

If the scroll is real, the stories about Zel-Kar creating such a sword may be real. I now believe the sword does exist, and Slayer has the ability to take it. But the scroll also foretells the coming of one who bears the mark of a sword on his back. The scroll proclaims that if evil should ever reach the sword, the one with the mark of the blade shall rise to face that evil for control of the weapon."

*How does she know about my back and how does she know so much about this scroll?* "Have you seen this scroll? How do you know what's in it? How do you know it talks about some Chosen One?"

Sarah paused before she spoke. "I've never laid eyes on the scroll, but I've heard the stories, like all conjurers. When I discovered Slayer had found a scroll that might guide him to the Sword of Zel-Kar, I had to try to find the Chosen One if one existed. When I reached out with my magic one name and one face filled my thoughts. Your name, Samuel Every! Your face! My magic led me to find you, Chosen One! And if I found you, I fear Slayer also knows of your existence. I pray he doesn't know I've brought you here."

"Wait, there's one thing I don't get. In my time, this is all in the past. This Slayer dude couldn't have gotten the sword because he never conquered the world. Jeez, he's not even one of the pirates in history books. We should go back to my time and forget about this. Let me get on with my life."

"I know this is hard for you to understand but where magic is involved, there's more than one reality. In different timelines, Slayer never obtained the sword, but in this timeline, he has discovered it. If he succeeds, the future shall be changed. You, your mother and father may even cease to exist. The world you know shall be no more. You must believe me. This has become the pivotal moment in time that shall forever change all realities."

Sam rubbed his head, which hurt even more now. "And I guess somewhere along the way, I'll figure out what my abilities are and how to stop him?" It seemed unlikely.    "You must. I found you for a reason. Only you can stop Slayer's dark magic, and allow good magic to protect the world."

The thought of saving innocent children and protecting his world—most importantly his family—was enough for Sam to want to stop Slayer, but he still had questions. "You said there are others with magical abilities. What about them? There must be others much more ready for this than me."

Tears formed in Sarah's eyes. "Slayer has killed most of them and the few who remain, for the most part, are loyal to him," she explained. "I don't know of any person who is willing to stand against him."

"You are."

"Yes, but I lack the power." Sarah took a deep breath. "Chosen One, do you believe me?"

Sam sighed. "Yes."

"And you'll help me stop Slayer?"

With a long sigh, Sam stared off as if he looked beyond the hut, past the harbor to the open sea and to a ship commanded by a sorcerer pirate he was expected to stand against. *This still can't be real. Any moment I'm going to wake up safe in my bed. Then again, even if I do wake up, I have to go to sleep again at some point, and this girl will still probably be there haunting my dreams. What the heck? Maybe I should stick this out. See where this all leads me. If I finish this dream and stop Slayer, I'll get this freaky girl out of my head. Besides, what's the worst that can happen? I can die, let down those kids, Slayer gets that sword and the future will forever be darkened by my failure. But it's all just a dream— isn't it?* "Uh, yeah, I'll help," Sam decided. "After all, I'm the Chosen One."

# Chapter 12
## Some Magic Is Deadly

The setting sun cast the sky in a hazy glow and painted the string of clouds in shades of purple and orange. Sam walked beside Sarah along the dirt roadway filled with taverns and shops. Drunken sailors crowded the street as they enjoyed their shore leave, oblivious to the attack by *The Reaper*. Others talked of the kidnappings.

Sam and Sarah made their way toward the harbor. He considered the plan she had outlined at the hut while they partook of coconuts and foul-smelling dried meat from a jar. She had made hijacking a boat sound so simple, at the time. But now? Did she do this sort of thing all the time?

"That reminds me," he asked, "Don't you have parents? Are you on your own? How? Why?"

Sarah looked away, and Sam glimpsed tears in her eyes.

"I'm sorr—"

"No, it's all right. My father worked on a merchant ship that pirates raided. Cannon fire sunk his ship. Everyone on board was either killed or enslaved. Either way, I never saw or heard from him again."

"How long ago?"

"It would be five years now," she answered. "I was so very young—just a little girl really. I was eight."

"So you're thirteen now, like me." Sam examined her face. She seemed so much older, so much more mature, but she had been through so much.

"Yes."

"Was it Slayer? Was he the pirate who attacked your father's ship?"

"I don't know." Sarah tightened her fists. "It doesn't matter. I hate all pirates. They're scum, and I'd like to see them all hang by the neck until dead."

Sam nodded. "And your mom, uh, mother?"

"She was a great woman. She made this dress for me." Sarah embraced herself; her hands wrapped around the dress' sleeves.

The dress, which had been white, was now brownish and covered in little rips and tears. Still, on her, it looked right, like she and the dress were one, and she looked beautiful. "What happened to her?"

"She had magical abilities like me, but different. She used her powers to help heal the sick and injured. She absorbed a person's illness and her magic destroyed it, saving the person's life and protecting her own. When there was an outbreak of small pox, she tried to heal as many as she could, but in the end her own body couldn't fight off the disease as she absorbed too much of it."

"I don't know what to say."

"Forget it. It has no bearing on what we must do."

"You said your magic is different from your mother's. You don't have her healing abilities?"

"I guess I have some of her abilities, but I'm no healer—not like she was. She was so strong, so powerful, so good. Sometimes I think I'm dark inside—no bloody good—like Slayer."

Sam placed a hand on her shoulder. She must be hurting, and had to be strong to overcome such loss. Since losing her parents, she had taken care of herself and the hut had become her only home. She had learned to provide her own food, water and clothing and to survive in such a dangerous place and time. How much had she depended on magic to survive? He didn't ask the question out loud.

In the twilight they began their search for a boat.

Sam had replaced his clothes with items Sarah provided for him. He now wore a torn shirt and knee-length pants, which Sarah called breeches, along with some old boots. Everything was a size or so too big. Who had worn them before him? He didn't bother to ask.

They strolled into town on a roadway lined by flaming torches that ushered in the night. An orange glow settled over New Providence as townspeople and sailors mixed in the street—their laughter, shouts and insults sounded like the sounds of his school cafeteria.

Lost in his thoughts, Sam bumped into one man, or rather the man bumped into him. The man carried a mug filled with some liquid that smelled like paint remover. "Out of my way, boy," the man slurred.

"Sorry." Sam bowed his head. With more than a little disgust, and careful side glances, he eyed the man and the others who drank, laughed and fought. *Don't they know children have been kidnapped? Don't they care? Can't they show at least a little respect for the parents who have lost children?* Those parents held vigil by the shore, lit candles in hand, as the day gave way to night.

As Sam walked, a new question formed. "If you have this ability to move through portals, why don't you open one to wherever Slayer is going?"

"I wish I could," Sarah glanced toward the harbor, as if she didn't want to make eye contact. "He knows I'm on the hunt for him, and he may know I've sought your help. He's much stronger than I am, and I can feel him using his magic to block my power to reach him. If I try to open a portal to him, he might trap us in a netherworld forever."

"But how will we reach him?"

"You'll lead us to him. You know where the sword is."

"I do?"

"It's locked away in your mind. You just need to open the doorway to your most hidden thoughts."

"I don't—"

Sarah stopped and pulled him hard against the side of one shack. "We're being followed," she whispered.

"What?" The tingling in Sam's back returned, just like he felt in the library basement and at the pier. "Who's following us?"

"I think it might be one of Slayer's men." Sarah's words were hushed, her eyes wide.

"How do you know?" The tingling grew worse, like that time in dodge ball when some kid had smashed him at close range in the back with a rubber ball.

She peeked around the corner. "Worse! I think it's Maximilian Black."

"Who's that and why's he worse?" Sam's heart beat heavy in his chest. His back sizzled under his shirt.

"He's a swine—a killer—who serves Slayer. He wields his own dark magic," Sarah clenched her teeth. "Are you ready to run?"

"What? No!"

"Run!"

Before Sam could take one step, a blast struck the shack. Shards of wood splintered in every direction. The explosion threw him to the ground. Ringing in his ears deafened him. Confusion flooded his mind. He whirled around as the ringing faded and sounds of terror in the street reached him.

Women screamed all around and men drew their swords, or pistols, if they had them. Confusion filled the street. Mothers clutched their children. A man fired a pistol and the round struck a shack not far from where another group of men had gathered, their swords drawn. Fights broke out as sailor accused sailor of piracy. Sam guessed many of them were pirates, or reformed pirates. British soldiers, their muskets in hand, rushed into the street to quiet the mobs.

"Get up, Chosen One! He's coming! Get up!" Sarah dragged Sam to his feet. Dazed, he willed his legs to move, and together they raced past the shocked masses.

Sam looked back once to see a large bald man stomp toward them. A long sword was attached to a red sash draped over the man's hairy chest. The man, Maximilian Black Sarah had called him, didn't run, but for every three steps Sam took, Black took one. As he stalked them, Black formed a ball of red energy in his right hand and launched the projectile.

"Duck!" Sam called as he tackled Sarah. The energy blast sailed over their heads and struck another shack; its wood shattered all over the dirt roadway. More screams filled the narrow, dimly lighted street. This time Sam pulled Sarah up and together they fled again. Black charged after them, like a lion stalking prey.

"Over here!" Sarah dashed into an alley darkened without even a single torch to light the pathway. Sam couldn't see much beyond a few feet in any direction. *She knows this place. Have faith in her.* Sarah held his hand and led him along one narrow passage that connected with another, like a maze. They reached an opening that led to another path—this one vacant and abandoned. Their backs against a shack wall, Sarah peeked around the corner. "It looks clear. Let's—"

Another blast of red energy flew through the night and slammed into the ground just in front of Sarah.

"Girl, there'll be no mercy given to you today. Maximilian Black, scourge of the seven seas, means to kill you." There was a twang to Black's words, like he never learned to speak correctly. It reminded Sam of the bums back home on the beach who begged for money through toothless grins.

Sarah turned to Sam. "Chosen One, this is my bloody fault. I should've been more careful. You need to escape and stop Slayer. I'll hold off Black. You run."

"What? No."

"Do as I say. There isn't time. He comes."

"Little girl, who is that boy by your side? Boy, that girl shall be the death of you." Black was close now—too close.

"Please!" Sarah pleaded.

"I can't leave you." Sam ignored the searing pain in his back. He stood his ground as another blast struck the wall just over their heads.

"Go!" Sarah shoved him deeper into the alley then pointed her hands at the giant man. Something like a red laser shot from each fingertip and Black cried out in pain. "Go now!" Sarah shouted.

Sam shook his head in protest but turned and ran away from the battle. *What am I doing? How can I abandon her like this? Turn back! You have to turn back!* He skidded to a stop, took a deep breath, and ran back toward Sarah. He had to help her, but how?

# Chapter 13
## My Back Is On Fire

Sam reached the edge of the alley and dove into the dirt, like a baseball player sliding head first into second base. Pressed against the corner of a shack, he peered around the corner toward the vacated street. He was too late. Black held Sarah by the neck against the side of a shed; her feet dangled inches off the ground. *He's killing her!*

"You shouldn't have defied Captain Slayer." Black's twisted grin revealed yellow teeth even the darkness couldn't hide. His scratchy voice caused Sam to shiver and step farther back into the alley's protective cover. "You shouldn't have brought the boy to these parts. You have angered the Captain. He shall reward me well for returning with your head."

"I've no interest in Slayer. Only with a common boy from a trading ship. Your attack... unnecessary." Sarah labored to speak but continued her lie even as Black squeezed her throat harder. "The boy... no harm to Slayer." A weak gurgle escaped her throat as Black lifted her higher.

"No!" Sam stormed from his hiding place and threw himself at Black. He slammed into the giant man's back, but it might as well have been a brick wall. Sam fell to the ground, the air knocked out of him. He gasped as he tried to move air in and out of his lungs. While his offensive did little to move Black, the pirate dropped Sarah. She slumped hard onto the dirt, her body as limp as a Raggedy Anne doll.

"You shouldn't have come back, boy." Black lifted Sam by the shoulders with hands as thick and hairy as a grizzly bear's claws and tossed him into the middle of the street. Sam yelped as he struck the ground. He fumbled to his feet and backed away as Black strolled toward him, eyes aglow as if on fire.

Black laughed. "This girl shouldn't have brought you here. This world is not yours. Now I have to kill the girl and you. It's a deplorable action, and I take no pleasure in it. Maybe just a little."

"Leave her alone." Sam's legs shook. His voice quivered. "I'm the one you want."

"Is that so?" Black raised his right hand and a red energy ball formed. Without hesitation, he hurled it. Sam rolled to the side to dodge the blast as it kicked up dirt and mud from the street. He scampered to his feet when another blast raced toward him. The blast whizzed by his head and singed his hair.

"You are wasting my time, boy." Black spoke as if this were a game, and he were a child in a giant man's body playing pirates. "I think I'll just kill the girl—what do you think, boy? Shall you watch her die, or save her? Either way, sooner or later 'ol Maximilian Black shall hunt you down." Black turned toward Sarah, who remained motionless, and raised his right hand to throw an energy ball at her.

"I told you to leave her alone!" Sam lifted himself, but an explosion of pain in his back, like flames, had burst through the skin, dropped him to the ground. He screamed and reached under his shirt, sure his fingers would find charred, blistered skin. Instead, his hand passed through the flesh, like passing through water, until it reached bone. *What's happening to me?* On his knees, eyes wide, he dislodged something from his back and slowly drew the object through his skin. The pain, so intense seconds ago, vanished.

When he brought the object close to his face, his eyes bulged and he tried to release it. But his grip on the object locked. *This can't be! How is it possible?* In his hand was a fiery sword! A long, thin flame formed the blade instead of steel. The burning blade rose from a handle made of bone. Where had it come from? Could it be from the sword-shaped birthmark on his back? *Can it be?* Sam shook away the question. His life and Sarah's were still in danger. He had to stop Black. He grasped the bone handle with both hands and lunged at the pirate as Black lobbed an energy ball at Sarah.

Sam blocked the blast with his fiery blade and slashed at Black. The pirate took one step back and raised a hand to his face to block Sam's blade. The fire sword still found a target; it carved a searing gash into Black's arm.

"Ayyy!" Black winced as he fell to one knee. "So, boy, you discovered your ability." The pirate stood painfully and glared at Sam. "Good, killing is no fun unless there is some fight in the prey."

"Back off, dude," Sam raised the fire sword over his head.

"The boy shows guts." Black unleashed a deep guttural laugh and flung one more energy ball, then another. Sam's skinny arms trembled and his hands throbbed, but he still blocked each of Black's blasts. *I can't keep this up. I can barely hold up this sword.*

He pointed the fire blade at the pirate's chest then charged at Black, but the pirate unsheathed his own blade and slashed it toward Sam's head. "If it is a duel you want, a duel I aim to give you." Black challenged.

Sam blocked the blow; sparks leaped from his blade. Though his sword was seemingly made of glowing flames, when the two blades clashed, a great *ching* echoed through this quiet, deserted stretch of the town.

Though he panted with exhaustion, Sam slashed and ducked and did his best to block each thrust of Black's blade, but he was outmatched. Panic froze his limbs. *What am I supposed to do? I can't beat him! He's going to kill me and then Sarah!* The thought of self preservation took over. He wanted to drop the sword and run. *No, you can't leave her! You have to stay and fight! Oh, please let this be a dream!* With labored breaths, he sucked in as much air as possible. *This is a dream, nothing more. You won't really die, so keep fighting.* One more deep breath and he lifted his sword.

"Still got some fight in you," Black grunted. "Let the dance continue."

Sam rushed at Black, and their swords struck several times. Flames erupted from Sam's sword; each crash of steal against flame lit up the street. The fight continued until Sam ducked one slash of Black's sword only to have the pirate deliver an unexpected kick to his chest. Lifted off his feet, Sam flew back and slammed against a wall. The impact forced the swords from his hand. As the fiery blade fell to the ground, it vanished as if it had never existed at all.

The kick had not felt like a dream. It rattled his bones and robbed him of air. Unconsciousness hovered over him. Stunned, Sam struggled to push air through his lungs. He coughed and gasped as he tried to climb to his feet, but he slumped back into the dirt as Black strolled toward him. The fight was over. He had failed before his journey to face Slayer had begun.

Black wrapped his large hand around Sam's neck and squeezed. Sam kicked and twisted as he was lifted off the ground. "Now, boy, time to die." The tip of Black's blade pointed directly at his heart.

# Chapter 14
## Death Arrives

The death strike Sam expected never came. Instead, a deep and threatening voice spoke from behind Black. "My friend, I think it would serve you best to challenge someone your own size. Put down your blade, or else the tip of my sword you feel against your back shall pierce your heart."

Sam couldn't see who spoke the words behind Black's large and wide frame. He struggled to free himself from Black's grip, but the pirate refused to release him, despite the stranger's warning. Black's eyes glowed brighter red at this unexpected interruption in his deadly plans.

"Stranger, I don't recognize the voice, but this fight is between me and the boy," Black's words slithered from his throat like a snake's hiss. The crimson radiance from his eyes revealed pulsating veins in his forehead. Black seethed. "Move along. This is not your concern."

"I am afraid that just would not be right." The stranger spoke in a formal English accent, like he was well educated, each word as precise and sharp as the blade held to Black's back. Someone's blood was about to be spilled. Sam prayed it wasn't his own.

Black eased his grip on Sam's neck. A gutteral laugh slipped from his lips, but it sounded more like a wild dog's growl. "I mean no harm. I'm just having a bit of fun, that's all. I swear I'm not going to hurt this boy. I'll take my leave from you now." Maximilian Black lowered his blade. Sam gazed into the large pirate's smoldering eyes. Black was not about to give up that easily.

With a quick pivot, Black swung his sword around to slash off the stranger's head, but the stranger ducked the attack and thrust a blade deep into the pirate's back. Black winced and gazed at the blade, where the steal had sliced through his body and protruded from his stomach. His sword tumbled from his hand.

Sam stared up at Black as blood spilled from the pirate's mouth. Black released a soft gurgled laugh and his eyes rolled up until only the white shown. He took a last few breaths and slipped off the blade down into the dirt. Black landed with a thud and was motionless.

Sarah ran up and knelt beside Sam. "Are you all right?"

"I think so. What about you?"

"I'm not hurt, but you shouldn't have come back for me."

"I had to." Sam reached for her hand.

"My lord and lady, we, should make ourselves scarce from these parts," said the stranger who had just saved Sam's life. "There are likely more of these miscreants who seem to mean you harm."

In the darkness, Sam couldn't see much of the stranger—this savior—who was little more than a shadow against the night sky. Sam guessed the stranger was a man, at least the voice seemed male. "Wait, who are you? Why'd you help us?"

"I think now is not the time for introductions." The stranger wiped blood from his sword and sheathed it. His proper English was laced with urgency. "We must go."

Sam wasn't sure he could be trusted. *But he did save my life.*

"I suggest you both come with me. I mean you no harm. I only wish to help a couple of young ones who right now seem alone and in danger."

Sam faced Sarah who nodded ever so slightly. "All right," Sam agreed. "We'll follow you, but where?"

"To my boat, where else?" the man answered.

Sarah's eyebrows raised and her lips parted in a slight smile. She probably thought this could be their chance to begin their journey after Slayer. Sam, however, wasn't so sure. The three left the body of Maximilian Black and moved silently from the town toward the shore. They made their way through the town unnoticed since most people had cleared the roadways and doused the torches. A few men still roamed the town, swords drawn, but most had returned to their rum. Passage across the beach was much more difficult. A unit of British soldiers, maybe twenty in all, lined the shore, their muskets pointed out toward the sea. A number of other men, most armed with swords, some with pistols, joined the soldiers. Any hope they could slip away quietly was quickly dashed.

"Far too many red jackets," the stranger uttered. "It seems your run-in with Black stirred up quite the mess. So much for an easy escape, I would say." The urgency in his voice now seemed almost playful, like he enjoyed the challenge.

"Do we hide out and wait for them to leave?" Sarah asked.

"I think not." The man scanned the beach. "No, Black would not have been working alone. If we wait, you could be facing worse than our friend, Black."

"How do you know Black?" Sam squinted through the darkness into the man's face, but the man wore the night like an impenetrable mask that hid his features, all except for his eyes, which were icy blue marbles.

The man knelt to one knee and leaned in close enough for Sam to finally see what he looked like. He was an average build. Layers of loose-fit clothing—a long tattered coat covering a baggy shirt—concealed his frame. His boots were dark and cracked. A wide belt, which held two knives and his sword, encircled his waist.

A shaggy, slightly graying beard covered his face. Beyond that his face was rather featureless, at least that's how the night made it seem. His hair was pulled back and crowned with a three-cornered hat with large brims pointed up. Impatience filled the stranger's blue eyes.

"I know scallywag pirates, like Black." The man spit into the sand. "One needs to be wary of such unsavory types if one is to survive. Now follow me." He snaked his way through the white sand toward a far outcropping of brush that touched the shoreline. Sam's stomach churned and his heart raced, but he and Sarah followed. They soon reached the brush unnoticed and all three crouched low.

"I assume you both can swim." The man gazed over the water. Sam nodded. Sarah did as well. "Then follow me. We are in for a long swim clear across the harbor. We can make our way among the longboats, get out far enough and dash to my sloop."

Sam eyed the water. He guessed the longboats were the smaller boats closest to the shore that had been used to move goods. In regards to the sloop, the man had to refer to one of the smaller sailing vessels in the harbor. So far, the man had proven a help, but Sam wasn't ready to follow him into the water. "Uh, why should we follow you? We don't even know who you are."

"That is right, lad—you do not," the man said gruffly. "And right now seems not the time to brood over that. You must either trust me or not. It makes no difference to me."

Sarah placed a hand on Sam's shoulder. "I don't sense he's evil like all these other harbor hogs in New Providence. I say we trust him. If he proves a mutinous parrot, he'll be the worse for it."

"Lad, I do not understand the content of all her words, but you should listen to her despite her rather callous use of the King's

English." The man's blue eyes glared at Sarah. "While I am an ally, time is not."

Sam relented with a nod. *But what does he mean by her abuse of the King's English. Is it because she abbreviates words, like me? Or is it because she curses?* He glanced at Sarah, who held her tongue. Rather than deliver her own insult, she turned her eyes to the ground and blushed.

"Good." The man slapped Sam's arm then slid on his belly into the water. Sam and Sarah again followed. They crawled in the muck and mud from one longboat to the next. Once far enough from the shore, they swam carefully toward the larger boats with masts and sails. They made sure not to splash as they navigated through the water. One by one, they passed the sailing vessels. Hulls creaked, ropes squeaked and pulleys clacked as if the swaying boats talked to each other.

"Over here." The man directed them toward one craft that, though small in comparison to other anchored vessels, still seemed impressive. It looked sleek and fast. The man reached for a rope attached to the boat and pulled himself up onto the deck. "Come aboard, my friends. Welcome to my boat, *The Mutineer*. She is not a ship—she is not a three-masted vessel—but *The Mutineer* is a fast sloop.

"Who are you?" Sam asked again.

"There is no time now for questions. We must weigh anchor and be on our way. The danger remains very real." The man scanned the beach. Red jackets, as he called them, still patrolled and other scruffy, ragged men remained along the shore as if they waited for a fight.

"But—"

"You must decide now whether you trust me. If not, it shall be to your detriment, but it is your choice." The man extended his hand. Sarah eyed Sam once more as if she trusted him to make the decision.

"Okay," Sam lamented.

The man smiled. "Ah, there you are. That is a wise choice."

Sarah was the first to climb aboard and Sam quickly followed.

"Keep watch, the both of you, on that beach." The man prepped his craft for launch. He used a crank to slowly raise the anchor. The steel links that formed the anchor's chain banged together as they wrapped around a wooden bar on deck. Sam cringed with each clank of the chain and stared toward the shore, but still no one paid attention to the sloop. *How is that possible? They must hear.* He let the question go and just held his breath until the anchor reached the deck.

The man never rested. He hurried to the mast at the center of the sloop's deck, untied a triangular sail, gripped a rope and hoisted the sail to the top of the mast. Sam motioned to help, but the man snapped an order. "Do not touch anything on my boat until I give the command." He returned to his work and unfurled two smaller sails—they too were triangular and extended toward the front of the vessel. "Which one of you knows a thing about sailing a sloop such as this?" The man panted heavily and sweat dripped from his brow.

Sam was silent. Sarah was not. "I do, sir," she answered in a more proper English accent, as though she had shifted from a commoner to nobility. *Is she trying to match the stranger's sophisticated tone?* Sam wondered.

"All right then, lass. Take the tiller. You'll steer us out." The man's eyes fell on Sam. "I need you to follow me." He led Sam to one side of his boat where a large oar—it must have been about twenty feet long—was tethered to the side of the hull. The man untied the oar, placed it into some kind of locking device on the hull, which held the oar in place.

"Take this oar, stick it in the water and begin to row. The oarlock should keep it steady for you. I am going to do the same over there." The man motioned to the opposite side of the boat. "We have get to get *The Mutineer* moving, so she can find the wind."

Sam guessed the oarlock was the locking mechanism. He took hold of the oar and lowered it into the water. While the oar was heavy wood, the oarlock eased some of the strain in his hands.

"What are you doing, lad—row!" the man whispered loudly.

"I'm trying!" Even with the oarlock, Sam's hands shook against the weight as he forced the oar to slice through the water. It was tough at first but became a bit easier with each stroke. The boat started to move. *I'm doing it! I'm doing it!* His hands quickly weakened and his arms and shoulders burned, but he was not about to stop.

"All right, let us get *The Mutineer* turned around and haul wind." The man tipped his head to Sarah. "Danger is still close. I can feel it. Lass, come about to get us pointed toward the far passage around Fog Island."

Sam gazed at the island that seemed to be a doorway into and out of the harbor; Fog Island, as the man called it, divided their safe escape into two narrow passages and who knew what evil might lurk in the shadows of the island.

The man continued to give quiet orders. "Once we get beyond the island, there should be a spot of wind that I mean to catch." In just a matter of moments, the boat swung around to face the island and the sails expanded toward a bit of wind that flowed through the harbor. The wind, little more than a breeze, was just enough to guide the boat toward the passage out to sea.

"Lad, pull up your oar and take a position aft," the man ordered. "Keep watch for pirates—anyone following."

Sam strained to lift the oar, but his arms no longer worked. With a grimace, he tried a second time, but to no avail. A third attempt failed as well. His hands, weak and exhausted, lost their grip. The oar started to slip away.

"I got it." The man suddenly stood next to Sam. He caught the oar and lifted it onto the deck.

Sam's face warmed, but the darkness hid his blush.

"It is all right. Now head aft and keep watch. Stay sharp."

"Uh, where's aft?" Sam shrugged his shoulders and lowered his eyes.

"By God, you are a landlubber."

"What—"

"Back… go to the back." The man pointed to the rear of the boat. "Keep your eyes focused on the shore."

Sam did as ordered, but lost his footing as *The Mutineer* rocked back and forth in the water. The motion dropped him to the deck, but he quickly picked himself up and stumbled toward *The Mutineer's* aft. Once there, a glance toward shore revealed two longboats filled with men, possibly British soldiers, rowed toward *The Mutineer*. The man's sloop had been noticed. "We're being followed!" Sam hollered.

The man, armed with a musket, joined Sam. "Red jackets—do not worry over them. Keep watch for unsavory types."

Sam glanced again at the longboats. The soldiers, if that's what they were, cut quickly through the water. One soldier, a sword in hand, stood. "Captain of the sloop, you are commanded, on orders of the Crown, to remain in the harbor. If you do not heed, you shall be fired upon and boarded."

"Uh, what do we do?" Sam gripped *The Mutineer's* aft railing.

"We keep moving." The man studied the island at the harbor's entrance. "We have bigger concerns—namely whether we shall be fired upon from Fog Island." He positioned on the side of his boat closest to the island; the musket he held was cocked and ready to fire.

From behind, a crack sounded. A musket from the soldiers had been fired. The shot whizzed by the sloop. If it struck anything, Sam had no idea. He ducked behind a barrel. Several more rounds of musket fire interrupted the quiet of the night. All had been fired from the longboats.

The man kept his focus on Fog Island. The sloop started to pick up speed and left the red jackets behind. Sam held his breath as *The Mutineer* moved through the shallow waters just off Fog Island. No attack came. All was calm, except for a few more cracks of musket fire from the soldiers. Sam released a lungful of air as the sloop slipped beyond the island and caught more wind. The sails grew rigid and the boat cut faster through the water as it raced away from Fog Island and New Providence.

Sam's muscles relaxed. He breathed normally. Perhaps the danger was over. "We've made it."

"Not yet," the man warned.

A thunderous explosion filled Sam's ears. Seconds later, there was a splash to the right of the sloop. The man was right. They were not out of danger. "Cannon fire!" the man cried. "They are after us!"

# Chapter 15
## Racing The Wind

Thunder erupted again in the distance. The splash of a second cannonball, closer than the first, rocked *The Mutineer*. But had the cannon fire come from Fog Island or another vessel? "Who's after us?" Sam shouted.

The man who had saved them sprinted to the tiller to take control of the sloop before he bothered to answer Sam's question. He pulled sharply on the tiller. The sloop lurched to the right until the deck nearly touched water.

Sam fell and rolled against a crate. Seawater spilled into the boat and drenched him. His back tingled again. The burning blade! Did it call to him? If so, he ignored it. A fire sword magically embedded in his back would not stop *The Mutineer* from capsizing, which the boat was about to do. It didn't. Instead, the sloop's speed doubled as the man brought the craft in line with a stronger windstream.

"Look!" the man pointed to the right of *The Mutineer*. Sam, now back on his feet, stared in the direction he pointed. Through the darkness was the outline of a large craft three stories high. "The way I see it," the man shouted over the crash of water against his ship's hull, "if Maximilian Black is after you, you must have angered Captain Jem Slayer. Slayer is a bloodthirsty pirate with his own fleet and enough wealth to command an army of pirates; and Black is Slayer's right hand."

Sam held onto the railing for balance and inched closer to Sarah. She watched the mystery man from the side as if... *as if she doesn't want to make eye contact. Maybe she doesn't trust him as much as she said. Maybe she senses something.* Sarah grasped his hand and gently squeezed. He nodded to her. "It's going to be all right," he lied.

The man continued to shout his explanation. "Since Black failed, I assume Slayer has sent a warship to do what Black could not. Kill you!" He looked at the sails of his sloop. "Hang on, young ones! We are going to race the wind!"

One more explosion cut through the night. A cannonball screamed as it hurtled toward them. "No!" Sam mouthed moments before the cannonball splashed into the sea yards from the hull. Water sprayed onto the deck.

"Ha, you bloody heathens! You shall not catch *The Mutineer* tonight!" The man held the tiller with one hand and shook a fist with the other. As they pushed farther out to sea, the moon emerged from behind a cloud and revealed the pursuing ship. The glow showed a vessel with three masts topped with squared sails. Two rows of dark squares dotted the length of her hull—gunports. *So this is what a warship looks like. We're dead.* A cloud began to eclipse the moon, but before it did, Sam saw the mark emblazoned on the flag that soared above the ship—a skull and bones. "Pirates!"

"Did I not already say that?" The man pulled harder on the tiller. His sloop tore through the water as it raced away from the pirates. But the pirate ship started to rip its own trail as it picked up speed.

"Can we outrun them?" Sarah's question was lost against a chorus of wind and waves.

Somehow the man still heard her. "Careful, girl. Hold your tongue. She shall save us yet. Never faced a pirate ship *The Mutineer* could not outdistance."

"Yeah well, they're still getting closer!" Sam cried as an invisible fire seemed to scald his back. It had to be the fire sword's call to him, but he still did not reach for it.

The man rammed the tiller against his stomach and the craft turned sharply to the right, which brought his vessel into an even stronger wind stream. *The Mutineer* shot forward. The pirate ship fell farther behind. The man thumped his chest and bellowed, "I told you, did I not?"

He was right. Sam released a long breath as the pain in his back eased. Then a cannonball smashed through the left side of the boat. Shards of wood zipped in all directions as the vessel shook and groaned. A splinter stabbed Sam's thigh, and he crumpled to his knees. Blood seeped from the wound.

Sarah was quickly by his side and applied her hands to his injury. A blue light engulfed his leg and when she removed her hands, the splinter and wound were gone, as if they had never been there. The pain vanished. "What did you…?"

"Magic." Sarah offered a slight smile.

"Another pirate ship port side!" the man, still at his helm, roared as blood dripped from his forehead. "She came out of nowhere. Slayer must really want you two."

Sam rose to his feet as a hoard of pirates clustered along the rail of a much larger ship. They shouted and menacingly waved their swords and muskets over their heads. He gulped. Where had the ship come from? He swore she hadn't been there before.

Thunder erupted from the new ship. This time, a cannonball struck one of *The Mutineer's* sails, but the mast remained in place. Gunfire from the pirates ripped through the smaller sloop. Several shots struck the deck near Sam.

"Get down, boy!" the man ordered. "Both of you, stay down. We still have a chance."

Sam didn't think so. Desperation had slipped into the man's voice for the first time. *What will it be like to be captured by a pirate? If they're working for Slayer, will they even take us prisoners or kill all three of us immediately?* As such thoughts filled his mind, Sarah glided to the front of the boat. She did not bother to dodge the bullets that flew by her.

"What? Girl, get down!" the man yelled.

As gunfire tore into the sloop, Sarah raised her hands over her head and chanted quietly at first, but her words grew in strength until her voice boomed louder than the whizzing bullets. Her words were strange. Not English—not any language Sam had ever heard.

*It has to be a magic incantation, like in the hut.* He took a few steps toward Sarah, but stopped when her body rose over the deck and hovered in the air. A small wind vortex engulfed her in a maelstrom of swirling mist. Sam blinked. *What's happening? How is she doing—?*

The vortex exploded off her body and smashed against the sails. The craft shot forward with unnatural speed. *The Mutineer* became airborne as it warped away from both pirate ships and headed far out to sea.

"What is this witchery?" The man clutched the tiller as his craft was magically pushed through the air just above the water at speeds he clearly had never experienced.

Sam stared wide-eyed at Sarah. Her feet back on the deck, she drew back both her arms and swung them toward the mast as if to fling one last blast of wind to propel the boat forward. The pirate ships quickly disappeared. New Providence became a distant point of land, no bigger than a spec.

Sam struggled to stay upright as the sloop glided above the water. He scrambled to Sarah's side, but she didn't seem to know he was there. "Sarah, we're safe. You can stop now."

"Boy, I can hear the deck cracking!" the man cried out from his helm. "My boat cannot take much more. Stop that girl before she goes from saving our skin to killing us."

Sam grabbed Sarah's hands. A sudden jolt ran through his body and flung him against a railing. Sarah was propelled over the side of the boat. "Sarah!" Sam scanned the sea for her as the wind died and *The Mutineer* splashed into the water, but she must have slipped beneath the surface.

Without hesitation, he jumped in after her.

# Chapter 16
## When Will This Nightmare End

The warm, salty water stung the small gashes over his body caused by flying knife-like shards of timber. He ignored the pain as he scanned the sea. *Where is she? Come on, find her!* He swam from the ship, dove down, but under the cover of night, he could not spot her.

"Sarah!" He shouted as he resurfaced and twisted his head in every direction. "Sarah!" Hope faded. He screamed wildly and punched at the water. "Sar... As if someone had set him ablaze, the burning sensation returned. It arced from his back and spread through his body. He thrashed about in the water as if to stamp out the fire that baked his insides. *It's happening again, just like it did with Black.* The flaming sword, through the agony it caused, called to him. *Maybe it could help!*

He slipped beneath the water and pulled off his tattered shirt. With his right hand, he reached behind his back until his fingers pierced the skin and found the handle of the fiery blade. With one yank, the sword rose from his flesh. Sam resurfaced and brought the blade to his face. It glowed like a beacon. The water could not douse the dazzling light. The more he waved the sword, the stronger it burned; its flames spread light over the sea.

*There!* Sarah floated about twenty feet from his position. She didn't move. *Please be all right,* Sam quietly pleaded as he swam to her. It took ten strokes to reach her. She was face down in the water and when he turned her over, her eyes were shut. The skin on her face was as green as when she had first appeared to him. *No, you're not dead!* He wrapped one arm around her shoulders and released the fire sword to free his other hand to tread water. The sword disappeared into the night as soon as it left his hand. *I shouldn't have done that. How is the man going to see us, if he hasn't already abandoned us?*

Sarah remained motionless. "Breathe, Sarah!" he cried. "Don't give up!"

Something splashed beside his head. "Grab the rope, boy!" the mysterious man shouted. Sam swiveled around. The boat was still there. The man hadn't sailed away—he hadn't abandoned them to the sea. *Maybe he really does mean to help us.* Sam grabbed the rope with his right hand and held onto Sarah with his left. The man pulled and in a couple of tugs managed to bring Sam and Sarah back onto his boat.

"She's not breathing!" Sam looked to the man as if he might be a lifeguard.

"Stand back." The man knelt over Sarah and slammed a fist into her chest. She spit out a lungful of water and sucked in air as her eyes flickered open. Color returned to her face.

"Sarah!" Sam grabbed her shoulders.

"Y… yes." Her words were little more than a whisper. She coughed out more water. "I'm still here."

"Thank you." Sam reached up to shake the man's hand.

"Thank me later if we live," he answered with a frown. "The way you and this witch are behaving, I am not so sure we shall survive to see daylight."

"Yes we will." Sam took a deep breath to fill his own lungs as he gently helped Sarah to a sitting position. "We have to. We have to stop Slayer."

"That is a foolish idea." The man touched his fingers to his forehead wound. "I think we have some talking to do about Captain Jem Slayer, about this witch of yours and about that fiery blade you wielded in the water. Surely, you have brought a curse onto *The Mutineer*."

The man who had saved them from Maximilian Black and Slayer's warships stood in the doorway of his cabin with two plates of food. Just a single candle illuminated the cabin. It was difficult to see the food, but Sam didn't care. He didn't realize how hungry he was until he saw the plates. As he sat with Sarah on a hard bench by a wooden table, his stomach growled.

The man roughly placed the plates in front of them and spoke to Sarah first. "I do not know how, but you saved us. You may be a witch, but I wish to thank you for my sloop."

Sarah did not answer. Dressed in an old, oversized shirt with a tie string in the front and loose pants down to her knees, she somehow looked smaller and weak, like the use of her magic had sucked away a bit of her life. Or maybe she had yet to recover from the near drowning. Sam nudged her to eat and she reluctantly reached for a piece of meat.

After she took the first bite, Sam attacked his own plate, filled with a small portion of dried meat and a piece of bread that might have been a biscuit or thick cracker. He quickly snatched up the meat. As a chunk of tough beef slid down Sam's throat, the man poured a brown liquid into two bronze mugs and placed them onto the table.

"You, lad, are either quite brave or quite taken by this maiden. I would say you fancy her. I have seen many fool-hardy young men die in proving their courage to a pretty one such as this girlie." The man's face was hidden in the dim light of the single candle, but he seemed to grin. *He's mocking me*, Sam thought. He expected Sarah to protest the man's use of the word *girlie*, but she was silent, maybe because she was still weak.

"Twice I have seen you save her now," the man persisted. "Yes, you two are quite the pair." He settled into a seat on the opposite side of the table. "But now I need answers. You two are very different, and I think I have interfered where I truly should not have. Now I can count Slayer as an enemy thanks to you two. So how is it you are mixed up with the likes of him, especially you, boy, as you seem to be the target?"

Sam took a gulp from the mug. The liquid, likely some kind of alcohol, burned as it slid down to his stomach, and he decided not to drink any more. "Thanks for everything you've done, and for the clothes." Sam said as he coughed and cleared his throat. He wore the same loose fitting shirt and knee-length pants as Sarah.

"Never mind the thanks. You shall repay me for the damage to *The Mutineer*. In fact, if I choose to help you more than I already have, it is because you now have a debt to me. Now answer me."

Sam eyed Sarah. Once she had taken the first bite, she quickly devoured her food and even swallowed whatever liquor the man had given them. The man filled her mug a second time. "Uh, well, I'm Sam and she's Sarah." He stumbled over the words. "We—"

"Right you are, lad," the man interrupted. "Introductions are long overdue. I am Lieutenant Thaddeus Milan of His Majesty's Navy. At least, that is who I once was before I was declared a mutineer for disobeying my captain. But that is a long story." The man ran his hands through his long, greasy black hair. "Today, I am captain and sole crew member of *The Mutineer*. The reason for the name of the boat should be quite clear."

"Are you a pirate?" Sam asked as he finished the last of his food.

Thaddeus huffed. "Bite your tongue. Don't you know that miserable fellow Governor Rogers has forced pirates to denounce their ways or face the gallows? Perhaps I did not exactly come by this sloop in an honest way, but I am no pirate. I do not raid, plunder or harm anyone if I can help it. I take what I need and keep to myself. I live on the sea because it is the only home I have ever really known."

*Technically, he's a pirate.* Sam kept that thought quiet.

Thaddeus leaned forward. "Now, tell me your sad tale. And let us be clear. Your next words may lead to a parting of our company. There are plenty of islands in these parts where I may strand you both. And believe me, I have no interest in keeping a witch aboard, even if she did save my boat. Then there is you, with that fire blade of yours. What kind of beast might you be?"

"Stop calling her a witch!"

"Do not raise your voice to me." The man removed a dagger from his belt and studied the blade as it reflected the candlelight. "Now speak and I expect the truth from you."

Sam nodded. "You're right about Slayer. We're after him to save children he kidnapped, and he knows it. He sent that dude Maximilian Black and those ships to stop us."

"You think me ignorant? I know of the kidnapping. Everyone knows of the kidnapping. The entire British fleet in these waters is after him. What makes a young man and a witch chase after Slayer? And why would Slayer care? No, there is more to your story, and I am determined to hear it."

"You wouldn't believe me if I told you."

"After what I've seen this witch do tonight, there is no telling what I might believe."

Sarah placed a hand on Sam's shoulder. "It's all right, Chosen One, tell him."

"That right there." Thaddeus twirled the dagger in his hand as if in play. "Why is she calling you the Chosen One?"

"I keep wondering that myself." Sam took a long breath before continuing. "What you saw Sarah do with your sloop is magic. She has magical abilities, but she is not a witch. Slayer has abilities, too. And maybe I have my own magic."

"Madness!" Thaddeus drove his knife into the table. "You shall not take my soul. Do you hear me? I'll sooner cut out your throats."

"What?" Sam's back burned. He wanted to reach for the sword but forced himself not to. "We're not here to take your soul!"

"We shall see." Thaddeus pulled his knife from the table. "Continue your story."

Sam swallowed. "I'm not from around here."

"Oh, then for sure you are a landlubber," Thaddeus chuckled.

"You said that before. What's a landlubber?"

"One who has never been to sea. You are from the mainland—London, I guess—but you speak with a strange tongue."

"Uh, I'm not from London." Sam shook his head. "I'm not even from this time. Thaddeus, I'm from the future—I mean a long time from now. With her magic Sarah brought me here to this time because she thinks I'm some Chosen One who can stop Slayer."

"He is the Chosen One!" Sarah added.

Sam waited for Thaddeus to throw them overboard, but he didn't. Not yet anyway. He didn't even act with surprise. "And what are you supposed to stop him from doing?" Thaddeus pointed the tip of his knife at Sam. "I expect there is more to this than saving some children."

"You're right." Before Sam continued he wondered whether any of this was real. This could all still be some dream and he could be safe in his bed right now. *If this is a dream, why can't I wake up?* "Slayer took the children for a reason. There's some super powerful sword he wants called the Sword of Zel-Kar, and he needs to sacrifice them to get it."

"I have not heard of such a weapon." Thaddeus rubbed his cheek with the edge of the blade. "Is this sword worth much?"

"Forgive me, Captain Milan, but it is no prize to be won or lost," Sarah answered quickly. Sam noted the polite way in which she spoke. It didn't sound like her. Maybe Thaddeus' insult from earlier in the night had really stung her. "The Sword of Zel-Kar has no value to you. You are not a conjurer."

The captain of *The Mutineer* stared at her, and she lowered her eyes. Sam watched them both. Sarah didn't strike him as someone who would be easily intimidated. *Strange,* he thought.

And if Slayer gets the sword?" Thaddeus asked.

"He'll try to conquer the world and change history, I guess," Sam answered.

"And you, not much more than a boy, can stop him?"

"I guess. I hope, but I don't know."

"He can!" Sarah spoke forcefully, more like herself—less formal. "There's more that I haven't told you, Chosen One. The Sword of Zel-Kar can only be found on a hidden island. It's an island only conjurers can see."

"So that means the British Navy will never find Slayer," Sam reasoned.

She nodded in agreement.

Thaddeus scratched his beard. "I take it Slayer knows you are after him and knows you have powers like him. That is why he sent Black after you and that is why his ships attacked."

"Yes, Captain, but there's more yet to tell." Sarah rose and walked to the cabin door. She stopped in the doorway and breathed in the cool night air before she spoke again. "Even conjurers have no idea where to find the island and the sword. But that beast Slayer's found a scroll that shall lead him there. The only other person who knows how to find the island is you, Chosen One."

"What? I don't know where it is. I'm still not even sure I believe any of this."

"You know, Chosen One," Sarah affirmed. "Look deep within yourself, and you'll know I speak the truth."

Sam threw up his hands. "Great. Just great. This just keeps getting better and better."

"All right." Thaddeus sighed as if he grew weary of the discussion. "So this boy is supposed to lead you to some hidden island about which he knows nothing?"

Sarah pushed her hair away from her face. "Yes."

"And I guess you want me to help you reach this island." Thaddeus grew silent. Sam stared at Sarah until Thaddeus unleashed a hearty laugh. "This is a fool's errand. Slayer shall kill you."

"We have to try," Sarah responded.

Thaddeus grumbled under his breath and sighed. "I know this is a mistake, but this is personal now. No one harms *The Mutineer*. I shall join your quest for Slayer, but I expect a prize—if not that sword, something else."

"Any treasures we find shall be yours," Sarah offered.

Sam pounded his fist on the table. "I don't know if I can get us there. I don't know if I can do any of this."

Thaddeus grasped Sam's arm. The touch was icy, and Sam shivered. "You must lead us there. It would be wise to start believing in yourself, Chosen One."

Sam lowered his head to the table. "I really don't—"

Thaddeus interrupted. "Lift your head. Keep the spirits high. Our quest begins. Before we set out, though, you need to learn about sailing. This sloop might be hurting, but together we can keep her afloat and on Slayer's trail… I pray."

## Chapter 17
### The Sword Won't Obey

Forty-eight hours ago life made sense. Sam had woken up in his own bed, ready to launch into an average day in his average life. Then a visit to the pier, a stupid bet and a mysterious girl who nearly drowned him. Two days later, nothing made sense. With a sigh, he shifted his body on the hard, wooden deck where a few hours earlier he had given into exhaustion. He had hoped when he awoke he would be in his own bed and the dream would have ended, but the dream lingered.

A warm morning breeze smacked against a taut sail. The sea sloshed against the hull. Salty water and damp wood mixed in an odor that hung heavy in the air. All of it was a reminder he was still in this world and this time, whether it was a dream or real.

*I'm aboard a boat in the middle of the Caribbean in 1718, and I'm supposed to stop some mad man from reaching a magical sword that will allow him to conquer the world and change history.*

Sam shifted one more time. His body ached and his neck creaked. He stared at a pink sky, the first sign the sun was ready to awaken. His thoughts turned to the fiery blade in his back. *What the hell is this thing? How did it get into my back? How does it work? How do I control it?* Sam lifted himself, but the slight exertion caused his head to pound and his stomach to churn. *What did I drink last night? What did I eat?*

"Is that you stirring, lad?"

*Thaddeus.* Sam rolled over on his stomach. He glanced toward the tiller. Thaddeus stood at the helm, one hand on the tiller. *He must have been there all night.*

"Get up, Chosen One." There was a slur to his usual proper English. A jug that might have held wine or rum was tipped over at his feet. "You have much to learn, and we have little time. While you and the girl slept, I kept watch. So far, none are following close, but they cannot be far. Of that I am sure."

Sam blinked several times and forced himself to stand. For the effort, his stomach erupted. He dashed to the side of the boat and vomited. When the heaving was over, he leaned against the railing and steadied himself.

"What are you doing? We have no time for such foolishness," Thaddeus scolded.

Finally, Sam stood. "If we don't have much time, why waste it teaching me?" He rubbed the sides of his head. "Just let me find the Sword of Zel-Kar."

"Since you are now part of my crew, you best know something about *The Mutineer* and about sailing before you wreck her and drag us down to Davy Jones's locker."

"What is Davy—"

"Ah yes, you don't know Davy Jones's locker. It means a sailor's death, to die at sea, to rest at the bottom of the sea. I won't allow your lack of seamanship to cause my death, so you shall learn."

Sam lumbered over to Thaddeus. "All right, teach me."

Thaddeus released his hand from the tiller and nearly fell over, but he managed to catch himself before he slumped to the deck. When he hauled himself up, he belched and yawned. Sam, still a bit nauseous, resisted a slight smile. These were more the behavior of a pirate than a British Naval officer.

"Look at *The Mutineer* and tell me what you see." Thaddeus stretched and this time he released a bit of gas from his backside.

Sam shook his head and tried not to judge the man who so far had proven himself courageous and trustworthy. "I see the mast and sails and a bunch of lines holding up the sails."

"Ah, those lines are the halyards. Those lines are *The Mutineer's* life. If you cannot control them, you cannot control the sail. You cannot run before the wind."

"I understand."

"Good. And how many masts do you see?"

"Uh, just one."

"Right, you are a smart one. That means *The Mutineer* is not a ship. It is a boat—a small sloop to be specific—so do not ever refer to her as a ship. Ships, like those pursuing us, have three masts and squared sails. Our sails are triangular."

"Gotcha."

Thaddeus glared at Sam. "Now, do you see the tiller?"

"Yeah."

It controls the rudder, which controls our direction."

"Duhh."

"I do not know that phrase, but watch your tongue, boy."

"Sorry."

Thaddeus frowned then seemed to doze off. His eyes closed before he snapped back to attention and continued the lesson. "As I told you earlier, *The Mutineer* is a sloop built for speed, and she must be sailed carefully. The one who handles the tiller must understand that if we are to outmaneuver those warships."

"Why don't I see cannons?"

"Oh, she can hold about ten guns, but I ditched them, save a couple stored below. Have no need for them. I want her to be as fast as possible, which means carrying little weight."

"That seems dangerous."

Thaddeus stood silently and crossed his arms.

"Sorry again." Sam lowered his head.

"Where you stand now is called aft—the back—ahead of us is the fore—the front—to the left is port and to the right is starboard.

You must remember this. If I give a command, you best know how to respond."

"But—"

Sam stopped when Sarah walked on deck. She had slept in a hammock in Thaddeus' cabin while he remained awake on watch through the night.

"How are you, lass?" Thaddeus stood straight up as though he weren't drunk.

"I am all right, Captain, but I think you should know I have a name. It is Sarah. I hope you can remember that." Sarah nodded to Thaddeus.

*The Mutineer* captain raised an eyebrow. "Right you are, girlie—I mean Sarah. I shall strive to remember your name. I suppose you have earned that respect.

Sam smiled. *All right, Sarah.*

Thaddeus bowed to Sarah before he spoke again. "And please, call me by my name—Thaddeus. No need for such formality as to refer to me as captain."

Sarah turned her attention to Sam. "Thank you for saving me twice last night, Chosen One."

"The way I see it, you saved us and you risked your life for me." Sam's face grew warm and he couldn't hold Sarah's gaze.

Thaddeus stroked his beard. "Truth be told, I saved both of you, so if you mean to give thanks, I think it should be offered to me. But enough of this jabbering. Lass… Sarah… do you feel well enough to take the helm?"

"I think so."

"Lad, follow me. There is more to talk of."

"Uh, my name is Sam."

Thaddeus shook his head and grabbed Sam's arm. Still a touch drunk, Thaddeus stumbled once, before he led Sam away from the helm. They made their way down to the hold, packed with crates, barrels, and extra sails, ropes and poles. The jugs probably contained water or liquor. *I wonder if they're stolen supplies.* Sam sniffed the air. It was musty with the slightest foul scent, as if the odor of rotten eggs hung in the air.

Thaddeus must have noticed. "Smell it, do you? Get used to it… the mix of stagnant water seeping into the bilge below and a bit of rot. That is why you do not see much in the way of supplies. When I run out, I go in search of fresh supplies. But I would have you know this odor is nothing. On the large frigates, the smell below is something awful. You never shake it."

Sam expected some lesson to come from Thaddeus about storing food, but instead the former lieutenant unsheathed his sword and pointed it at Sam. The sword shook in Thaddeus' unsteady hand.

"Hey, what are you doing?" Sam backed away from the blade.

"Boy, draw your weapon." Thaddeus' eyes were serious.

"Look at me, I don't have a sword."

"Don't play games." Thaddeus stepped forward with his sword pointed at Sam's heart. "I have seen you wield that strange blade. It burns like the fires of hell. You used it against that scallywag Black. And I saw its glow when you used that same weapon to find your girlie in the water. I have never seen its like."

"I don't—"

"I mean you no harm. I know it is a weapon of great power, but you must learn to use it. If you do not, you shall lose more clashes, like the one with Black, and maybe next time I shall not be there. Now draw your weapon and try to strike me with it."

Sam sighed. "I really don't know how it works, but I'll try." He steadied himself, reached underneath his shirt and tried to retrieve the weapon. Nothing happened.

"Well?" Thaddeus' eyes blinked several times as if he fought to stay alert.

Sam shrugged. "I told you I don't know how it works. All I know is when I'm in danger, my back starts to tingle and that's the first sign the sword is… I don't know… calling to me. I guess the sword knows I'm not in danger with you."

Thaddeus sheathed his sword. "You best learn to control the sword rather than have it control you, Chosen One. You must become the master of the weapon. Until you do, that special sword of yours shall do you little good. You shall never defeat Slayer." Thaddeus didn't say another word. He led Sam back up onto the deck to where Sarah still had the helm.

Sam stood next to her, his eyes downcast. She nudged him, but he did not respond.

Thaddeus spoke; his words followed a long yawn. "I think we shall be safe for a spell. I am going to rest in my cabin. Maybe by the time I return, this Chosen One shall know our course. For now, take care of *The Mutineer*." Thaddeus disappeared into his cabin.

Sarah placed a hand on Sam's shoulder while she kept her other hand on the tiller. "Would you like to take the helm?" Sam moved away from her touch. "Chosen One?"

"You know I wish you'd stop calling me that." Sam stared out to sea. "The more I think about it, the more I think you found the wrong person. I'm not some Chosen One. I don't even believe any of this. It's all some dream."

"Why are—?"

"Thaddeus knows it. I see the way he looks at me, the way he makes fun of me. Just now he told me to pull the fire sword from my back, but I couldn't do it. I don't even know what this thing in my back is."

"It's the mark of the Chosen One. That you can create a fire sword is yet another sign I have found the true Chosen One. It means that one day you shall wield the Sword of Zel-Kar."

"Is it like this crazy fire sword in my back?"

"If the legends are true, the Sword of Zel-Kar is so much more." Sarah shifted the tiller slightly. "The one who wields it has the ability to bring peace or war to the world."

"None of this makes any sense, and I just want to go home."

"Chosen—"

"Stop it. Just stop calling me that."

Sarah again stroked his shoulder, her eyes filled with understanding. "Don't be upset about failing to call your fire sword when Thaddeus asked," she urged. "When it comes to magic, it doesn't always work the way we expect it to until we unlock its secrets."

"Whatever that means."

"It means you must learn to understand how your powers work, and you shall… soon. I'm sure of it. When you do learn to control your powers, you shall truly see that you are the Chosen One."

"There you go again." Sam moved away. "Just leave me alone." He walked to the front of the sloop, leaned against the railing and focused on the horizon. There was nothing but water stretched ahead until the ocean met the sky. It should have been peaceful, but it wasn't. *Think, Chosen One. You're supposed to know how to find this island, but you don't. Think. Think.*

He closed his eyes and forced himself to quiet his thoughts. He focused on breathing in the sea air, allowed it through his nose and mouth and into his lungs. At first, the rhythmic beat of the water against the hull and the slap of sails in the wind filled his ears. Sam breathed deeper and the sounds began to slip away as silence surrounded him. But the answers still didn't come. *I don't know where this island is. I just don't know!*

"Uhhhhhh!" he shouted and pounded his head with both fists. When he opened his eyes again, the world around him was different. Gone was the railing he had leaned against, the deck beneath his feet—the entire sloop. Sarah and Thaddeus had vanished and his own body had also disappeared. He had a sense of nothingness—as if he was a breeze that blew aimlessly over the sea.

He wafted slowly above the water. Then, he shot forward along an airstream. In some ways, he didn't move at all, rather the world beneath him raced by. Day turned into night as the sun passed from east to the west. The stars rushed high into the night sky as twilight gave way to the stillness of midnight. Morning rushed to replace the night as the first rays of the day shown in the east. The journey continued as the sun climbed. Up ahead a wall of clouds reached down from the sky and touched water. They were dark, foreboding—like an impenetrable barrier.

Sam tried to stop but had no control of himself. Closer and closer he soared toward the dark goliath. It reminded him of a sandstorm his family was once caught in as they traveled through the desert. The dust cloud had come of out of nowhere and cocooned them in an endless shadow that forced his dad off the road. He had been eight years old then and was terrified. This was worse. *If I enter, I might never find my way out.*

In the next heartbeat, he crossed through the barrier. Where he expected to be trapped in a fog, he emerged into a dazzling world where half the sky was filled with an orange sun larger and brighter than the sun he was used to. Its golden rays were visible against an emerald cloudless canvas. The other half of the sky held a full moon—twice the size of the moon back home—against a deep black night dotted by brilliant stars.

Sam gazed upon the water. The reflection of both the sun and the moon bounced off a crimson sea. In the distance were two islands. They were like twins, each with identical peaks, multi-colored greenery and long golden shores. The islands rested nearly side by side with the narrowest of passages between them. The highest point of each island peak formed an archway that connected both islands. From that archway gushed a great waterfall that flowed red, like blood that gushed from a wound.

Sam passed through the waterfall and just beyond it was another island, this one larger than the first two. He crossed from the water onto the shore, up through the lush plant life onto a mountain high above the shoreline. He couldn't be sure, but the mountain seemed to be in the shape of a human skull. *Like my vision when Sarah first brought me here. The sail under the water became a skull!*

Though scared, he continued until he reached a cave—the mouth of the skull. He moved into the darkness until he saw a doorway with the markings of a sword—the one Sarah spoke of— the Sword of Zel-Kar. It had to be.

In that moment, his eyes shot open and he was back aboard the sloop. His head pounded, but he still had a clear vision of that other world he had just experienced. *I don't know what just happened, but I know how to get to the island! I can't believe it, but I know!*

"Thaddeus, Sarah," Sam declared. "I know the way!"

# Chapter 18
## Visions Of The Way

"Lad, that cannot be right." Thaddeus stretched and slung on his three-cornered hat.

"I know what I saw." Sam drew himself up straight and raked his fingers through his hair.

"If we head due east we'll run into nothing." Thaddeus stumbled from his cabin onto the deck. His breath still stunk of rum. "This is what you stirred me for—to guide my boat to uncharted waters where we most assuredly shall become stranded and probably die."

Sam pointed east. "Look, I don't understand this power I'm supposed to have, but it's telling me that we will find the island and the Sword of Zel-Kar in that direction."

"You are daft." Thaddeus threw his hands in the air. "I am not taking my boat to the middle of nowhere. She is limping along as it is. She may not even be seaworthy much longer. No, we need to head southwest. That must be the direction Slayer is heading. We follow there and we shall run into the Windward Passage. It is a dangerous way, for sure. The waters are treacherous, but that is all the more reason Slayer would head that way. There lies a chain of islands. You have Hispañola, Tortuga Island, Cuba—I would wager your magic island is hidden among them."

Sam took one step closer to Thaddeus. "Listen—"

"Captain Milan... Thaddeus," Sarah interrupted, "we owe you so much. You have already done more than anyone could rightly ask. But we still need your help. You must believe in the Chosen One's gift. He is the only one who can lead us to the sword—the only one who can lead us to Slayer. We must go due east." Her accent turned formal, as it had after Thaddeus insulted her. She took hold of Thaddeus's arm. "Besides, Captain, if we succeed, we shall find a great deal more treasure on the island—and you are welcome to it."

Thaddeus slid away from Sarah's touch. "How much treasure?"

"Enough to buy any ship you want. Enough to buy a fleet of ships. Enough to choose whatever life suits you."

"I know what you are doing." Thaddeus sneered. "I am no fool."

Sarah shook her head. "I am not lying."

"I am not suggesting you speak with a spiked tongue. In fact, I believe you. So out of the goodness of my heart, I shall help you stop Slayer and save the children. But I shall hold you to your offer of treasure." He patted Sam on the back with a couple of heavy swats. "Lad, I hope you are right and do not strand us in the middle of the sea. I swear I shall slice your throat if you lead me wrong."

Sam swallowed. "I'm not wrong."

"Then let us set our course due east. I'll take the helm."

"But your drunk." Sam stood in front of the tiller and blocked Thaddeus.

"That may be, but that just makes me a finer sailor." Thaddeus leaned in close, his hand on his sword's handle. His next words were spoken in a whisper. "If you ever stand between me and the helm of my boat, my blade shall pierce your heart."

Sam nodded and backed away. Thaddeus grabbed the tiller with both hands and pulled it into his body. The boat responded immediately. With a creak and shudder, the hull dipped and rocked and *The Mutineer* turned due east.

His eyes locked on Thaddeus, Sam walked to the front of the boat. When he reached the bow, he contemplated the horizon where the water touched the sky. *I hope I'm right. Then again, if this is all a dream, what does it matter? And who is this Thaddeus? There has to be more to him than he is telling us. I'll have to watch him closely. Then there's Sarah. She seems to believe in me so much. Why? I've done nothing to deserve her trust. What if she's made the biggest mistake of all in finding me? What if the real Chosen One is still out there somewhere? Man, I wish I could just go home.*

Sarah joined him; she stood beside him, but did not say a word.

"You know, I could be wrong." Sam peered at a seagull that flew over the boat.

"You're not."

He huffed. "How do you know?"

"I don't." Sarah smiled as she gazed out to sea.

"Then—"

"I trust in my own magic. It has never deceived me. It led me to you, so I know you're the Chosen One. And your magic is telling you where to find the island and the Sword of Zel-Kar. I believe in your magic as much as my own, so I trust you're correct. We'll reach the island. I just hope before Slayer."

"What if your magic hasn't deceived you? What if you just didn't understand what it was trying to tell you?"

She glanced away from him. "I never thought of that."

"You never—"

"Ship approaching!"

Sam jumped at Thaddeus' words. *Oh no, Slayer!* Sam ran aft with Sarah quickly following.

"Three points forward on our starboard!" Thaddeus pointed off the right side of the boat.

Sam followed Thaddeus' finger. "What? Where? I don't see anything!"

"Wait, lad. Wait for *The Mutineer* to pitch." *The Mutineer* dipped on a small wave and when it rose, a black dot became visible in the distance. "There she is just as I said."

Sam strained his eyes. "I see it, but it could be anything."

"It is a ship all right, and she has sight of us."

Sam gasped and clasped his hands. "Is it Slayer?"

Thaddeus kept his eyes on the ship. "I do not think so. I doubt Slayer would allow his ship to be seen. No, this one wants us to know he approaches. He wants to see if we shall run. No, this one likes the chase."

"You know all that already?" Sarah asked. "Captain, you cannot possibly be so sure." Despite his fear, Sam snickered in silence. Every time Sarah addressed Thaddeus now, she matched his formality—his use of the *King's English*. Why did she have to prove anything to him? *Stupid question right now*, he realized.

"You have so much faith in this boy," Thaddeus responded. "When it comes to the sea, you must trust in me. I am right about this. Even more, I think I know who leads that ship. Sarah, take the helm, and, again, I invite you to call me Thaddeus, but if captain suits you, by all means—continue."

As Thaddeus disappeared into his cabin, Sam noted that he had used Sarah's name. *He still won't use my name. I still haven't earned his respect—maybe I never will.* Thaddeus quickly returned with a simple brass telescope, which he held to his right eye with one hand while he extended the device with his other.

"Well, sink me," he chuckled.

"What?" Sam asked.

Thaddeus did not answer. Once more he slipped into his cabin and this time he returned with a flag—a British flag, which he quickly attached to a line on the mast and hoisted to the mast's highest point.

"Thaddeus, what is it?" Sam squinted at the flag.

"It is as I thought." Thaddeus took the tiller from Sarah. "That ship sails under Captain Benjamin Hornigold, a pirate turned privateer. He now hunts pirates under orders from Governor Rogers."

The distant ship was now a bit more visible as it sailed closer. "Is that good or bad?" Sam wondered aloud.

Thaddeus laughed. "We shall see."

"What does that mean?" Sam's back tingled. "Why don't you just outrun him?"

"Boy, did you not hear me? That is Captain Hornigold. As a pirate, he taught Blackbeard before the two went their separate ways. He is smart and he knows these waters. If we see him that means there are at least two other warships under his command close by we do not see. No, we do not run. If he is in these waters, like us he is after Slayer. So we shall be friendly."

Sarah stepped closer. "So what do we do?"

"Heave to and wait. Let him know we do not mean to run. Let him see we are a friend."

"Is that the reason for the British flag?" Sam again stared at the flag above their boat.

"It is well known Hornigold does not attack British ships. That is part of the reason he and Blackbeard parted." Thaddeus nudged the tiller, so that *The Mutineer* turned away from the wind and came to a stop.

"Now what?" Sam walked to the starboard railing and watched Hornigold's ship.

"Now we wait and pray he does not think us pirates." Thaddeus laughed again and winked. "If he believes us to be pirates, he most certainly shall bring out his ship's 6-pounders."

"6-pounders?"

"His cannons," Sarah answered.

Sam gulped.

The massive ship was close now, maybe a football field away. Her port side cannons were visible. Sam counted eighteen 6-pounders, as Thaddeus had called them. And those were just the ones he saw on the port side. There had to be more on the starboard side. "We're in trouble," Sam mouthed. The ship's hull must have housed at least three levels. Her three masts and stacked, squared sails rose high into the sky.

Nearly two hours had passed since they first sighted the ship. For those two hours, he had paced *The Mutineer* in silent protest of Thaddeus' decision to do nothing but wait.

During that time, Thaddeus had returned to his cabin to sleep with the order that he be awakened when the ship's guns were visible, and not a moment sooner.

"Well, I see them now," Sam said to Sarah. "Do I wake him up?"

"No need." Thaddeus bounced onto the deck. He seemed more alert as if the effects of the rum had worn off. "I can smell his cannons. All right, let us see if Captain Hornigold wants to be friends."

When the ship got within half a football field from *The Mutineer*, her crew lowered most of her sails and dropped anchor.

"*Ranger* is quite the grand ship," Thaddeus announced.

"What?" Sam asked.

"The name of Hornigold's ship is *Ranger*. It is a vessel I have long admired."

"That's a better name than *The Mutineer*." Sam smiled slightly and a bead of sweat fell from his forehead.

"I swear I shall cut out your tongue one day." Thaddeus wrapped an arm around Sam's shoulder. "Wipe that sweat away. Do not sweat, do not stumble over your words and make sure you look Hornigold square in the eyes when you address him. If you give him any reason to suspect you are lying, we are dead."

Thaddeus' words made Sam sweat more. He wiped his forehead and rubbed his hands.

"Ho, there," a booming voice called from the ship called *Ranger*. A number of sailors lined the side of the ship, but one stood out from the rest. He was a large, hulking man. But any more than that was hard to tell. From this distance, he was a silhouette against the sun. That had to be Hornigold and the voice had to belong to him.

"Greetings!" Thaddeus answered.

"I see you fly British colors," Hornigold shouted. "You would not be trying to practice any treachery would you?"

"Most certainly not. This is a British vessel." Thaddeus' voice was strong and direct. If he was shaky, he did a good job of hiding it.

"Do you know who you are adressing?" Hornigold asked.

"The great Captain Benjamin Hornigold, I presume." Thaddeus removed his hat and bowed.

"Aye, so if you are a pirate, I shall claim your sloop and make you my prisoner."

"As would be your right, sir."

"You look like you have already seen battle."

"It is the work of Slayer."

"I see." Hornigold grew quiet. He gestured to his men. "You speak as a gentleman, so I shall grant you the opportunity to address me directly. I shall send a longboat over to you, so you can come aboard and we can talk in a more civilized way, but I shall keep my guns on you just the same."

"Thank you, Captain Hornigold." Thaddeus waved his hand.

"So we're good?" Sam's back tingled, but the sensation wasn't worsening.

"Not yet." Thaddeus moved slowly, carefully into his cabin. He picked up two knives and hid them inside his boots.

"But, Thaddeus, we are on the same side." Sarah eyed the outlines of the knives, barely visible inside Thaddeus' boots.

"We still have to prove that to Hornigold. Do not think him so trusting. Take a close look at his ship. What do you see?"

Sam stared closely at *Ranger*. A dozen sailors, all little more than shadows, guarded them. "They have muskets pointed at us."

"I would imagine they are good shots, too," Thaddeus warned. "We still have to be careful."

From *Ranger*, a longboat, large enough to hold ten sailors, was lowered to the water. One sailor was to row the boat. A second sailor held a musket. It took just moments for them to cross the sea and reach *The Mutineer*.

"Good afternoon, gentlemen." Thaddeus tipped his hat to the two men.

"None of that, now." The man with the musket frowned. Of the two, he was the younger one. At least his face was young, though it was scruffy. Strands of brown hair slipped out from a bandana over his head. His eyes were angry, full of distrust. "Just get aboard. Captain's waiting on you."

He placed his musket over his shoulder with a strap and from his breeches produced a long-barreled pistol. He pointed it at Thaddeus.

"I assure you that is unnecessary." Thaddeus raised his hands as if to show he was unarmed.

"Just as well, no tricks, you hear," the young man barked. "The Captain is still not convinced you are not pirates. And I trust you even less."

"You are right to be careful." Thaddeus smiled.

Sarah climbed down to the longboat. The sailor eyed her closely, too closely. The other sailor, an older man with slightly graying hair and a rounded stomach, stole a quick glance at her and quickly crossed himself as if to ward off any danger through prayer.

Sam, the next to leave *The Mutineer*, noticed the second sailor's reaction to Sarah. *Is he scared of her?* Once aboard the longboat, he positioned himself between the two sailors and Sarah.

Thaddeus hesitated, scanned *The Mutineer* one last time, then slowly climbed aboard the longboat. "Gentlemen, again, I thank you. Let us be off then."

"You best not be armed," the younger sailor aimed his pistol at Thaddeus' head. "Turn around and let me see."

Thaddeus spun. "I dare not take a weapon aboard your ship."

As they cast off, Sam stared at Thaddeus. *The Mutineer* captain played a dangerous game.

# Chapter 19
## The Great Captain Hornigold, Pirate Hunter

"So you would have me believe that after Slayer damaged your boat in the harbor at New Providence, you set out on your own after him." Captain Hornigold paced along the deck of *Ranger*, scratching his long, brown beard, tinged with gray. His voice was loud even though he spoke in close quarters. His accent was unmistakably British, and he spoke like he was educated in the British Royal Navy, but he could not disguise his pirate past. His voice was rough, maybe from all the years he downed rum and commanded tough men.

"That is the truth, Captain," Thaddeus answered.

"These two scrawny beings, this girl and little man, demanded that they be allowed to come with you, for their younger kin was among the kidnapped?" Hornigold stopped pacing. Sam held his gaze as Hornigold's large eyes focused on him.

"True, again, Captain." Thaddeus was quick with his response.

"And you agreed to take on these young ones as your only crew?"

Thaddeus took a deep breath. "Captain, they were very persuasive. The lad there held a pistol on me. And while I could have overpowered him, I decided if it meant enough to them to help me track Slayer, I would be cruel not to let them join me."

"I see." Hornigold huffed and grew silent.

Sam studied him. A large man, Hornigold had a good-sized gut and arms and legs as thick as tree trunks, but he carried the bulk well. His mustache, which accentuated his rounded cheeks, hid his mouth. He carried a large sword with an elaborate gold handle. His clothing was clean and crisp but simple. A long, dark coat covered most of his frame and spotless black boots reached up to his knees.

A knife was tucked into his breeches under this coat. A pistol was tied to a ribbon, which hung from the back of his neck. A black, three-cornered hat covered his head.

His crew, a motley bunch of fifty men or more, stood behind him. They were dirty, unshaven, for the most part—the kind Sam wouldn't want to run into in a darkened alley. Most wore a basic shirt and wide-legged breeches that stopped about mid-calf. But others, maybe those with more authority, were dressed like Captain Hornigold.

Sam turned his attention to Hornigold's ship, *Ranger*. It dwarfed *The Mutineer*. The deck on which he stood was three stories above the sea and the sails were so high on the masts that the tops were hard to see through the sun's glare. Instead of a tiller, like Thaddeus' sloop, this ship had a large wheel at the helm.

Heavily armed with cannons not only on the deck, but in the hull where black iron barrels protruded from square portholes, *Ranger* could easily blow *The Mutineer* out of the water. The next few minutes would probably decide if that, in fact, was what Hornigold planned to do. Sam's stomach ached at that last thought. He forced himself to breathe easy.

Finally, Hornigold spoke through gritted teeth. "You think me a fool!"

"What?" Thaddeus asked.

Hornigold whipped out his sword and pointed it at Thaddeus. "I know a pirate when I lay eyes on one. Men, over the side with these three! Then we destroy their vessel." His crew shouted their excitement.

"What? No!" Sam backed away, but two men grabbed him and lifted his feet while a third tied his hands behind his back. The same was done to Thaddeus and Sarah.

"Thaddeus, do something!" Sam cried as his back started to sizzle.

"Captain, I implore you. I speak the truth." Thaddeus did not raise his voice, even as he was pushed toward a gangway on the side of the ship.

Sam struggled against the men who held him by the arms. *This can't be happening! This can't be real! I mean, this is too much like the movies! Sam, wake up! Time to wake up from this dream!* He glanced at Sarah. She remained quiet and still; her eyes imploring him to do the same. *How can she be so calm?*

"The little man goes first," Hornigold ordered. Sam was about to plead for his life, but he locked eyes with Thaddeus. The former Royal Navy lieutenant mouthed the words, "Steady, lad."

As two of Hornigold's sailors pushed him onto the edge of the gangway, Sam did as Thaddeus directed. He said nothing, but his mind raced as the magical blade in his back continued to summon him. *Maybe I can reach for the sword. Why should I just let myself be pushed into the sea when I could fight?* Sam resisted the blade's call. He had to trust Thaddeus. *The Mutineer*'s captain would find another way out of this. *I hope.* Besides, a sword—even one made of fire—wouldn't be enough to defeat an entire crew armed with muskets, swords and knives.

Hornigold walked forward and pointed the tip of his sword at him. "Boy, for your treachery I condemn you to a death at sea. If you want to save yourself, confess your acts of piracy, and I shall consider leniency."

Sam peered at the water. From the deck it would be a longer fall than when he jumped from the pier. *Please wake up—now! This is all way too crazy!* "We have not lied." Sam stared into Hornigold's eyes, voice firm. He tried to mirror the *King's English*. "Kill me if you must." *What am I saying?*

Hornigold sighed. "Off with you then. Jump like a man and accept your fate to the sea."

Sam nodded then turned toward Sarah whose eyes started to glow green while Thaddeus raised an eyebrow.

"Jump, boy," Hornigold ordered.

*Wake up, dude! Wake up!* Sam shook his head as if it might stir him from this dream, but it didn't work. *Fine, let's see what happens.* One last look at Sarah and he stepped off the gangway. As his body fell, he tightened for the impact with the sea, but his fall was cut short. A rope snaked out of the sky and snared him around the waist. He slammed into the hull as laughter erupted from the deck. *What the...*

"Well done." Hornigold peered over the rail. His laugh bellowed louder than the others. "Quite a good show."

"What's going on?" Sam's eyes followed the line of rope up to the deck. A rather large sailor held the other end. Several other sailors grabbed the rope and roughly hoisted him onto the deck.

"Just having a little fun with you all." A much-more jovial Hornigold motioned to his crew to untie the ropes. "Forgive an old, reformed pirate for giving his crew a laugh. I do not know if I completely believe your tale, but I sense you speak the truth about hunting Slayer, so let us talk."

Sam rubbed his shoulder where he had struck the hull. He filled his lungs with air. At first it hurt to breathe, but the pain faded. Sarah's eyes no longer glowed, but they were angry.

"Quite funny, Captain." Thaddeus smiled.

"Please, join me in my cabin." Hornigold wrapped an arm around Sam's shoulders and motioned for Thaddeus and Sarah to follow. Sam suppressed a whimper as Hornigold's thick arm pressed against his sore shoulder. He also fought the desire to hold his nose against the *Ranger* captain's heavy odor, a mix of beef, sweat and liquor.

"Again, my apologies to you all. No harm was meant." Hornigold sat at the head of an ornately carved, jewel-encrusted wooden table. He filled three tarnished and dented mugs with a liquid that smelled like paint thinner. Hornigold filled his own mug, gold and twice the size of the others, to the brim. "Please, my friends, lift your tankards and drink with me."

Sam eyed his mug, which Hornigold called a tankard. Although unidentifiable bits and pieces floated around the edges of the thick, brown liquid, he picked up the mug. He would drink so as not to be rude.

"Captain Hornigold, before we drink, I think we need to strike some truth between us." Thaddeus pushed his mug to the side.

Sam frowned at Thaddeus. *What's he doing?*

"Speak your mind." Hornigold leaned back in his chair and crossed his arms.

"What you did out there—with this boy, this little man—that was no game." Thaddeus leaned forward, his elbows pressed against the table. "It was a test I would wager. You wanted to see if he, under threat of death, would declare himself and us pirates."

Hornigold sat silently for far too long. Then his cheeks rose as if he smiled, though his thick mustache disguised the Captain's expression. "Aye, it is as you say, but the boy did not crack, and I now believe you are pirate hunters. That is to say, I believe some of your story, but I do not know you, sir, and I am well acquainted with most in these parts."

Thaddeus drank from his mug. "Captain, allow me to introduce myself then." Sam's eyes grew wide. *No, Thaddeus, don't tell him about your past. He'll think you a pirate for sure.* "I am Thaddeus

Milan. I once served as a proud member of the Royal Navy. I sailed under Captain Blake Niles, a scallywag if there ever was one. He was cruel and knew nothing of sailing or commanding men." Thaddeus slammed his empty mug onto the table. "When I challenged him, he branded me a mutineer. He locked me away in the brig, but I escaped. I now roam these seas as my own man— and occasional pirate hunter."

Sam shifted his stare between Thaddeus and Hornigold. Silence filled the room. With a jittery hand, Sam lifted his mug to his mouth and sipped the liquid. It burned his throat and made his stomach tighten.

Hornigold broke the silence with a chuckle as he raised his golden mug to his lips. "I know of this Niles—only now he is Admiral Niles. You are correct, sir. He has a reputation as a fool."

Sam exhaled and unclenched his stomach.

"Fair enough," Hornigold continued. "If you are after Slayer, then—"

"We are after Slayer!" Sam spoke quickly. "He's going after a mag—"

Sarah kicked him under the table and scrunched her face. Thaddeus shot a glance at him. Sam closed his mouth and lowered his head. He took a long swig of the liquid inside his mug and allowed too much to slip down his throat. He coughed and chocked. His mug dropped as he struggled not to spew up the liquid.

"Ahh, the half man cannot handle a little rum." Hornigold laughed and took a long drink; his eyes again shifted back and forth between Sam and Thaddeus. "I have no need to know the whole truth of your run-in with Slayer. I do know your little boat is not seaworthy. I suggest you join my crew and help me on my hunt for that dog Slayer."

"That is a fine offer, Captain." Thaddeus leaned back in his chair. "And what direction are you heading?"

"Why southwest, of course." Hornigold answered as though it were obvious. "Slayer must be headed toward the Windwards."

"You're wrong!" Sam shouted.

Thaddeus pointed a finger at Sam. "Manners, lad."

"What does the little man mean?"

Thaddeus sighed. "Captain, I know it is foolishness, but he thinks Hornigold is headed due east."

"What? There is nothing out there."

"You're wro—" Sam started to say.

"I know that, Captain," Thaddeus interrupted, "as does any man who has ever sailed these waters. But he believes what he believes, and I swore an oath to him."

"Plain foolishness." Hornigold shook his head. "You shall strand yourselves in that pitiful boat in the middle of the sea and die."

"If that is our fate, so be it," Thaddeus lamented.

Hornigold filled Thaddeus' mug with more rum. "I guess there is little else to do but have another drink and part ways. Yet I have to say, pirate hunter to pirate hunter, I hope for your sake the lad is wrong."

"Captain?" Thaddeus asked.

"That Slayer is a savage one. If you are right and find him out there in the middle of nowhere, and you attempt to square against him with nothing but that tiny boat of yours and these young ones for a crew, he shall skin you alive."

Sam forced one more swig of rum. He held it in his mouth for a moment before he swallowed. It burned less this time.

Hornigold continued his warning. "I think it would be better if your boat sinks before you find him. Better to die at the hand of the sea than by the hands of Slayer. Poor souls you shall be, for sure, against the likes of him." Hornigold's laughter echoed throughout his cabin. "Then again, what do I know, right?"

# Chapter 20
## We're Sinking!

Water seeped into the bilge through the hull. The seawater lapped at Sam's knees, and despite Thaddeus' best efforts to repair his boat, the water still rose.

"We're in trouble, right?" Sam already knew the answer.

"She has given her best, but she is hurting." Thaddeus stared at his boat. Pain filled his eyes as he slowly lost *The Mutineer*—his only real love—to the sea.

"We're not going to make it, are we?"

Thaddeus shook his head. "Perhaps we should have joined Hornigold's crew."

Sam lowered his head and bit his lip. It was his fault they were in the middle of nowhere in a boat about to sink. They had lost sight of Captain Hornigold's ship two days ago, and yesterday, the first crack in their boat appeared. It radiated from a hole in the hull, the remnant of a cannonball fired from Slayer's warships just off New Providence.

The crack spread like a spider's web from the upper hull down to the waterline and below. The sea's pressure soon eroded one of the cracked planks. As bits of wood gave way, the water spilled in until Thaddeus hammered in a new plank. But there was no way to completely block the leak. Sarah refused to use her magic to save the boat because she feared it would alert Slayer to their current location. If he found them, he would kill them. So *The Mutineer* slowly sunk.

"Sorry, Thaddeus." Sam kicked at the water. "I didn't mean for this to happen."

"I know, but nevertheless, it is happening." He hammered in the last nail in one more extra length of wood to seal the leak. "As

I warned before, we find ourselves stranded in the middle of the sea, taking on too much water." Thaddeus wiped sweat from his forehead. "It shall not be long, maybe a day or two, before the sea swallows us."

"But we can't give up!" Sam took a step toward Thaddeus. "Slayer is still out there somewhere."

Thaddeus smiled. "Who spoke of giving up? If I am to lose *The Mutineer*, I shall have Slayer pay with his blood."

"Great. So what do we do?"

"I cannot say as I know yet. I need to think awhile. But of one truth about the sea I am sure. She may take your soul, but sometimes she shall surprise you."

"Captain Milan, I mean Thaddeus…Chosen One, come and see!" Excitement filled her words.

Thaddeus patted Sam on the shoulder. "You see."

"Yeah, but you don't know—"

"I see a boat and an island!" Sarah shouted.

Thaddeus shrugged and hurried out of the hold. Sam followed. As he emerged on to the deck, he squinted from the brightness of the mid-afternoon Caribbean sun. Thaddeus was already beside Sarah at the tiller. She handed him a spyglass—what Thaddeus called his small handheld telescope—and pointed off the starboard side of the boat. Thaddeus aimed the spyglass in that direction.

"By God, you are right!" He lowered the spyglass and grinned.

"What… what is she right about?" His eyes still not quite adjusted to a glare, Sam tripped and stumbled as he rushed to join them.

"See for yourself, if you can manage to stay on your feet." Thaddeus handed him the spyglass.

Sam placed it to his right eye and panned right to left in the direction Sarah pointed. There! He saw it! A ship anchored off an island! Was the discovery reason to hope? Or could it be Slayer? He couldn't tell the size of the vessel, but it seemed to have only one large mast with no sails visible. That meant it was no warship. At least he hoped that's what it meant. He also couldn't tell the size of the island, but it couldn't be the magical island where they would find the Sword of Zel-Kar. What about the cloud barrier? No, this was not the island of his vision. *But at least we might be saved!*

Thaddeus grabbed the spyglass. "It is as I say. The sea sometimes chooses to give. Perhaps she finds favor with our cause."

"How do we know this is a good thing?" Sam's eyes narrowed until he spotted the boat and island without the spyglass. "That could be Slayer out there."

"Not likely."

How do you know?" Sarah asked.

"That is no warship." Thaddeus raised the spyglass once more. "No, that is a sloop. Maybe a small trader off course. Not sure. But it would not be one of Slayer's. He would have no use for such a vessel unless he is setting a trap."

"Yeah, I bet he is." Sam cleared his throat to hide the quiver in his voice.

Thaddeus shook his head. "My bones are telling me this is something else, and since we are in need of a boat, I would say our path is clear."

"No!" A knot formed in Sam's stomach. "I don't like what you're thinking."

"Chosen One, we have no choice." Sarah clearly understood what Thaddeus contemplated.

"We need that boat." Thaddeus nodded to Sarah who returned the gesture.

Sam paced back and forth. "How are we supposed to just take a boat, especially if it has a full crew, most of them probably armed?"

"There is moisture in the air," Thaddeus lifted a hand toward the sky as if his fingertips could touch the hovering dampness. If a good mist forms tonight, we can hide our approach. I cannot be sure, but judging how she is anchored, there is not a full crew on board. Most must be on the island—just not sure why. Anyone still aboard shall be drunk tonight. They shall never see us."

Sam stopped pacing. "We can't just kill—"

"There shall be no need to kill." Thaddeus once again stared through the spyglass.

Sarah touched Sam's shoulder. "We must, Chosen One. It is the only way."

Sam glared at both of them as he took a few steps toward the starboard side. They were right, of course. *The Mutineer* still took on water—its fate was inevitable. It would sink. If they didn't do something, they would die. And they still had to stop Slayer and save those children. *Why can't this just be a dream? Why can't I just wake up? Wake up, man! Wake up*! He closed his eyes then opened them again. He remained aboard *The Mutineer,* and Sarah and Thaddeus still stared at him. "Why do I feel like I'm becoming a pirate?" Sam offered an uneasy smile.

Thaddeus grasped the tiller and pointed *The Mutineer* toward their target. "There are worse things you could become."

Night had fallen. Just as Thaddeus had predicted, a mist—heavier than Sam expected—had snaked in over the sea. Thick and green, it surrounded their boat. For the first time since he arrived in the Caribbean, Sam shivered from the cold. Or maybe he was just scared. Sure, the mist hid their approach, but it also hid any warship—maybe one of Slayer's—that might attack. He recalled the thunderous rounds fired as they escaped from New Providence. He never wanted to hear it again.

Stationed on *The Mutineer's* bow, Sam scanned the water in every direction. He listened for any ship hidden in the mist. Timbers creaked. A sail cracked. A line smacked against a mast. Water splashed against a hull. But these sounds came from *The Mutineer*. If Slayer was out there, the mist absorbed any sign of his presence.

Sam shivered again. He steadied himself and turned toward the stern. They sailed with no torches or candles in the dank pitch black of night. The mist cloaked Thaddeus in a ghostly shroud. Only his two bright eyes betrayed his presence at the tiller. *Man, I have the creeps bad. Get a hold of yourself. Don't wuss out now. You're the Chosen One. Remember?* It made perfect sense to sail without lights. Darkness was their best weapon. Surprise their only chance at success. *Besides, there's no danger yet. My back's not on fire. The sword's not calling to me."*

A tap on his shoulder startled him. "Chosen One, you are quiet. Are you all right?"

For the first time tonight he welcomed the darkness. His face was warm, and he knew he blushed because he had jumped at Sarah's touch. "Hey, I'm fine. I just have this feeling we're sailing into a trap."

"Captain Milan does not think so."

"Stop talking like that."

"What do you mean?"

"That formal stuff. You used to curse and talk—I don't know—differently." Sam looked way from her. His eyes searched for Thaddeus through the mist. "It's because you're trying to impress him, isn't it? Why do you trust him so much?"

Sarah leaned closer. "Why do you not trust him?"

"I… I do, I guess." Sam grasped her hand. "You know we wouldn't have to steal that boat if you used magic."

"I told you I bloody can't." Sarah snatched her hand away as she spoke more like herself. Sam figured her anger brought it out. "He'll know and find us. You'll suffer. He'll kill you."

"Slayer?" Sam asked.

"Yes."

"You could be wrong. Come on—"

"If you two are done bickering, we have arrived." Thaddeus spoke in a loud whisper. "But if you want to go on jabbering and give us away, by all means—continue."

With her face downcast, Sarah slipped away. Sam returned his focus to the sea. He couldn't see either the boat or the island through the soupy mist. "How do you know? I can't see a thing."

Thaddeus didn't respond. He moved stealthily to lower *The Mutineer's* sails then disappeared into his cabin. When he returned, he held two pistols and two canvas pouches, one shaped like a ram's horn.

He handed Sam one of the pistols. With a shaky hand, Sam grabbed the rounded wooden handle of the pistol and lifted the weapon to his face. It was lighter than he expected even though it had an iron barrel about nine inches long. The pistol had obviously been used many times before. The wood, faded and nicked, cradled a barrel marked by scratches and blotches of what might have been dried blood. As he studied the weapon, which reminded him of the toy pirate gun he once played with as a child, one question bounced around his head. Whether shot or bludgeoned, how many people had Thaddeus killed with this weapon?

Thaddeus finally spoke. "I trust you know how to use it?"

Sam shook his head.

"By God, I hope you are not useless in a fight. This is called a flintlock pistol." Thaddeus grabbed the weapon. From the pouch shaped like a ram's horn he poured a black powder into the barrel. From the second pouch he pulled out a bullet and loaded it into the barrel. "You see this. It is the lock cock." Thaddeus pointed to the firing mechanism above the handle. He pulled back the lock cock half way. "Now it is half- cocked. Leave it that way. But be careful. When we board the boat, pull it back all the way, and be ready to fire. You shall have just one shot. After that, flip the pistol around so you are holding the barrel. Strike someone if need be. They do not call it the skull crusher for nothing."

Sam gulped. "You said we wouldn't have to kill anyone."

"I have no wish to kill this night, but raiding is dangerous. You have to be ready. I need you by my side."

"What about me?" Sarah asked. "I know more—"

"You are coming, too, but I want you out of the way, you hear, unless I order otherwise. Take this dagger. I sense you know how to use it." Thaddeus handed her a thin blade atop a curved handle. It looked more like a miniature sword than a knife. "But I mean it. Stay out of danger's way."

"I shall not—"

Wait, Thaddeus, you never answered my first question. Sam purposely cut off Sarah. "How do you know we're close?"

"Listen."

Sam closed his eyes and listened. At first, the slight splash of water against their hull was all he heard until music, faint but there, slipped through the mist. Though the music had melody, it sounded a lot like fingernails scratched against a chalkboard.

"Hear it?" Thaddeus asked.

"Yeah," Sam whispered.

"That is the music of bagpipes mixed with yodeling. They are good and drunk, just as I said." Thaddeus gazed in the direction of the music. "This raid shall be easy."

"I hope you're right." Sam eyed the pistol in his hand. *Yeah, easy! We could all die tonight, just as easily.*

# Chapter 21
## The Raid

Sam didn't dare blink. He pressed a hand against his chest to calm the wild beats of his heart. Thaddeus faced him as he paddled *The Mutineer's* tiny rowboat through the mist and icy Caribbean waters to the sloop they planned to raid. Sarah clutched the dagger Thaddeus had given her and cleaned the blade with a rag. No one spoke.

*The Mutineer* slipped out of view as a wall of fog engulfed it. Sam lowered his head. *I'm going to miss that boat.* Thaddeus also peered one last time at his vessel; his bright eyes dimmed. *He must blame for having to abandon his boat. Why is he still willing to help us?* Sam let that thought fade away as their rowboat emerged from the mist. They were no longer concealed. With the sloop they intended to raid anchored twenty feet ahead, the crew would easily be able to see them. *Please be drunk. Please don't see us.* They certainly sounded drunk. The bagpipes still played and the yodels were slurred.

The sloop, similar to *The Mutineer*, had one important distinction. A 6-pounder! A cannon's barrel pointed at them from the deck! *No! They're going to fire on us!* Sam ducked his head.

"Easy, lad," Thaddeus whispered with a slight chuckle. "They do not see us. That 6-pounder was there long before we arrived. We have not been discovered yet." That last word hung in the air as they reached the anchor line, a thick rope covered in muck and seaweed.

Sam closed his eyes and tilted his head toward the sloop's deck. The men aboard still yodeled. Clumps echoed across the deck as if the sailors danced. The bagpipes screeched some strange happy tune.

"Lad, you have your pistol?" Thaddeus placed a hand on Sam's shoulder.

"Yes."

"Remember, what I told you. Once on board, cock it all the way and be ready to fire if it comes to it. Once you fire a round, swing that weapon around and strike anything that moves. Our lives might just depend on it."

"What?"

Thaddeus didn't respond. Instead he turned his gaze on Sarah. "You stay here until I give the word."

"No." Sarah raised her voice. "Captain Milan… Thaddeus… I can fight."

With a finger to his mouth, Thaddeus glowered at her. "Do as I say. We shall need you on deck soon enough."

Sarah remained silent, but her hand tightened around the knife.

Thaddeus winked at both. "Be steady, young ones."

*The Mutineer* captain grasped the anchor line and climbed. It took him just seconds to reach the deck. With a quick glance around, he slid on board and motioned for Sam to follow.

Sam trembled. His chest hurt and his stomach heaved, like he might throw-up. What would he face on the deck? Hand to hand combat? Other than his duel with Maximilian Black, he had no fighting experience, and his battle with Black had not gone well. If not for Thaddeus, he would have died that night instead of Black. And Sam had never fired a weapon. Was this what it felt like to go to war? Would he be a coward in combat?

Thaddeus gestured to him once more. Sam urged his limbs to climb, but they failed to heed his command. *Come on, Thaddeus needs you! Get up there and fight! Prove you're the Chosen One! But what if I'm not?*

"Chosen One, do you want me to go in your place?" Sarah's eyes lit up. "I know how to use that pistol. I've used one before. I'm a pretty good shot, actually. Let me—"

"No, I can do this. If I'm this Chosen One, I have to do this. Thaddeus told you to stay here and wait. Stick to the plan." Sam gazed into her eyes one last time. Even through the darkness, they comforted him.

With his right hand, he reached up and gripped the slimy rope to begin his climb. Hand over hand, with his legs wrapped around the rope, he inched toward the deck. Half way up, he stopped to steady his breaths. That proved a mistake. His hands started to slip from the rope. *No! No!* If he fell, those aboard would hear the splash and the gunpowder in his pistol would be worthless. *Hold on! Keep climbing! No! I'm slipping!* First, one hand slid from the rope then a leg slipped. He gritted his teeth as he strained to hold on with his other hand. His muscles ached in protest; even though he was skinny, one tiny, rubbery arm and a thin leg were not enough to hold up his body. The other hand started to slip. *Have to hold on!*

"Chosen One, I've got you!" Sarah hung beneath him on the anchor line. She held on with one hand and with the other she lifted his loose hand back onto the rope. "Keep going. You can do it."

Sam shook his head as he swung his dangling leg back onto the rope. *Saved by a girl!* Thaddeus would never let him hear the end of it. Then again, by now it should be no surprise to have Sarah save him. She was stronger than him in every way. He shook his head one more time and took a deep breath. *Forget about it. This raid is just beginning.* He continued his climb up the anchor line until he reached the deck. Cautiously, he eased himself onto the sloop and slid next to Thaddeus behind a barrel.

"You are a landlubber for sure," *The Mutineer* captain whispered.

"Hey, this pirate stuff is new to me."

"I told you, I am no pirate."

"I still get the feeling this isn't your first raid since you left the Royal Navy."

Thaddeus was silent for a moment. "Follow my lead if you want to live. We can get through this without firing a single round if we move fast. If you must shoot, do so at close range. Now pull your lock cock back all the way and be ready for anything."

With pistol in hand, Thaddeus crawled away from the barrel and crept toward the bow where the music played the loudest. Sam took one more deep breath. With a finger poised on his pistol's trigger, he followed.

They edged their way along the deck until the legs of the sailors became visible. They danced and, by the sound of it, they clanked bottles or mugs together. What had Hornigold called the mugs? Tankards? Sam guessed most likely they contained rum as the sailors' voices still sounded slurred.

Sam listened carefully to the words chanted to the playful music of a bagpipe. They sang of a beast of the Caribbean waters called a *lusca*. *"A mix of shark and octopus, it comes from the deep to drag you down toward endless sleep. Oh many a sailor cry for upon the whirlpool they spy, they knowth come the lusca and they most surely shall die. Still, to seek a treasure's might is worth the bite of the terrible, terrible lusca."*

Thaddeus smacked Sam in the head. "Stay alert. The time has come. They most surely are drunk. They shall be slow and clumsy, but in their drunkenness they may put up a fool's fight. Be ready?"

Sam nodded. He blew out quick breaths of air and gripped the pistol tighter as his muscles tensed and his heart pounded. His back started to burn, as if the fire sword beckoned to join in the action. He fought the urge to reach for the burning blade, but its presence strengthened his nerves. It might just save his life if this raid failed.

Thaddeus slowly unsheathed his sword so he held the blade in one hand and the pistol in the other. "Move!"

In the next heartbeat, he sprang from his hiding place and struck one sailor over the head with the handle of his sword. The man fell to the deck. Three others, one who held the bagpipes and two armed only with tankards, whirled around to face Thaddeus. The piper, a rather pudgy man with a thin beard and patch over one eye, dropped the instrument.

"My friends, do not move or a *lusca* is not the only beast you shall have to fear tonight," Thaddeus warned.

Sam stood next to him, his pistol aimed at the three sailors as he tried to conceal his shaky hand. He squirmed against the heat that rose up his back.

"I am here to take this sloop." Thaddeus moved a step closer to the three men. "I hope you decide she is not worth dying over."

One of the sailors, a tall, thin beardless man with long hair and a bandana over his forehead, laughed. He stumbled and took a swig from the tankard he held. When he spoke, he sounded like a weasel, his threat uttered in a high-pitched squeaky voice. "One man and a half man plan to steal this here boat. You are a fool—a dead fool."

The tall sailor lunged forward and swung the tankard at Thaddeus' head. But his attack was off-balanced. Thaddeus easily side-stepped the sailor and kicked him in the stomach. The man slumped to the deck and Thaddeus followed with a kick to the man's head. The man fell unconscious. Sam cast his gaze down at the man. *Is he dead? Thaddeus swore there'd be no killing.*

The pudgy musician and the third sailor in the group, who was clearly younger than the rest but still older than Sam, backed away. Thaddeus stepped toward both. Sam struggled to keep the pistol steady as he shuffled his feet closer to the two sailors. He focused on the young sailor's eyes. They showed no desire to risk death. The pudgy musician must have felt the same. His body quivered and he might have peed in his pants—then again, it might just have been liquor that had spilled on his pants.

"All right, who is the captain of this vessel?" Thaddeus asked. The two sailors glanced at each other but remained silent. "Come now, friends. Answer." Thaddeus stuck the point of his blade against the musician's stomach.

"Captain Charles Vane, sir." The musician answered quickly, his eyes zeroed in on the blade.

Thaddeus laughed quietly. "Vane! Of all the scallywag pirates on the sea, I would not have expected to have a run-in with the likes of him. And where are Captain Vane and the rest of the crew?"

"On the island, sir, gathering food to replenish our stock." The musician gulped loudly.

"Very well, then. Musician, what is your name?"

"Jim Holley, sir."

Thaddeus removed the tip of his blade from the man's stomach. "Mr. Holley, if there are shackles and chains aboard please bring them to me at once. Consider yourselves my prisoners... no, my guests... for now. I mean to visit your Captain Charles Vane on that island."

Thaddeus stepped back and placed a hand on Sam's shoulder. "Keep your pistol squared at—"

The click of a pistol being cocked sounded behind them followed by a raspy voice. "Drop your weapons. If not, this round shall find one of your backs. No telling which one, though. Guess we shall just have to see."

Sam froze. Who could have snuck up on them? All four men—the two still conscious and the two fallen sailors—were accounted for. He and Thaddeus had failed to see a fifth man. They were caught. *Oh no! What do we do now?* Flames crackled underneath his birthmark. The time had come for the fire sword. *Have to reach—*

A thud followed by the thump of a body as it fell to the deck stopped Sam as he reached for the sword. He and Thaddeus turned. There stood Sarah, a club in her hand. At her feet was the unconscious fifth sailor. "I told you I was good in a fight."

"I never doubted it." Thaddeus bowed.

Sam smiled as the sensation that flames seared his back eased, but his ears still rang with the crackle of the magical sword's flame.


"This is a really bad idea, Thaddeus." Sam huffed as Thaddeus made him paddle their small rowboat toward shore. "We have their sloop. We should just take it and go after Slayer. This is crazy."

Thaddeus pointed his spyglass toward a group of men who stood by a bonfire on shore. "Lad, Charles Vane is a pirate not to be taken lightly. If he is out this way, so far from the Windwards, there is a reason for it. I must know his secrets. You might say I am compelled."

"Those pirates on board told you he's gathering food."

"Lies!" Thaddeus spit into the sea. "It is unheard of for a captain to embark on such a tedious duty. I am sure there is more to this."

"You're going to get us killed."

"Maybe, but not this night. Vane is reasonable. I just wish to talk. No more. I swear by the pirates' articles."

"What?"

"The articles are a code that a pirate crew swears to. It is what keeps such bands of misfits and miscreants from killing each other over their bounties."

"You said you're not a pirate."

Thaddeus lowered the spyglass. "Nevertheless I respect the pirates' ways. Now quiet yourself and quit your rowing. We are close to shore. As before, follow my lead and no one need get hurt."

"Sure." Sam wished Thaddeus had chosen to bring Sarah onto the island. She was back at the sloop they had raided. Her orders were to fire the cannon at the shore if she heard three rounds fired from the island. He had chosen Sarah for the task because she knew how to load a canon. Sam did not. *It seems like I don't know how to do much lately.*

A pistol in one hand and a second pistol tucked into his belt, Thaddeus slid over the side of the rowboat into knee-deep water. The second pistol had come from the pirate Sarah had knocked unconscious. Sam also clutched a pistol as he gently slipped into the water on the opposite side of the rowboat. Together, they dragged the boat onto shore then crouched like lions about to stalk prey. A nod from Thaddeus and they tread softly farther up shore, pistols aimed at the group of sailors—maybe ten—huddled around a fire just up the beach. The group's attention was focused toward the fire, their eyes cast away from the water. The pirates' shadows spread over the sand as flames leaped and spiraled into the sky.

The site of flames awakened Sam's fire sword. A peak over his shoulder revealed an orange glow from underneath his shirt. Still, he ignored the blade. *Why? Am I afraid if I use it, Slayer will know? Why should I be scared of that? I'm out here to face him, so if the sword brings him to me, that makes my job easier. I can kill him sooner than later. Or he can kill me. That's what I'm afraid of.*

Thaddeus tiptoed a few steps ahead and stopped about twenty feet from the pirates. A quick glance at Sam, a confident wink and he cleared this throat. "Gentlemen, if I may."

The pirates spun around. One man, armed with a musket, raised his weapon and fired one round. It struck the sand between Sam and Thaddeus. Sam fell on his back. He stared wide-eyed as Thaddeus fired his pistol. The round smashed into the stomach of the pirate who had fired the musket. That man slowly dropped his weapon and slumped to the sand. He lay motionless. Dead!

"Thaddeus!" Sam rose to his feet. "What—"

"Quiet!" *The Mutineer* captain dropped the pistol he had just fired and snatched the second pistol from his belt. He aimed it at the outraged pirates who drew their swords and cursed loudly. "That is two shots, you dogs." Thaddeus warned. "If a third is fired, my gunner shall fire your own 6-pounder on this island. We shall all die. Yes, my friends, I have seized your vessel. Need you proof, just force me to fire another round."

Sam shook his head. *What is Thaddeus doing?*

Laughter erupted from behind the pirates. It was the laugh of a man who didn't seem to have much fear of Thaddeus' threat.

The pirates parted down the middle to reveal the man who laughed. He had to be Captain Charles Vane. He wore finely tailored clothing, as though his outfit had been cut to fit his rather tall, thin frame. A red coat with a thick black belt covered him. A pistol hung from what could have been a silk scarf tied around his neck. A second pistol was tucked into his belt. He wore knee breeches and a dark three-cornered hat. Long, curly hair fell down the sides of his face, though it could have been a wig. If he had a beard, it was little more than stubble.

He sat on a chest in the sand, his legs crossed. He fingered what might have been a gold coin in his right hand. The flames behind him seemed to make the coin glow. Vane didn't bother to rise before he spoke.

"Quite brash of you, my dear fellow." Vane twisted a strand of hair. His manner of speaking was undoubtedly British. He spoke like a member of high society rather than a pirate captain. "Am I meant to be frightened of a man armed with a pistol with only a half man at his side and a declaration that my vessel now is under your lead?"

Thaddeus smiled. His British accent and tone of superiority matched Vane's. "No, I do not seek fear from you, sir. I simply wish to know whose sloop I have raided, and why you are so off any rational course and with so few men."

Vane stood. "And who dares questions me? I believe the lad called you Thaddeus."

"Captain Thaddeus Milan is my name. And I believe you are Captain Charles Vane. But you are known to command a warship, not a sloop."

Vane inched toward Thaddeus. "You have me at a disadvantage, for you are right—I am Captain Vane. But your name is unknown to me. Never mind that. Might I inquire as to why you have seized my vessel?"

Thaddeus shook his head. "You must first answer my questions as I have the upper hand."

Vane laughed again. "Yes, it would seem so. Yet—"

With a quick nod of Vane's head, another pirate lifted a pistol and fired off one round. Thaddeus dove, rolled along the sand, then came up and fired his own round. It was a pinpoint shot that struck the pirate's pistol. The weapon flew from his hand as he yelped in pain and fell to his knees.

A crack of thunder sounded from the sea. Sarah had fired the 6-pounder. The shot screamed toward the island. Sam lay on the beach. Thaddeus had told him, back aboard the sloop, to do this rather than run.

The pirates scattered; most dashed toward the tree line just beyond the beach. That proved to be a mistake as the shot flew overhead and crashed into a grouping of trees with an explosion that shook the beach. Sam peered up in time to see the pirates who had run thrown backward from the explosion's shockwave. They moaned as they lay on the beach, but they were alive.

Vane stood tall on the shore. He had not run, not moved at all as far as Sam could tell. He just continued to twirl a strand of hair.

Thaddeus also hadn't run. He rose from the sand and stood about ten feet from Vane. The two men studied each other. Sam was sure they would draw swords, but both chuckled as if they had told some inside joke known only to pirate captains. Vane spoke first. "You cannot blame me for testing your threat."

"Certainly." Thaddeus unsheathed his sword and grabbed the one remaining unfired pistol from Sam. "And so it is clear, if one more pistol or musket round is fired, my gunner has orders to fire at will at the island."

Vane nodded and walked back to the chest he sat on earlier. He lifted the lid to reveal a mound of gold coins. "If you follow a pirate's articles, you shall leave me a fair share since this find is mine."

Thaddeus' eyes bulged and he slid along the sand toward the gold as if in a trance. He licked his lips once. Sam rose to his feet and followed. *Oh no. This is all he wants. Gold. Treasure. He's going to abandon us. He's going to forget about Slayer.*

"How did you know this treasure was here?" Thaddeus fell to his knees in front of the chest.

Vane held up what might have been a scroll. "This gold was seized by Sir Henry Morgan in his raid on Panama in 1671."

"So it is true! Not all of Morgan's gold was found! Morgan hid some of it!"

"Aye, and this map led me to it." Vane held the scroll to his chest. "But it has come at a price. We were sailing in the Windwards when I told my crew I possessed Morgan's map. They doubted its authenticity. When we mistakenly fired on a French man-o'-war, I knew we would lose the battle and I might lose this map, so I broke off the attack. My crew branded me a coward and mutinied. My quartermaster, that villain John Rackham, took my ship. I and these men loyal to me were cast off in the sloop you have now seized."

"Your choice was wise. Rackham and those who followed him are fools." Thaddeus remained on his knees. He kept his eyes on the gold.

"There is more to tell," Vane continued. "This is not the only gold the great Morgan hid. There is more hidden in Honduras, which is where I shall sail come morning. If you are kind enough to leave me my sloop, perhaps you and your crew could sail under my colors and share any riches we find."

Sam started to back away. Thaddeus had what he wanted. He would join Vane and sail for Honduras to seek more gold. *I have to get back to Sarah. We can still escape with Vane's boat. But I have to move now.*

With a deep sigh, Thaddeus lowered his sword to the sand and picked up a handful of gold coins. He eyed the coins for a while before he let them slip through his fingers into the chest. When the last coin fell, he reached for his sword and rose to his feet.

"Captain Vane, it is a most generous offer, and a wise man would follow your lead. But I cannot."

Sam stopped. *What did he just say?*

Thaddeus carried on. "You asked me before why we seized your vessel. We are after the pirate Jem Slayer. I, the boy and others wish to bring him to justice."

Vane closed the lid on his gold. "I know of Slayer's attack on New Providence. Yours is a fool's errand. Slayer shall destroy you."

"That is true enough, but I swore an oath to this lad, and we need the use of your sloop as Slayer damaged ours. But, sir, I do not leave you stranded. My sloop, *The Mutineer*, sits out there just beyond the mist. She is a fine boat but in need of repairs I do not have time for. She must be careened on shore to carry out repairs. You and your men are welcome to her."

"That is mighty kind of you." Vane bowed. "And what of my gold?"

"I leave it to you and your men." Thaddeus bowed as well. "And wish you strong winds as you sail for Honduras."

Thaddeus walked up to Sam and placed a hand on his shoulder. "Ready?"

Sam took a deep breath. *I can't believe it.*

Vane approached them from behind and handed Thaddeus a cloth filled with gold coins. "You should take this," he offered. "Perhaps if you share it with Slayer, he shall have pity on you and kill you quickly rather than torturing you. Then again, he does indeed like to torture his prisoners, does he not?"

Thaddeus snickered as another explosion erupted from the sea. Sarah had fired another round. It whizzed through the air until it smashed into the rowboat they had brought to shore. Splintered timber flayed in all directions as the explosion shook the shore.

Sam fell to the ground but Thaddeus didn't blink. "I guess we shall have to take your longboat to sea as it appears my gunner misfired. *The Mutineer* shall await you when you find your way to her. I bid you adieu, Captain Vane." Thaddeus tipped his three-cornered hat.

Vane did the same. "Pray our paths never cross again, Thaddeus Milan."

# Chapter 22
## A Missing Barrier

Sarah was distant. She leaned on the railing of their new sloop, which carried the name *Striker* but which Thaddeus had re-christened *The Mutineer II*. She stared at a point where the sea and sky touched. Sam hesitated to approach her, but he had to. It was too quiet—had been since the raid three days ago. Even the seagulls that flew overhead had long since disappeared.

*The Mutineer II* sailed due east, but a calm sea and soft wind barely pushed the boat forward.

Thaddeus sat on a barrel as he helmed the tiller. How much longer would he follow this course? Sam shook his head and focused on the eastern horizon. *I don't understand. In my vision, only a day passed before I reached that strange fog barrier. We should be there by now. Where are you? Why aren't you here?*

He brought his attention back to Sarah. Slowly, he walked along the deck until he stood beside her. She did not turn to him. Sam licked his lips and tried to build some spit in his dry mouth. "You're quiet," he mumbled as he squinted into the mid-day sunlight.

"What? Oh, I'm sorry." She slightly shifted her gaze toward him but quickly looked away. "I'm just thinking about those children with that scum dog Slayer. I pray they're all right. I pray we reach them in time."

Sam struck the railing with his fist. "Sarah, it should be here. I just don't understand why we haven't reached the barrier yet. My vision was so clear, and even now I feel like this is right—like this is the direction we should be going. I just don't know why we're not there yet."

Sarah did not immediately respond. She blinked several times. "Maybe you didn't understand your vision?"

"Huh?" That was the first time she had doubted him.

"Maybe Thaddeus and Captain Hornigold were right. Maybe we should have followed the Windward Islands."

"Sarah…" Sam lowered his head and moved away.

"Wait, I'm sorry, Chosen One." Sarah grabbed his arm. "I'm just scared. I didn't mean it. Maybe in your vision you were traveling much faster. Maybe if we were traveling faster—"

She released his arm and ran to the main sail where she raised her arms and started to chant.

"What is she doing?" Thaddeus jumped from the barrel and moved toward Sarah. "Boy, what is she doing?"

Sam ran to her side. "Sarah, wait!"

Her eyes became green orbs and concentrated on the sail as her body lifted from the deck. A visible gust of wind encircled her. Faster and faster the wind swirled then it exploded off her body. The blast of air slammed against the sail; *The Mutineer II* creaked and shuddered in protest.

"Boy, this boat is going to break-up! I can hear it happening!" Thaddeus fell onto the deck as *The Mutineer II* shot forward through the water—or actually just above the water. "We'll drown for sure!"

Sam grabbed the mast. "Sarah, stop!"

If she understood his words while in her magical trance, she didn't listen. Her head tilted back, and her green eyes peered skyward. Her chants intensified as strange dark words flowed off her tongue and a stronger wind surged from her hands.

The boat skimmed above the water, faster than when she had used her powers to escape Slayer's attack off New Providence. Chunks of wood broke off from the hull. The mast cracked.

"Boy!" Thaddeus shouted over the unnatural wind's roar.

"Sarah, you have to stop! This is too fast!" Sam still held onto the mast until—split, crack, rip—the mast toppled and flew back behind the boat into the sea; the sails flew away with it. *The Mutineer II* came to a jolting stop. Without the mast to hold onto, Sam was thrown aft. He crashed against Thaddeus and together they rolled against the tiller with such force that it fractured and fell to the deck.

Sarah collapsed to her knees.    Sam climbed off Thaddeus and ran to her. "Sarah, are you all right?"

"Forget about the witch!" Thaddeus barked. "She has condemned us all!"

Sarah raised her head. "Oh, what I have done?"

"Witch, I should kill you." Thaddeus withdrew the sword at his side.

"Stop!" Sam rose to face Thaddeus. "Don't call her a witch. This is my fault. She did this because of me. She did this to try to help us."

"Maybe I should just kill the both of you and be done with this." Thaddeus raised his sword.

A pain rose up Sam's back. He knew exactly what it was. "Stay away from her!" He reached behind his back and retrieved his burning sword. "Thaddeus, I'm warning you." Sam pointed the fiery blade at *The Mutineer II* captain. "Don't make me use this sword against you."

"Ahh, there it is." Thaddeus sneered. "All right, boy, try to use it against me, but I swear I shall have your heart."

"Please, stop!" Sarah put herself between them. "Don't do this. I can repair the damage. Please, we need each other."

"Too late, girlie." Thaddeus swung his sword at Sam.

A thunderous explosion echoed over the water and disrupted their argument.

"Down!" Thaddeus ordered. A cannonball flew over *The Mutineer II* and struck water off the port side. Another explosion soon followed, but the cannonball splashed down off the starboard side. Silence followed except for a continuous whoosh and an ominous creak—signs a large ship approached. Thaddeus glanced over a railing on the starboard side. "It is a frigate—a warship—and I think it is one of Slayer's."

"Another one!" Sam pointed to a second ship, just as large as the first, off the port bow.

"My magic," Sarah whispered. "Slayer must have felt when I used my magic. I brought him to us."

His hands tightened around the fire sword, Sam brought the burning blade close to his face, but even the blade's warmth couldn't quiet his fears. His arms shook and his body trembled. He glanced at Thaddeus. "We're dead, aren't we?"

"That is a true enough statement." Thaddeus sheathed his sword and removed the pistol from his belt. "We are dead in the water. If you have an idea to save us, by all means, let us hear it. Lass, use your witchery. Get us out of here."

"I'm sorry, my powers are drained." Sarah bowed her head. "I'm so sorry."

Sam peeked again at the two ships. They sandwiched the sloop between them as marksmen, armed with muskets, aimed to prevent the sloop's escape. "I say there," a voice—more like the hiss of a snake than Hornigold's booming voice—assaulted Sam's ears from all directions. "Thank you for the use of magic. I had lost your trail until that little sorcery. Who among you lighted the way for us? Speak now."

Sam grabbed Sarah's shoulder and shook his head. "No. Don't answer." He tried to signal Thaddeus, but to no avail. Thaddeus rocked back and forth, his pistol clutched to his chest. Would Thaddeus fight with them? Or did he intend to turn them over to Slayer to save himself? A shiver ran down Sam's back.

The snake-like voice returned. "I say, who led us here?"

Thaddeus finally snapped to attention as though he had reached some decision. "Steady, both of you." He buried the pistol in his belt, winked and stood. "Who do I have the pleasure of addressing and why have you fired on my boat? I assure you I have nothing to offer, and your time would be greatly wasted in attempting to claim this vessel as a prize." He spoke meekly and with a stutter, clearly an act to show fear. Then again, maybe it wasn't an act.

"Such audaciousness in the face of death." The voice slithered across the sea to reach *The Mutineer II's* deck. "Do you think me a fool? You have a certain boy aboard with a unique quality and a very bad little girl who must be punished."

Thaddeus raised his hands. "What is this foolishness? I am a simple merchant who deals in the movement of goods and wares. As you can see pirates have badly damaged my boat. Offer help or leave me be so I might limp to a safe port."

"You shall hand over to me the two very special beings you have aboard your vessel or you shall most assuredly die a slow, painful death," the voice threatened.

"And who would carry out this awful deed against an unarmed boat?" Thaddeus shifted his stare from one ship to the other.

"I am Captain Slayer."

Sarah started to rise, but Sam held her down as he released the fire sword and watched it vanish. "Sarah, no. I'm not going to let you do what you're thinking. You're not going to sacrifice yourself."

"I have to," she whispered.

"Listen, we can get through this if we stick together." Sam forced a slight smile across his face. It didn't last.

"Captain Slayer." Thaddeus picked up his three-cornered hat, which had fallen to the deck, and placed it back on his head. "I believe I have heard of you. You are indeed a fearsome individual. I praise you, sir. Seems all that has been said about you is true." The stutter in Thaddeus' voice disappeared.

A bone-jarring laugh cascaded down from one of the ships—Slayer's ship—and seemed to swirl around the sloop like a fog.

"Oh, my dear friend, I do not know you." Slayer sang his words more than he spoke them. "But it does not matter. You have mistakenly intervened in events that are far beyond your understanding. And you must die for your effort."

Thaddeus knelt and lowered his voice to a whisper. "My friends, I am sorry we had words and that I raised my sword against you. I would ask for your forgiveness, but it no longer matters. It looks like our journey has reached an end, but since I do not much like this Slayer, let us have a little fun. I think we should load this boat's 6-pounder. It shall not do much, but never let it be said Thaddeus Milan died without a fight. Care to join me?"

Sam's jaw tightened and his teeth clenched. His eyes watered as he fought back tears. He couldn't be a coward. Still! *I don't want to die! I'm not ready! This can't be real. I know it's a dream. It just has to be.* How many times had he told himself that? Yet, he hadn't woken up—ever. If this was a dream, he seemed trapped in it until the dream reached an end. Maybe this was the end, and he had to die to be free. That didn't make the thought of death any easier. He steadied himself and placed a hand on Thaddeus' shoulder. "Let's get him."

Thaddeus stood again. "Slayer, you vile beast, I'll never—"

"Captain Slayer, here I am." Sarah's voice was loud, as if magically enhanced. With a wave of her hand, she pushed Sam away and stood. "I give myself to you. But you have no need for the boy. I made a terrible mistake. He is not the Chosen One. His magic is weak and useless. He has led us astray. I give myself over to you. Do as you shall, but leave these meaningless beings alone to die on this ruined vessel."

"Ahh, child, your words move me," Slayer mocked. "Perhaps you have failed in your attempt to reach the Chosen One. Then again, perhaps your words are trickery. I think the latter."

Sarah quickly turned to Sam. "Jump! Get off the boat!"

"Sarah!" Sam reached for her with both hands.

"Jump now!" In that instant, she disappeared from *The Mutineer II* as if an unseen force snatched her.

"No!" Sam clutched the air where she had stood.

"We best do as she said." Thaddeus grabbed him.

"Boy." Slayer's voice surrounded Sam. "I thought I might like to meet you, but my mind has changed on the matter. I think I shall just kill you now."

A blast of invisible energy slammed into Sam and knocked him against the railing. The energy held him there like a vice. The same occurred to Thaddeus. Sam strained, but could not move.

"Good-bye, boy." Slayer's voice faded, replaced by a chorus of thunder from both ships. At that second, Sam's back erupted in searing fire. He would have screamed if there was time, but volleys of cannon fire rained down on *The Mutineer II*. The boat disintegrated into shards of timber. The ear-shattering explosion engulfed Sam, as if a sudden barrage of hundreds of fireworks lighted up the sky. Then silence cocooned him.

He tumbled over and over across the sea; his body twisted, like a torn paper bag thrown about by a strong wind. Everything around him went dark.

*He stood back on the pier and stared out to sea. His friends were next to him, their attention on a couple of cute girls who strolled by but paid them no attention, as usual. He gazed at a bright, blue sky filled with an array of white clouds. A strong, warm breeze blew from the ocean and brushed against his face.*

*"It was a dream, wasn't it?" Sam asked. "I'm home again, where I belong, on my pier, with my friends, looking out over my ocean."*

*"Who are you talking to?" John leaned against the railing.*

*"Huh... oh, no one." Sam turned from the water. "Hey, let's hit the mall. I'll get us a pizza. We can play some air hockey."*

*"Sounds good," Greg agreed. They started to walk away from the pier railing.*

*A hand fell on Sam's shoulder. He glanced at the fingers. They were bone thin. He peered farther back until his eyes reached the glowing outline of a man—an elderly man, more skeletal than flesh with a long white beard and eyes buried deep within the skull. He wore the clothing of that pirate age Sam had dreamt of, only his clothing was all white from the long coat that covered his bony frame and his knee-high boots to the three-cornered hat upon his head. He wore a sword at his side with a silvery handle shaped like a bird.*

*"Let me go!" Sam begged.*

*"Your task is not complete, young Samuel Every," the old man whispered. "It falls upon you to finish what I began. Our family bloodline demands it. Return…"*

*"What? Who are you?"*

*"I am an Every…"*

*The old man's words trailed off, and he vanished. Sam twisted back to see if his friends were still there. They were gone, too, as was everyone else on the pier. He was alone. Drops of blood dotted the concrete at his feet. Sam glanced all around and above him to find the source. Uhh! His head erupted in pain, like the worst brain freeze he had ever experienced. His ears rang as if he had stood too close to an explosion of firecrackers. He clutched his ears to quiet the noise. When he removed his hands, blood dripped from his fingers. He was the source of the blood on the concrete. He fell to his knees and screamed, but heard nothing. Silence surrounded him, just like—*

Sam's eyes shot open and he stared into the bloodied face of Thaddeus. The captain of *The Mutineer II* spoke, but Sam couldn't hear the words. For that matter, he couldn't hear the ocean or the burning, crackling remnants of the sloop, which surrounded them.

Then sounds started to penetrate the quiet. They were hushed at first, broken, like the intermittent sound of a bad connection on a cell phone.

"Lad, can you hear me? We're alive." Thaddeus' words came in pieces, but the message was clear.

"Sarah." Sam couldn't hear his own voice. He brought the palms of his hands to his ears and pressed as hard as he could to force more sounds through whatever barrier had him locked in silence. As he stared at his palms, blotches of warm blood covered them—blood that had clearly come from his ears.

*What's happening to me?* He shifted his head to the right and the left and realized, for the first time, he lay on something solid but wet. In either direction, burning debris from *The Mutineer II* littered the sea.

"Sarah!" he weakly shouted and this time he heard his own voice. He raised himself onto his elbows and vomit overtook him. When he was finished, he rolled onto his back; his head spun, but he could hear.

"She is gone." Thaddeus reached for a jug. "Here, drink this. It is water I salvaged from the wreck. Come on—up with you slowly and have a drink."

Sam did as Thaddeus directed. The water was warm, but it helped clean out his mouth and calmed his stomach. "How did Slayer get her?" Sam took another drink and forced air through his mouth and nose.

"She just vanished. I have never seen anything like it." Thaddeus took a swig from his own jug. Was it filled with water or liquor? Sam guessed liquor. "She did it for us, you know. She gave herself to Slayer to save you."

Sam sighed. "I know."

They sat quietly. Sam surveyed the deck that had become their life raft. It was a large section of *The Mutineer II*, about the length of a mid-sized car. Pools of blood—their blood—mixed with seawater on the deck.

Thaddeus must have pulled him to safety and found some supplies, as there was a chest of what looked like food and either more water or rum aboard. A couple of pistols, knives and swords were tied to the deck. A hammer, some rigging, shredded portions of sail and lose timber were also aboard.

Sam thought back to the explosion. They had been trapped by Slayer's magic on *The Mutineer II* and the boat had basically disintegrated around them and yet they had survived.

"How are we alive, Thaddeus?"

"I cannot say for sure. All I know is that your back, where that fire sword of yours seems to come from, started to glow bright orange and that glow engulfed you and then me. Best I can figure is that you somehow saved us with your magic. You must be stronger than you know."

"I didn't do anything."

"I cannot explain it. I do not even know if it is true. But it is the only answer I can think of because you are right. We should be dead. Your magic seems to come when you are threatened and the greater the threat, the greater your power. We can use that against Slayer. That and the fact he thinks you are dead. He did not even stay around to see your body. He thinks you disintegrated into nothing."

Sam whirled in each direction. The sea around them revealed no trace of Slayer. He slipped away in his search for the Sword of Zel-Kar, with the belief the Chosen One was dead. *But I'm not dead!* Sam turned his attention back to the wreckage. "I'm sorry I let this happen. I'm sorry you lost your boat—well, both boats."

"Do not waste a moment on feeling sorry. Rather, tell me what you now wish to do."

Sam rose shakily. "I have to save her, Thaddeus. I have to save her and stop Slayer. I know that now more than ever. Dream or no dream, I have to do something. If I'm this Chosen One, it's time I get to it."

Thaddeus smiled. "That is all I need to hear."

"But we've got no boat. It looks like even the longboat we stole from Vane is destroyed. We're stranded in the middle of nowhere."

"All I need to get us anywhere in this great sea are a few pieces of timber and a bit of sail." Thaddeus stood as well. "Now, let us make ourselves a mast and go save your witch."

Sam frowned but nodded. As they got to work, one thought weighed on him. What was it the old man in his vision said? *It falls upon you to finish what I began. Our family bloodline demands it. And he called himself an Every.* Sam wanted to share the vision with Thaddeus but decided it was best not to—for now. It was probably nothing more than a hallucination anyway. He could think about it later.

Right now, they had to rescue Sarah and the children.

## Chapter 23
### The Barrier—At Last

He couldn't focus. Whether from the sun, the heat or the cuts and scratches that covered his body, Sam's head pounded. Sweat saturated his brow. His stomach danced around; he thought he might spew. Again. Thaddeus's work didn't help. Each strike of hammer against timber shattered his skull. Sam just wanted to close his eyes and submit to the darkness that threatened to tunnel in on him. *No! If Thaddeus isn't giving in to his injuries, I can't either. Sarah needs us. She needs me.*

Sam craved another drink of water, but Thaddeus had said they needed to conserve their supplies. He was right. Sam knew that. It had been hours and Thaddeus hadn't touched a bit of water despite his labor under the sticky unforgiving Caribbean sun to build a makeshift mast with nails and timber he had salvaged from the wreckage.

*I should be working too.* He had started to work but soon tired and crumpled to the deck. Thaddeus had ordered him to rest. Sam tried to lift himself but couldn't find the strength. He glanced at Thaddeus. *The Mutineer* and *Mutineer II* captain worked despite serious injuries. A large gash in his side still bled through his shredded clothing. Gaping cuts covered his right leg where splinters of timber had sliced through him. As Thaddeus moved aboard their makeshift vessel, that right leg didn't budge. When he did try to take a step with that leg, he limped. *I should never have doubted him. He's a good man.*

"I think she is just about ready to sail." Thaddeus finally sipped from a jug of water and offered it to Sam. Bits of dirt danced around inside the jug, but the water looked inviting. Still, Sam shook his head. He hadn't worked and didn't deserve any more water.

"Aye, lad, take some water." Thaddeus ordered. "You are hurt, and we need you and that magic of yours strong if we hope to save that girl."

"What about you, Thaddeus?" Sam allowed himself just a drop of water. "I think you're hurt pretty bad."

"This is nothing." Thaddeus smiled, but winced at the same time as he tried to move his injured leg. "In the Navy, I was in some scuffles you would not believe. I have been shot and stabbed but nothing ever takes me down. I am tough. You have to be to live on the sea. Tell yourself that. It shall make you stronger."

Sam nodded.

"All right, let us set sail. We stay here much longer the sharks are sure to be on us." Thaddeus unfurled the sail, which quickly caught wind and the deck—their life raft—began its journey. Thaddeus knelt on the deck and controlled the sail.

Sam rose to his knees, took a deep breath and forced away the desire to vomit. He placed a hand on Thaddeus' shoulder. "I can't believe how you built a mast and sail on this deck in the middle of nowhere."

"When you sail alone, you best know what you are doing. You never know what the sea has planned for you."

*But that doesn't explain how this deck is even staying afloat.* Sam wanted to ask, but what was the point? Perhaps this remnant of *The Mutineer II* desired revenge as much as Thaddeus and was determined to stay afloat until they reached Slayer.

They sailed for hours in calm seas as the hot sun bore down on them. Sam dipped his head into the ocean and though the water was warm, it did help him cool off.

"I would not be so quick into that water." Thaddeus grabbed Sam's arm. "There are all kinds of sea creatures ready to drag you down to Davy Jones's Locker. I once saw a shark take a man's head clear off for doing just what you are doing now. And the sharks are nearby. I can feel them. They are tracking our blood."

After that, Sam did not dunk his head. His clothes dried around his body as if he was covered in plaster that weighed him down and sapped his strength. He could remove his shirt, but the clothing was protection against the sun. The heat didn't seem to bother Thaddeus. He had removed his long coat and vest and loosened the strings around the collar of his shirt, but he seemed at ease in the sun.

Sam forced himself to stand up. He blinked away the daze that threatened to knock him unconscious. "Thaddeus, can we save her?"

"I do not know, but I promise you we shall make Slayer regret he ever crossed our paths." Thaddeus touched the gash at his side, which no longer bled, but he squinted as he pulled his blood-stained shirt away from the wound. "I have revenge on my mind, and I mean to follow Slayer to the world's end if need be. I aim to take his fleet as my own."

"How do you plan to do that?"

"By getting you, the Chosen One, face to face with Slayer so you can kill him as is your destiny?"

Sam was quiet until his eyes caught a dark object in the distance. He crawled to the edge of the deck and strained to focus on what appeared to be *a wall*. "Could it be?" he asked.

"What?"

"There, in the distance, don't you see it?" Sam gazed at a shadowy form that rose from the water, like a dark cloud—like the cloud barrier he had seen in his vision.

"I see nothing but water and clear skies on the horizon."

"What? No, it's there. Look closer!" Sam pointed to the barrier.

"The sun and the sea are playing tricks on your mind." Thaddeus reached for the jug of water. "Take a drink and rest."

Sam shook his head. It was there. He was sure of it. He grabbed Thaddeus' arm and pulled him to the edge of the deck. "I'm not crazy!"

Thaddeus kept silent until a smile crossed his face. "By God, I see it! I do not know what it is, but I see it, and we are heading right into it!"

Sam eyed Thaddeus then focused on his own hand, which still held onto Thaddeus' arm. "Wait a second."

He released Thaddeus and the reaction was immediate. "It is gone! I cannot see it anymore. What trickery is this?"

One more time Sam gripped Thaddeus's arm. "Do you see it now?"

Thaddeus nodded. "What game is this?"

Sam kept his eyes on the wall of clouds. "I know why only those of us with magic can reach the island where the Sword of Zel-Kar is supposed to be. The island isn't part of this world. To reach it, you have to cross through a magical barrier, but even that barrier only exists for those with magic abilities. That's why you can only see it if I'm touching you. That's why the British Navy will never be able to stop Slayer. They can't pass through to that other world."

Thaddeus slumped down to the deck and sat crossed-legged. "I have seen many things in my travels, and I fear nothing, but why do I get the feeling if we cross through that barrier of yours, we are never coming out?"

"Get me to the edge of that barrier and I'll cross through myself. You've done enough."

Thaddeus took a deep breath and stood again. "My desire for revenge has not softened. If Slayer is in there, then my future lies within that new world. So find a way to get me in there as I have no intention to turn back."

Sam nodded as he rested a hand on his lower back, over the birthmark. *Hang on, Sarah, we're coming for you. Hang on.*

The barrier loomed like a wall to some dark castle that extended to the clouds. The sky just before the barrier was blue and clear with just a few white puffy clouds. But where the sea met the barrier, a wall of dark, murky storm clouds rose from the water to the heavens and extended north and south as far as he could see. It stretched so far that it reminded him of the Great Wall of China. While the water just before the barrier was calm, a storm raged beyond the wall. Flashes of lighting lighted up the clouds and thunder roared deep inside the barrier.

"My God," Thaddeus gasped. "How about you let go of me so I do not have to see what we are facing?"

Sam shook his head and tightened his grip. "If I let go, I'm not sure you'll be able to cross through the barrier. I'm not even sure you'll be able to cross with me holding onto you. I'm not sure I can even cross through."

"What are you sure of?" Thaddeus kept his eyes on the barrier.

"Nothing," Sam admitted, "except if this is real, that's where we have to go to save Sarah and stop Slayer."

"So there is a chance this is nothing more than witchcraft?"

"There's a chance."

"But you think it is real?"

"Yes."

Thaddeus placed a hand on Sam's shoulder. "By all means, take us in, lad."

As the floating deck moved closer to the barrier, the tiny craft picked up speed. "We're being sucked in!" Sam yelled as he grabbed onto the mast.

"Aye, I can see that." Thaddeus did the same. "Hold on!" Their craft picked up more speed. They were close—very close. Sam held his breath and counted. *Five, four, three, two…*

Before he counted down to one, they burst through the barrier, and the world around them went crazy. Winds blew. Water thrashed. Clouds swirled. Lighting flashed. Thunder followed. A wave slammed the deck and knocked Sam down. He slid toward the edge of the makeshift boat, but Thaddeus grabbed his collar.

As the wind screamed, the mast snapped in two. Ripped free, the sail vanished in the darkness. A fog surrounded them while hail pelted them. Sam could barely see Thaddeus' face.

"We're going to die!" Thaddeus shouted. The wind's cry nearly drowned out his voice. "You have to do something!" Thaddeus was right, but what? A piece of the deck splintered off as another wave struck them. "Lad!"

Excruciating pain radiated from Sam's lower back to his shoulder blades. Smoke rose around him. His shirt disintegrated into ashes. He wished to fall into a snow pack to ease the inferno that assaulted his back, but at the same time he was thankful. *The fire sword!* He reached into his back until his hands found the flaming blade. *Yes!* He quickly freed the sword from his back and held it with two hands. For some reason, he uttered the words, "Sword, guide my way." He repeated the mantra over and over as he pointed the fire blade straight ahead into the fog. From the tip of the sword, a single flame shot forward; it paved a blazing line through the fog and created a cavern through which they could pass.

Sam held onto the sword as tightly as he could and kept the blade pointed forward. Like his fishing rod back home, the flame hooked their destination and the sword reeled them toward wherever the barrier would take them.

His arms shook as the sword grew heavy, but he refused to let go. All around them, the wind blew and the water thrashed, but within the cavern the sword had created, all was calm.

"Look!" Thaddeus pointed. "Is that an opening?"

Sam blinked several times to steady his vision. Yes, there did seem to be light that pierced through the darkness. His arms wavered and the sword drooped.

"Steady, lad." Thaddeus grabbed hold of Sam's arms. "Stay strong. Our survival depends on you."

Sam gritted his teeth. Even with Thaddeus' support, his muscles screamed and his wrists felt like they might break. But they were closer. The light grew brighter. *Hold on! Hold on!*

In another heartbeat, they burst through the barrier.

# Chapter 24
## What Is This Place?

"Where in all the world have you delivered us?" Thaddeus' eyes were wide. His hands crushed his three-cornered hat. "I have never seen the likes."

The burning sword vanished. Sam slumped to his knees. His arms throbbed and his hands pulsated with a reddish glow. His head throbbed, like an explosion had ripped through his skull. All he wanted was to close his eyes and give in to the darkness that hovered over him.

"Boy, stay with me." Thaddeus placed his hands on Sam's shoulders. "You did it. You saved us, but we are in a strange place, and Sarah is still out there somewhere. If you truly mean to save her, you cannot stop now. Not when we are so close."

Thaddeus was right. Sam took a deep breath. He opened his eyes and slowly, painfully rose. Sarah was out there, and she deserved to be saved along with the kidnapped children. Once on his feet, Sam focused on the world they had entered, and his jaw dropped. Silence descended over their deck until Thaddeus shattered the quiet. "I have not seen a sea bleed like this since the blood of a hundred dead men floated against the wreck of a French merchant ship pirates raided." The sea did seem to bleed. The water that surrounded their deck was a deep crimson for as far as Sam's eyes could see.

Sam squinted against an orange sun in the West, the crown over an emerald sky. But, as he turned to the East, the green gave way to a purple nighttime sky spotted by stars and an array of large planets seemingly close enough to touch, as if their raft floated through space instead of within a crimson sea. It was as if day and night coexisted here.

The cry of a creature split the sky. "What in all the seas was that?" Thaddeus pointed toward the West. A beast, with a wingspan the size of an airliner, dove in their direction. "Is that a…?" Thaddeus asked.

"A dragon!" Sam finished Thaddeus' thought. "And it's coming right at us!" The dragon unleashed a terrible scream as it grew closer. Its neck was long and its head spiked. A long tail, spiked just like its head, whipped around ready to plunge into any victim the dragon chose.

"I think it best we not be here!" Thaddeus held the grip of the pistol tucked into his belt.

"What do we do?" Sam reached toward his back to again bring forth the burning sword.

"Into the water, boy, now!"

"The blood water?"

"Now!" Thaddeus dove into the water first. Sam eyed the dragon a split second longer before he followed Thaddeus. As soon as Sam was beneath the surface, the shadow of the dragon passed low over the sea before the beast disappeared with one last growl that, though muted by the water, still caused Sam to shiver.

Unsure if it was safe to surface, Sam stayed underwater where the warm crimson sea energized him. *What is this!* His exhaustion slipped away, the pain from his wounds, which should have stung in the salty water, faded. His strength grew. Finally, short on air, he cautiously surfaced. He rose just enough out of the water to keep most of his head hidden by the deck. From there, he scanned the emerald sky for any sign of the dragon. It had vanished as if it had never been there. Also gone was the cloud barrier they had passed through.

Thaddeus emerged from the sea and quickly climbed onto the deck. He had a wide smile and his eyes beamed. "Lad, look at me!"

Sam climbed onto the raft. "What?"

"I'm healed! All my wounds have just gone away." Thaddeus spun around and danced."I have no recollection of any time I have felt this good." He was right. Though blood still stained his clothes, the gashes and holes in his body were gone, and his eyes were sharp, no longer marked by the red lines of hidden pain. "Look at yourself."

Sam scanned his own body. His wounds had disappeared, too. "It has to be the water."

"Maybe this is not such a bad place you have led us after all." Thaddeus' laughter spread over the sea, but it didn't last. Steam and a stench, like the engine exhaust spewed from an old car, came from behind them, followed by low, guttural breaths. Thaddeus turned slowly.

Sam didn't want to. "The dragon?"

"Aye." Thaddeus timidly reached for his pistol and sword. Sam couldn't bring himself to move. His body froze. But one thought filled his mind. *Why didn't the sword warn me? It seems to come alive when I'm in danger. Maybe...*

Sam peered toward the sound of the dragon. Its neck rose from the sea, its massive head towered over the deck. Its eyes were catlike, golden orbs surrounded by a sea of blazing yellow. Natural armor, a mix of shades of dark green, black and purple, covered the dragon's head and neck. Horns rose from the head and fangs as long as Sam's arms protruded from either side of the snout.

Thaddeus lifted the pistol from his belt. "No," Sam whispered. The dragon's eyes shifted once to Thaddeus and the lips at the end of its snout curled up—much like an angry dog—to reveal a mouth full of razor-sharp white fangs. Thaddeus didn't speak. He slid the pistol back into his belt and raised his hands to show the dragon they were empty. "What now?"

*What now? How am I supposed to know? Now, we pray fire doesn't come spewing from its mouth or it doesn't decide it's time for a meal.* "Just don't move." Sam kept his voice calm. "I don't think he means us any harm."

The dragon lowered its head to within a few feet of his face. Sam stared into two large nostrils. Sweat dripped from his brow at the steam the creature produced with each breath. The creature growled softly. It sniffed him from head to foot. Then it quickly snapped its head back and shook its head.

*Is he disgusted by my smell?* As if to answer, the dragon bared its fangs and hissed two words in a language Sam had never heard before but somehow understood. "Siiiisoosaaa Haaassiiii." The dragon didn't speak again. It lifted its wings from the water, spread them out, like a huge umbrella, and, with one mighty thrust, took flight. Once airborne it flew high into the western sky. Sam followed it as long as he could, but the dragon disappeared against the orange sun.

"The creature spoke." Thaddeus released a lungful of air.

"Yes, and I know what it said."

"How?" Thaddeus grabbed Sam's shoulder and twisted him around so they were face to face.

"I don't know how." Sam again stared at the emerald sky, but there was no sign of the dragon. "I just know."

"All right, then, what did its words mean?"

Sam glared at Thaddeus. "He called me Chosen One."

# Chapter 25
## The Rising Twins

"In my lifetime I have heard tales of the kraken and the lusca roaming the sea, but I have never seen the beasts." Thaddeus sat on their deck, breathless, like a child who has just seen a mall Santa Claus for the first time. "Truth be told, I have never believed in such stories. I always thought they were simply the creation of drunken men meant to scare young sailors. Now you bring me to a world with dragons. Talking dragons! I nearly relieved myself at the sight of the creature. I am no coward but it makes me fearful for what other terrible monsters we might face here."

"I think Slayer is the biggest monster we have to worry about," Sam offered as he took a sip of water from a jug.

Thaddeus shook his head. "I would much prefer to fight a man—even one endowed with magic. All it takes is a good sword and strong arm, and you can kill the likes of Slayer. A dragon—I am not so sure."

"That dragon is a friend, I think." Sam glanced toward the skies, but the beast had vanished.

"You keep strange friends." Thaddeus removed the vest that covered his shirt and handed it to Sam. It wasn't much more than threads, but at least it would provide some protection from this world's sun as Sam's shirt had burned away when the fire sword ignited. Thaddeus continued to speak. "Dragons aside, lad, I must say our time together has not been dull. If I had not abandoned *The Mutineer* and the witch… I mean Sarah… had not sacrificed herself, I would call this a grand adventure. Maybe it is the strange healing powers of this red sea, but I find myself with newfound hope that we shall survive this, save that brave girl, the children, and find our way back home."

Sam nodded, but he didn't agree. *I wish I felt that way.*

"I wonder what this world shall bring us next?" Thaddeus took the jug from Sam and swallowed just a drop of water.

"I don't know the answer to that, Thaddeus. There should have been an island here—really two islands that joined at their peaks and my vision showed me that those islands would lead us to a third island where the Sword of Zel-Kar should be, but there's nothing here."

"There must be a reason we came all this way. Your island must be around these parts somewhere." Thaddeus rose to his feet. "Do not lose heart now. Your little witch friend is out there waiting for you to save her."

"But where?" Sam's words echoed over the sea and the water rumbled back a response. It started low, but grew in intensity, like the earthquakes back home. The sound stirred from deep within the sea and brought waves that pushed against their floating deck.

"Oh my!" Thadddeus struggled to maintain his balance as the sea rumbled louder, the sea swelled, and their deck tossed side to side. "Hold on!" he called out.

"To what?" Sam's eyes caught sight of an object toward the distant western horizon. "Thaddeus, do you see it?" Whatever it was, it burst from the sea's surface and grew toward the sky, and like a ripple effect, caused waves—the largest yet—to crash toward them.

"God save us!" Thaddeus mumbled. He pointed to a wall of water, its crest several stories high. The tower of blood-red sea eclipsed everything as it raced toward them. "Lay down on the deck!" he barked.

The tidal wave sucked-in their raft, like objects are sucked into a black hole in space. Sam did as Thaddeus instructed. He laid flat on the deck as it rushed toward the massive surge of bloody water. But what was the point? There was no way to survive this.

"Stay down!" Thaddeus bellowed. "We are not done for yet. We are light. We can ride this to the crest, get over it, and slip down the other side. Whether we live or die, they shall sing of our glory for facing such a wave."

Sam lay on the deck, chin up, and faced the mountain of water. He thought of his mom, dad, brothers, friends, even his cousin Zack—the life he used to have. His thoughts shifted to Sarah, and this new life he had discovered. She still needed him as did those kidnapped kids. Thaddeus was right. They could survive this— they had to. *I'm the Chosen One.* Sam gripped the edge of the deck and tightened his hands, arms, and stomach. He held his breath.

The wave roared as it hid the sky and painted the world within Sam's view blood red. Like a giant hand, the colossal wave reached out to crush them. They would die for sure unless Thaddeus was right—unless they could ride the wave like some surfer back home. *Or maybe my fire sword can help!* Sam started to reach for his magic blade, but it was too late. The wave was upon them.

"You're not going to kill us today!" Thaddeus shook a fist.

"Not today." Sam echoed Thaddeus' words. A wind generated by the powerful tsunami wave howled back at them, and his confidence faded. *Mom, Dad... I love you guys. I'm sorry for leaving you,* Sam thought. He was sure death was upon them until the unexpected happened. As if someone cut a loaf of bread down the middle, the wave split in two from its highest point down toward its heart. The tear in the wave moved quickly. By the time the mountainous wave reached them, it had completely divided into two and formed a passageway between the two separate waves.

Thaddeus shouted and Sam covered his head. The two waves rushed past them and their little deck was slung, as if fired from a slingshot, through the passage. The timber shivered and creaked like it would break-up. *Please stay together*, Sam begged. Instead, a piece of deck Sam gripped snapped off and he flew back. Thaddeus snatched him from the air with one hand and held him by the wrist "I ordered you to hold on!" he shouted over the water's roar.

Sam cried out as his legs flailed behind him. "Thaddeus!" His wrist bone cracked and his shoulder popped. "I'm slipping!"

"I forbid it!" Thaddeus yelled as they emerged on the backside of the waves and their wild ride ended. The water calmed. The crimson sea grew silent. The air moved softly. Sam collapsed onto the deck and couldn't stop the tears that formed. He quickly wiped his eyes. *Why am I crying? Stop it!*

"It is all right. I shall not tell the lass." Thaddeus knelt on the deck and rubbed his arm as though it ached from the strain of saving Sam's life.

"Thank—"

"No words are necessary." Thaddeus shook his head. "I did nothing. Your magic is what saved us. How did you do it?"

Sam wiped another tear. "I don't know. Maybe I had nothing to do with it. Maybe it was me. I wish I understood my powers." He glanced toward the direction the two waves had traveled as he breathed in as much air as possible and slowed his heart.

"No reason to question it. The sea is on our side this day. Nothing else matters." Thaddeus patted the deck of *The Mutineer II*, their life raft. "We must give a proper thank you to the remains of *The Mutineer II*. She is not much, but she still has the heart of a boat. I imagine, though, we shall not be trading her back to Vane."

Sam turned in the direction the wave had originated. Two islands that hadn't been there before now filled the western horizon. "Thaddeus, look! Do you see them?"

"I do. They rose from the deep."

Sam swallowed saliva. "They have to be the missing islands! They must have caused the waves!"

"Aye. I guess they would be our destination." Thaddeus did not look pleased.

"They have to be. I'm sure just beyond them will be the island where we'll find the Sword of Zel-Kar. I know it."

Thaddeus sighed. "There are bad things under the sea. If that is where these islands come from, I foresee pain and death ahead."

Sam gulped. "I hope for Slayer and not us. Either way, what choice is there but to get to those islands and see what's on the other side?"

With a nod, Thaddeus grabbed a side of the deck and pulled with all his might until a plank broke off.

"What are you doing?"

"We have no sail. How do you think we get to your islands?" He thrust the plank in the water and started to row. Sam reached for a loose plank, wrestled with it until it separated from the deck. Though he panted from the fight to free the plank, he jammed it into the water and rowed along with Thaddeus.

There was no way to tell how long they rowed. For the longest time, no matter how much they paddled, they could not close the distance to the islands. His arms ached, but Sam rowed harder with each stroke to keep a rhythmic pace with Thaddeus. *Please, let us get there. I'm so tired. I can't go on much more. No! You have to push on.*" When his strength depleted, he slumped to his knees. "Thaddeus—"

"We are nearly there. Look. Listen."

Sam peered up and gasped. They were close—close enough to see waves crash onto the shores of the twin islands. Sunlight sparkled on the golden sand as the water ebbed and flowed. Beyond the beaches, rainbow colored walls of thick, lush tropical trees and brush rose toward each island's single peak, which slanted toward each other to form an archway high above the shores. A waterfall of the same crimson water as the sea cascaded from the archway down to the passageway between the two islands. A red mist from the waterfall spread over the tropical jungle. It gave Sam the sense that a fire storm covered the trees.

*Wait a second!* Sam squinted at the waterfall. "Thaddeus, am I crazy or is that water actually moving up from the sea toward the peaks?"

"I have never seen the like." Thaddeus shook his head. "How can water flow up?"

Sam smiled. "Magic."

Thaddeus snorted. "So you say. Now, Chosen One, where do we go from here?"

"We go between the islands through the waterfall."

"And what then?"

"I believe we'll find another island just beyond these two and that's where the sword is hidden." They rowed toward the passageway between the two islands. Sam strained to listen for any signs of life. He heard nothing, save the crash of the waves as they reached the two separate shores, and the flow of the sea as it surged through the passageway and magically ascended toward the archway that connected both islands. He also watched for any signs of Slayer.

"Careful," Thaddeus warned as they moved into the passageway. "This could be a trap."

"I don't think so. The skin on my back isn't burning. My sword isn't warning me of any danger."

"That may be, but caution is prudent." Thaddeus scanned the shorelines on either side of the passageway. He rowed with one hand and in the other held his pistol cocked and ready to fire.

Sam nodded. "You're right." Slayer had to be nearby. He had taken Sarah and left them for dead among the wreckage of *The Mutineer II*. He must have sailed for the barrier, but there was no way to tell how far ahead he was unless... *Slayer isn't really sure where to find the barrier. Can it be that he's lost somewhere back in the Caribbean?*

If that were the case, they could reach the Sword of Zel-Kar first, find their way back to the Caribbean, and use the sword to save Sarah and the kidnapped children. *Armed with the sword, I can kill Slayer and protect the future. Imagine all I can do with the Sword of Zel-Kar. Destroying Slayer is just the beginning. I can become immortal and go through time, stopping all evil in the world. I can create the perfect world—one I can control with the sword.* Sam shook those thoughts away. *What am I saying? That would make me no better than Slayer or would it?*

"You expect me to do all the work, do you?" Thaddeus nudged Sam with the barrel of his pistol.

"Huh?" Sam's focus returned to Thaddeus.

"You are no longer rowing. You are just standing there. What would you be gnawing on in that head of yours?"

"Nothing," Sam lied. He wasn't about to tell Thaddeus of his thoughts of world domination. He wasn't even sure where such thoughts had come from, but they had not yet vanished.

"Start your rowing," Thaddeus ordered, "and keep your eyes pierced. Your sword may not be burning your back, but I sense

Slayer is around here somewhere, and he shall not be too happy to see us alive."

Sam dipped his plank into the water and rowed. "Why do you think Slayer's not attacking, if he's here?"

"Fine question. He may think you are dead. That would be the most likely notion. But I have two other thoughts. First, he may fear you, so he is keeping his distance as he searches for the sword to use it against you."

"And what's your other thought."

"He may not fear you one bit."

"So he wouldn't bother to leave traps or any of his men to stop us then," Sam reasoned. "He'll just kill me when he feels like it."

"Kill us, lad. And I have no desire to die, so we best make sure we are ready for anything." They rowed on in silence. The islands remained largely quiet. But there was a mix of whispery noises—leaves that rubbed against each other, a hidden creature's soft cry, and the thud of a coconut as it hit the ground. Or were the noises something else?

A few more strokes and they arrived at the waterfall. Sam craned his neck as he watched the water flow up toward the archway. *That is freaky*, he thought. The weird waterfall also was strangely quiet—a mere whisper when it should have declared its presence with a thunderous cry.

Sam reached out with one hand toward the water as it inexplicably defied gravity. Slowly, cautiously his fingers extended toward the upward falls. When his whole body shook, he yanked his hand back.

"Go ahead—see what happens," Thaddeus urged. "What is the worst that can happen? You set off some Slayer trap that sends a million deadly arrowheads flying at us from the peaks above."

"Thanks, that helps." Sam frowned at Thaddeus, sucked in a lungful of air and reached again toward the surging flow. His heartbeat echoed in his ears like bass drums at a rock concert. He took short, shallow breaths. His muscles stiffened. A cold sweat dotted his brow. *You can do this.* With one final push, he thrust his hand into the falls and—nothing. He pulled out his hand and examined it front and back. He wiggled his fingers. His hand was fine. He peered upwards, but he hadn't sprung any traps. He plunged his hand back into the water. Again, nothing changed. "I think it's safe."

"Then let us be on our way. These islands are unnatural. The sooner we leave them behind the better." Thaddeus tucked his pistol in his belt and rowed forward into the falls. Sam did the same. He expected to burst through the other side to a view of the island where they would find the Sword of Zel-Kar. Instead, they became trapped in the falls.

"We're not moving!" Sam cried.

"I can see that!"

The water blinded Sam. It poured into his mouth, up his nose, and drowned all pathways to his lungs. He struggled to clear his eyes and to breathe. "What do we do?" he shouted as he coughed up seawater.

"You are the Chosen One!" Thaddeus covered his face with his hands. His words were lost in a gurgle. "She is your girl not mine. This is your rescue!"

"Think of something," Sam pleaded to himself, but he couldn't control his thoughts. He just wanted to break free of the water and breathe. He forced his eyes open just for a moment. They weren't just trapped in the waterfall. The upward rush of the water lifted their deck up toward the arch.

"Thaddeus—"

"I know! Hold on for your life!"

The deck ascended horizontally through the falls. Sam dropped to his knees and gripped the deck as it swayed side to side. He had to stay calm, had to hold on, but his lungs burned. Still they climbed. *When will it end? I can't hold on!*

Sam's head dropped forward as the flow of water filled his lungs and cut off air. He jerked his head up, but the water-clogged heaviness forced his head to sag again. His eyelids seemed glued shut. A gray fog flittered around the edges of his mind. The waterfall threatened to drown him. *No, you can't! You'll die! Stop it. Stay awake just a little longer.* The fight within his mind worked. He remained conscious, but if he didn't breathe soon—

The falls flung the deck into the air like a pebble shot from a rubber sling. The makeshift boat soared until it crash landed into another body of water. Thrown from the deck, Sam plunged headfirst into the water.

Underneath the surface, the water was cloudy. He couldn't see more than a foot in either direction. Disoriented, he twisted wildly. *Which way back to the surface?* Light—he had to find light. But a murky cloud of mud and the blood-colored water surrounded him in darkness.

Something snagged his shirt and yanked hard to lift him out of the water. He broke the surface, and before he could even focus his eyes, he coughed out enough seawater to fill three buckets.

"I have you," a familiar voice declared.

"Thaddeus," Sam rejoiced through coughs.

"We are alive—yet again." Thaddeus pulled him onto the deck. "But something tells me this adventure is far from over. We need to stay ready. The current is starting to move fast."

Sam coughed out the last bit of water, took a deep breath and rose to his knees. He peered back. They were at the top of the falls—the archway that connected both islands.

Still on his knees, he patted the deck. How had their makeshift boat survived? What kept it intact? *Thank you for staying together. You must want Slayer as bad as I do. Hang on just a little more, boat.*

When Sam looked ahead, something was wrong. Gone was any sign that there were two separate islands. Instead, they floated down a wide stream of what appeared to be a single island. Large, tropical brush—the craziest looking trees with corkscrew trunks and wagon wheel-sized flowers, hugged the shore on either side of the stream. Thick brush prevented glimpses of whatever lay beyond the stream.

Thaddeus was right—the waterway flowed faster by the second. "I may be mistaken, but we seem to be a flowing downhill," Thaddeus crouched and placed his arms in the water as if to slow their life raft.

"I don't understand. This isn't what I saw in my vision." Sam's ears detected a rush of water up ahead. He tried to climb to his feet to see farther downstream but slipped as the deck sped forward. "We should have come through the waterfall and found a third island, the one with the sword."

"Visions can be wrong, boy." Thaddeus took hold of the deck just like he did when they faced the giant wave. "Whatever may come, I suggest you hold on to something now."

Sam lowered himself and gripped the deck. The stream grew angry as if it wished to flip the deck. Swells of whitewater splashed skyward. The water slapped him in the face with the sting of an ice-filled snowball. *What's coming next? Is this world trying to kill us?* The water howled as it twisted and turned and smashed against rocks in the stream.

Sam sighed: "I just want off this deck. I miss dry land."

"I knew you were a landlubber." Thaddeus lowered onto his belly. "Here we go!"

The remains of the deck plunged into the rapids. It dove, twisted and turned as it wrestled the water. The rapids flowed to the right and curved to the left. The deck slammed against rocks. Pieces of wood splintered off and disappeared from view. Every few hundred feet the deck plunged down small waterfalls and each time the water seemed to push them faster and faster but toward what? *Is it ever going to end?* They smashed against another rock and even more of the deck gave way. There wasn't much left now of their life raft save a few planks that somehow managed to hold together.

"Look!" Thaddeus pointed ahead.

Sam followed Thaddeus' finger. The rapids vanished into the sky up ahead. That meant one thing—*another waterfall.* Only this one might send them down to their deaths.

"Get to shore!" Thaddeus ordered. They both paddled furiously with their hands. They tried to steer the deck to the shore on their right, but it didn't work. "It is too late. We are going over. Grab a plank. Brace yourself."

The deck raced toward the falls. A quick glance over the edge revealed a long drop. A white mist seemed to rise toward them, like the magic beanstalk in the old fairytale.

"I want to wake—" Before Sam could finish that thought, the deck plunged. He screamed and clutched the deck. Fast shallow breaths did little to fill his lungs. He forced his eyes shut. No reason to see the long fall that would ultimately smash them against rocks hundreds of feet below. But as their chorus of screams continued, the remains of their deck never pitched into a vertical fall. *Wait a second—we're not falling.* Sam cautiously opened his eyes. The deck remained horizontal and seemed to float downward gently. Sam peered beneath the deck. The white mist had formed into a ramp. *How—*

He let the question trail off. In this world where magic is clearly at work, anything is possible.

"Nothing makes sense here," Thaddeus asserted.

"Don't complain. We're alive, right?"

"Unless we are already dead and resting at the bottom of Davy Jones's Locker." The mist led them down to the base of the waterfall and softly deposited them back into a stream that led to the sea.

Not far ahead was an island—far larger than the twins through which they had just traveled. This island had a number of peaks and valleys, but the largest peak had a distinctive shape—the shape Sam had seen in his vision. He shuddered. "Thaddeus, is that what I think it is?"

"It looks like it. A mountain shaped like a skull."

"That's what I thought." Either nature or man had shaped the granite into a skull with deep-set eyes, a triangular nose, and a huge mouth filled with fangs. The eyes seemed to stare directly at him.

Thaddeus must have noticed. "I think they are staring right at you. This must be your missing island. Are you sure this is where you want to go?"

Sam answered, though he never looked away from the skull. "Like I said before, I don't have a choice."

# Chapter 26
## Skull Island Awaits

It didn't take long to reach the island. Once on shore, they pulled the remains of their life raft onto the beach and sat down in the warm sand. They stared at the deck—little more than a few planks barely attached to each other.

"Sorry, you lost two boats because of me, Thaddeus."

Thaddeus fingered a small piece of the deck that had chipped off onto the beach. "I do not grieve much for the loss of Vane's sloop, but *The Mutineer* served me well. I hope to one day be reunited with her."

"If I can help, I will." Sam placed a hand on his shoulder.

Thaddeus shook off Sam's hand. "I do indeed hope we find and kill Slayer as I aim to claim as many of his ships as I can. He owes me with his life. Let us hope your magic is stronger than his."

"I still don't know what my magic can do." Sam pounded the sand. "Besides this fire sword in my back, I don't even know if I have any magic."

"Nothing better than trial by fire and that burning blade has certainly brought its share of trials, though it is a great ally." Thaddeus stood and dusted away the sand from his soaked clothing. "We should be on our way. We have some climbing ahead of us."

Sam stood and peered at the skull. "You mean there, huh."

"Aye, lad."

"I still can't believe there's no sign of Slayer." Sam scratched his head. "It's like he just disappeared."

"Strange, yes, but do not doubt that he is close. We would do well to get off this shore and into that brush. We can use it to hide our trail and throw off Slayer."

They started toward the lush jungle just beyond the shore until a new rumble from the sea stopped them. The ground under their feet shook, slowly at first, then violently. Sam swung around to face the sea. Just as mysteriously as they rose, the twin islands plummeted into the ocean; a giant wave formed in their wake and rushed toward the shore where Sam stood.

"Run, boy! Get to high ground!" Thaddeus tripped over his own feet and fought to keep his balance as he bolted from the beach. Sam raced after Thaddeus in a dash toward the thick brush. They smashed through plant life until high treetops blocked the sun and encased them in darkness. The canopy of trees allowed only a few beams of light to illuminate their path.

"Don't stop!" Thaddeus pulled Sam through the undergrowth as an explosion that matched the deafening boom of cannon fire rolled over them. Thaddeus glanced back. "Here comes the wave!"

The rush of water filled Sam's ears as the wave crashed onto the shore. Massive trees cracked—a signal of the seawater's approach as it overcame the beach and flowed up the hillside. Sam glanced back as floodwater washed over their feet, their calves and up to their knees. *Oh, God! We're not going to make it!* "The water's on us!" Still, the water rose to their thighs and their waists.

"Keep running!" Thaddeus still gripped his arm.

Sam splashed through water, stumbled but fought to stay on his feet. "I can't make it!"

"Yes, you can!" Thaddeus dragged him through the water. "You have to!"

The direction of the water suddenly shifted. It flowed back toward the blood ocean. Sam breathed a sigh of relief as he realized the water level lowered, until the water began to drag him out to sea and toward death.

"Grab a tree! The water is going to try to suck us out to sea!" Thaddeus wrapped an arm around the tree in front of him. He grunted as, with his free hand, he pulled Sam toward the same tree. Teeth clenched, Sam grasped the tree with one hand then the other. He mashed his face against the trunk. "Do not let go!" Thaddeus commanded.

"Are you kidding me? Of course I won't let go!" He hugged the tree, like he used to hug his mom after a day of kindergarten. The water did its best to tear his grip from the tree. *You're not going to take me, sea! Not today!*

It took just seconds for the floodwaters to slip down the hillside. When the water disappeared, Sam eased his grip on the tree and fell into the mud. He gazed at the devastation left by the floodwaters. Many of the trees had fallen under the sea's crushing might. Those that stood were cracked and splintered. Mud replaced the thick brush.

Next to Sam, Thaddeus slid from the trunk and joined him on the ground. Neither spoke for several minutes. Sam blew out a lungful of air to end the silence. "I think we're safe."

"Are we now?" Thaddeus took a deep breath, reached for a low-hanging tree branch and pulled himself to his feet. "Slayer must still be around somewhere. Safe! I would not be so sure. We must keep moving."

Sam ran his hands through his hair and sighed. Thaddeus was right. The situation looked more hopeless by the minute. *I'm no hero. What am I even doing here? I don't belong here.*

Thaddeus extended a hand to Sam. "I see that lost look in your eyes. My words are not meant to discourage you. I just mean to point out the truth. I believe you have magic you have not learned to use yet. So it would be wise not to give up."

*The Mutineer* captain started to walk farther up the hill. Sam wiped mud from his clothing and followed. *Fine, hero or not, Chosen One or not, let's find that sword, save Sarah and the children, and get back home.*

Thaddeus bounded up the hillside. He nimbly dodged branches and brush, careful to make as little noise as possible and to not disturb the vegetation. That made sense. No reason to leave behind a trail for Slayer to follow. Sam moved less gracefully. Each time he crunched a dead leaf under his feet or broke a plant stem, he furrowed his brow. If Thaddeus was cautious not to make noise or reveal their path, *why can't I do the same*? He wiped sweat from his face. *What does it matter anyway? With my luck, Slayer already has the Sword of Zel-Kar. If so, I'll never save Sarah or the kidnapped children. I will have blown it and the world will suffer because I was too slow and weak.* He pounded one fist against the palm of his other hand. *Stop that! Don't be a baby. Just focus on what you have to do.* He raced to catch Thaddeus.

They made their way uphill through the brush in a heated climate that matched the Caribbean. He panted like a dog, and his skinny legs might buckle at any moment, but he refused to let Thaddeus know this. Intent on his objective, Sam would not stop.

Snap—a branch broke off to their right. Sam's head jerked up and he halted his climb. The slight burning sensation in his back signaled danger. *Could it be Slayer?*

Thaddeus glanced at him. "What is it?"

"Shhhh, stop moving—listen." The burning in his back worsened. He wanted to reach for the sword, if only to stop the pain. But he waited. Leaves on the ground just beyond their field of vision cracked as if someone approached. Sam's pulse quickened. *Am I ready for this? Am I ready to face Slayer? I have to be.* "Did you hear it?" Sam asked as the noise vanished.

"We are not alone," Thaddeus answered.

"Is it Slayer?"

"I do not think so." Thaddeus surveyed the tree line. The growth above of large, rainbow-colored plants and trees continued to block sunlight and left them in endless shade. The jungle made it impossible to see much farther than a few feet in any direction.

"So who is it?" Sam wondered aloud.

Thaddeus drew his pistol. "I believe that is the wrong question. Our pursuer is not a *who*. It is a *what*—perhaps one of your monster friends."

Sam started to reach for his sword. "Could it be the dragon?"

"Could be, but—"

The noise returned—louder. The crackle became a series of snaps as if tree limbs split under heavy weight. Sam closed his eyes and listened. Something slithered across the jungle floor. Then it stopped.

"I don't hear it anymore." Sam held his breath as he strained to hear the slightest crack of a stem or the breath of the person or beast that tracked them. "Let's keep moving."

"Wait," Thaddeus whispered.

"But—" Sam's back glowed, and he dropped to his knees. The fall saved his life. Something crashed through the jungle. The invader ripped tree trunks and brush in half as it cut a line through the air where Sam's head had been. Sam rolled several times. When he climbed to his feet, he gripped the fire sword and waved it in front of him. The flames swished through the air. "What was that?" He turned in every direction, but saw only fallen trees and broken brush.

Thaddeus aimed his pistol in one direction and pointed his sword in another. "My eyes failed me. I did not see it clearly."

"We better get out—" Sam's sword blazed bright. Without hesitation he dove to the right. A massive snake head sprung from the shadows and snapped at him. His sword burned even brighter, like the sun. He rolled again as a second snake head crashed down from atop the trees. When his sword blazed red hot, he threw himself behind a large tree. A third snake head launched straight toward him. It smashed into the tree and forced Sam to spin away as the tree fell. He ran to Thaddeus, and they stood back to back.

"I told you evil was awaiting us." Thaddeus held his pistol and sword directly in front of his body.

Sam gripped his fire sword with both hands. His eyes scanned the jungle around them, but all grew suddenly quiet. His sword's flame danced as it emitted an orange glow. "Should we run?" he asked.

"It would do no good," Thaddeus said, and Sam quickly realized he was right. The three snake heads burst through the jungle in front of Sam. They did not immediately strike. They swayed back and forth, up and down. Their eyes—solid black orbs—never blinked. Spiked tongues whipped out to reach for prey. Scales covered their heads, colored much like a tiger's orange and white stripes. The snake heads studied him as if they prepared for another attack.

"That's not something you see every day." Sam held his sword high and pointed the blade at each head. What first had seemed like three snakes was actually a single serpent with three heads. Its long body stretched endlessly into the jungle. The beast reminded Sam of the multi-headed serpent Hercules fought in Greek mythology. What was the monster called? Hydra? Yes, just like the constellation. "Well, they say snake soup tastes good, and I'm hungry. Let's kill this thing."

Thaddeus snorted. "Well done—a jest in the face of danger. I like that. It shows courage."

"How do we—" Sam started to ask.

The center head dove toward him. Thaddeus pushed Sam out of the way and fired his pistol. The round struck the snake head's open jaw and caused the beast to hiss in anger. It reeled its head up toward the sky. "Take that, beast!" Thaddeus fumbled with his pistol to reload it as the left head swooped down toward him. This time Sam stepped forward and swung his burning sword wildly, as if to hit a curveball. The snake dodged the blade and snapped again. Sam swung his sword one more time, but the snake avoided the blow. When it attacked a third time, he sliced across the beast's neck in a glancing blow that ripped at the snake's outer scales. The creature lurched back and whipped its tongue into the air. As it steadied itself, the snake head focused its cold eyes on him.

By this time, Thaddeus had reloaded. When the third snake head—the one on the right—leaped at them, he fired his weapon. The round struck that snake head in its right eye, and the beast cried out as it shook its head from side to side. Sam waited for that head to fall to the ground, but it recovered. Now one-eyed, the head joined the other two snake heads as they more cautiously prepared another attack.

"We are going about this all wrong." Thaddeus again reloaded his pistol. "We have to work together."

"How?"

"I shall draw one head down and you kill it."

"Gotcha."

Thaddeus lowered his pistol and approached the snake heads. "Come on, beast. I would make a fine morsel for you. Take a bite out of old Thaddeus." The center snake head launched itself at Thaddeus. Sam raised his sword and threw himself at the beast's neck. One mighty strike was all it would take. His burning sword could cut through the neck with ease. He was sure of it. He slashed at the snake's neck but his attack failed when the snake head to the right smashed into him and knocked him to the ground.

Before Sam could climb to his feet, Thaddeus jammed his sword into the center head's mouth. The snake whipped its head back and Thaddeus, who held onto the handle of the sword, was thrown over the trees and into the brush. He disappeared from view.

Sam stood alone. The left head lowered itself and twisted to grab the handle of Thaddeus' sword. It slowly pulled the blade from the mouth of the center snake then dropped it to the ground. Thick red blood fell from the center head, but all three heads remained alive. Sam searched for any sign of Thaddeus. There were none. Thaddeus probably lay unconscious somewhere.

*How am going to kill this thing by myself? Thaddeus where are you? I need you. Please don't be dead.* He took a few shallow breaths. *Get a grip man. You can't give up... not because of some killer snake.* He slowly backed away from the giant, Hydra-like snake. He kept his sword pointed at the beast and didn't stop his retreat until he backed into a tree trunk. "Fine, I'll fight you here!" he shouted. "Come and get me!"

The snake slithered forward. Each head dipped close to the ground as if to prepare for a strike. Sam's gaze shifted from one head to the next. Which would attack first? Would they all attack at once? Just yards away, the beast raised its three heads until they towered over him. The center one opened its mouth wide and bared yellow fangs the size of daggers. Blood dripped from its mouth. The heads to the right and left flicked their tongues. Sam focused on the center snake. "You won't take me easy. I swear I'll take at least one of you—"

A rustling from behind stopped him mid-sentence. Sam twisted around, but too late. The snake's tail curved around the tree and wrapped around his legs. "No!" All three snake heads hissed and snapped out their spiked tongues. The snake's tail encircled his torso and squeezed. Sam nearly dropped his sword as the air rushed from his lungs. His arms grew numb and shook uncontrollably. "Got to hold on to the sword." He willed away the shake in his arms and plunged the tip of his fiery sword into the snake's tail. Red blood squirted from the wound. The sticky, hot liquid covered Sam's hands, arms and clothing.

The snake loosened its grip, and Sam jumped away from the tail. He landed on the ground and rolled then rose to his feet, ready to defend himself again. With a whip of its tail, the snake slapped him in the back, just like when his cousin whipped wet towels at him at the beach. Each blow from Zack had stung. The slap of the snake's tail felt like ten wet towels struck him at once. Sam flew through the air until he crashed against a tree trunk and slumped to the ground. Darkness surrounded him, but he held onto his fiery sword. *Can't give up. Have to fight. Have to survive. Sarah is depending on me.*

He struggled to his feet and tried to lift his burning sword, but his arms were too weak. The blade dragged along the jungle floor. Sam peered into the eyes of the center snake. They seemed lifeless, but he sensed the snake's exhilaration, as if it knew its prey was defeated. The snake prepared to feast. With his last bit of strength, Sam lifted his fire sword. "Not done yet."

All three snake heads launched at him. He closed his eyes as he expected to be swallowed whole. Instead, a gust of wind blew him off his feet. A familiar roar echoed through the jungle. Just above the tree tops was the dragon—the one from the sea that called him *Chosen One.*

In its claws, the dragon dangled the three-headed snake. With one bite of its jaws and a twist of its massive head, the dragon tore the snake in two. Blood cascaded like a waterfall to the jungle. Sam's eyes locked once with the dragon. The creature then flew off, the two halves of the snake still within its claws.

Thaddeus burst through the jungle brush just as the dragon disappeared. "Did you see it?" Sam asked.

"Aye, lad." Thaddeus placed his pistol in his breeches. "It seems you have a pet dragon."

"I don't think it's a pet."

"Whatever it is, let us hope it continues to watch over you."

"I just hope we don't run in to any more of those three-headed snakes." Sam let go of his fiery sword, and it vanished. He dropped to his knees and forced himself to breathe carefully in and out. It hurt to breathe.

"Are you all right?" Thaddeus placed a hand on Sam's shoulder.

"I think so."

"If you are, we should be on the move. That snake may have family. Besides, we still have some climbing to do." Thaddeus offered his hand to Sam. "Come on, I shall help you walk."

"Thanks." He took hold of Thaddeus' hand.

Together, they climbed toward the skull-shaped peak. Sam turned back once and tried to peer through the jungle brush. *Where is Slayer? I can feel him. I know he's close.*

# Chapter 27
### The Cavern Of Shadows

Sam and Thaddeus trekked toward the skull quietly, and for the moment, without further interruption. If more three-headed snakes hid in the tropical jungle, they didn't attack. If more did exist, the dragon had frightened them off. A glimpse through the trees revealed no sign of the winged creature. "Please be there," Sam whispered.

Higher and higher they climbed, and their ascent soon changed from a gradual slope to a steep rise. Thaddeus showed his agility as he grabbed hold of tree limbs and hanging foliage and easily scaled what became a near vertical mountain. Sam scrambled to keep pace. A cold sweat drenched his hair and dripped off his temple onto his neck and shoulders. He grabbed hold of a tree branch to pull himself forward. It broke, and he started to slide down the mountain. He clutched at branches and plants, but couldn't find a grip.

Thaddeus caught him by the vest. "I have you. Do you want to rest here?" Sam wanted to say *yes*. Instead he just shook his head, wiped sweat from his forehead and continued the climb. Thaddeus chuckled. "See, you are becoming a man. Maybe you would even make a fine pirate."

"I thought you said you're not a pirate."

"I am not—least ways that is what I would have old Governor Rogers and the likes of Captain Hornigold believe."

Sam smiled slightly. "Well, pirate or no pirate, you've stuck with me. Thanks for all you've done."

Thaddeus winked. "Thank me when we save Sarah, stop Slayer and become heroes."

They climbed in silence. Thaddeus remained at Sam's side and offered a hand to help him ascend the steeper parts, some of which were like a wall. At times the climb mercifully leveled off only to quickly be followed by another barrier of brush. One particular hedge was exceptionally high. Thaddeus began his climb. Sam started to follow, but when a search revealed no top to the thicket, he stopped, slid back down and stared at his feet.

"Come on. Do not stop. Make the climb." Thaddeus hung on about twenty feet into the climb.

"I can't." Sam still eyed his feet.

"You scurvy dog, do not be a scallywag now, not when we are so close." Thaddeus began to climb down. "I cannot do this without you. I do not even know what to do here without you. This is your quest, remember. I am just the stowaway."

"Thaddeus—"

Sam's words cut off when branches rustled from behind.

"Lad, I think you should climb!"

"Another snake?"

"Not this time. Do not look back. Just climb!"

Sam didn't listen to Thaddeus. He turned to find a tidal wave of brush and trees rushed at him, just like the crimson wave that had pounded against the shore. "Oh my God!" Sam jumped onto the thicket and raced toward Thaddeus.

"Keep moving!" Thaddeus hastened his own climb.

Sam peered down just as the wave of greenery smashed against the wall and rose toward him. His eyes grew wide as the plant life formed a hand. The fingers stretched out to him. The sword in his back burned to life again. He quickly pulled it out from underneath his vest, and the blade blazed anew. As he climbed, he swung at the finger tips and sliced away the plants and trees, finger by finger. But each time he cut off one finger, a new one formed and the hand raced closer. From above him, Thaddeus yelled a war cry and threw himself into the hand.

"Thaddeus! No!" Sam stared wide-eyed as the hand formed a fist around Thaddeus and squeezed—as if to crush a bug. Before Sam could slash with his sword, the fist shook and lost its form. Branches and limbs fell to the jungle floor below. With the thud of steel against timber, the fist exploded. Sam shielded his eyes from the flying foliage. When he looked again, Thaddeus, his face scratched and bloody, climbed back up the wall.

"No time to waste, lad. I do not wish to do that again."

Sam nodded. Together they clawed their way up until Thaddeus suddenly stopped. "We made it!" He let out a cheer and extended a hand, which Sam gladly accepted. They finally stood on a ledge above the jungle. Sam couldn't be sure, but it was as if they stood on a grand shoulder. Just ahead was a thick granite neck that signaled yet another climb to the skull peak.

Below them was a panorama view from the tropical brush to the shoreline to the blood-like waters that surrounded the island. The skies above were a darker shade of green and the orange sun loomed even larger as it inched across the sky. On the horizon the emerald colors of day gave way to a starry space-like view filled with planets that now seemed closer.

Sam cast his eyes back to the jungle. Gone was any sign of the damage caused by the flood as if in a manner of hours new trees and plants had grown to full size. The island had somehow restored itself. *How is it possible?* Magic was the answer unless his eyes tricked him. Then again, maybe there had never really been a flood. Maybe there were forces at work on this island that twisted his mind. "Focus on what matters," he told himself. "And what matters is Slayer." There were still no signs of the evil pirate. *Come on! Not even one single Slayer ship around the island.*

"Maybe he really didn't make it across the barrier," Sam announced to Thaddeus.

"No, Slayer is out there hiding."

"How do you know?"

"You know I am right."

"Yeah, I know. Somehow I can feel him close by. It's like he's in my head watching me. It gives me the creeps."

"Then we must continue. Have you noticed where we are standing?"

"Near the peak." Sam's eyes traced the strange curvature of the peak that formed the massive skull. Four dark opening marked the peak: a fanged mouth, a triangular nose, and two circular eyes. "Why does this stupid rock scare me?" The skull's dark eyes, though lifeless, seemed to track him. He shuddered. "I know we have to go inside this skull, but I don't want to."

"We have come all this way," Thaddeus reminded him. "The fun is just getting started. You would not deny me whatever treasure lies inside now would you?"

Sam frowned. "I thought you wanted to save Sarah and those kids as much as I do. I thought you wanted revenge on Slayer. Is treasure all you want?"

Thaddeus fingered his sword's handle. "Do not get me wrong. I do wish to help you save that brave girl, and if children need saving, I shall help. But I expect treasure from this little quest. Along the way, I plan to drive my sword deep into Slayer's gut for what he has cost me."

"I understand. If there's treasure here, it's yours. But first we have to get up there to the mouth. I'd say it's about a hundred feet up. How are we supposed to get there?"

"Carefully." Thaddeus placed his fingers in a small crevice, just wide enough for his fingertips, and pulled himself up. He lodged his right foot into a second crevice as his hands searched for another place to grip. When he found none, he slipped back down to where Sam stood.

"You see, it's impossible." Sam threw his hands in the air and turned from the wall.

"After the wonders we have beheld, how can you utter such words?" Thaddeus placed a hand on his shoulder and forced him to turn. "Now, you try."

Sam swallowed a bit of saliva. He could never make this climb, but he had to try. When he touched the wall, a searing sensation crept up his back. His fire sword again beckoned him. Usually, it signaled danger, but not this time.

"Your back is glowing," Thaddeus took a few steps back.

"I know." Sam willed away the pain and drew the blade. He contemplated the fiery steel and the granite wall. He wasn't sure why, but with all his strength he plunged the blade into the rock wall. The blade sliced into the granite as easily as it had cut into the three-headed snake. The rocky cliff they stood upon shuddered. A low guttural howl emanated from the skull peak as if the fire sword had wounded it. The shudder grew in intensity and knocked Sam to the ground.

Thaddeus knelt beside him as small rocks from the skull rained down on them. Thaddeus shielded Sam with his own body. "Watch your head!"

Fractures radiated upward from the skull's nose. A loud crack echoed around them. The entire island seemed ready to split apart. A perfectly shaped, razor thin slab of stone shot out from the rock wall. A second slab followed, then a third, a fourth and fifth. Slabs continued to burst from the rock wall, each one just above the previous one, until they stretched to the mouth of the skull. Then the tremor stopped. The noise disappeared. All grew quiet, except for a few rocks that slid off the skull.

Thaddeus stood. "What did you do?"

Sam dislodged his fiery blade from the granite. He glanced at the stone slabs, which formed something of a stairway to the skull's mouth. "I don't actually know what I did. It just felt like I was supposed to do that."

"Cannot say as I understand, but we have stairs to climb, so enough talking and let us end this quest." Thaddeus clutched his pistol. "I shall go first. Stay close."

Sam stopped him. "I think maybe I should go first."

"Perhaps you are right." Thaddeus bowed. "All right, Chosen One. I shall follow you. Lead us to the sword."

His fire sword still blazed, an indication danger lay ahead. Sam took a deep breath and stepped onto the first stone slab. He paused. Would the slab give way? Would some new predator attack? Would the skull itself come alive and swallow them? Nothing happened. Air slowly flowed from his lungs as he took another cautious step and another. He turned back once. Thaddeus, who was right on his heels, offered a nod, and Sam continued his climb to the skull's mouth, one careful step at a time.

With his fire sword out in front, Sam soon reached the last stone slab. The ledge just above would bring him face to face with the mouth of the skull peak. Before he took that last step, he raised his head to take a quick peek. The ledge was deserted. What looked like the mouth of the skull from afar was really an oval-shaped cavern. It towered over them, the entrance shrouded in darkness. What had appeared to be fangs were cone-shaped stones that hung from the cavern entrance.

"What is it, lad? What do you see?"

In answer, Sam waved Thaddeus to follow and took the last step onto the ledge.

Thaddeus quickly joined him. "If I wanted to hide some magical blade with God-like powers on an island, this would be the place."

"I guess we have to go in there." Sam leaned forward and peered into the darkness. His eyes could not penetrate the shadows beyond the entrance. He pointed his fiery sword, but even the light generated by the flame bounced off the darkness—as though the shadowy layer was as solid as the mountain itself.

"If you choose, I can go in first and make sure it is safe." Thaddeus' eyes were large as they stared into the cavern.

"No, we go in together. We share the risk."

"Bravery fits you well." Thaddeus put his hand on Sam's shoulder. "I would be proud to sail with you, Samuel. Of course, I would be captain."

"Of course." *He called me Sam... well, Samuel! I can't believe it!* Sam hefted his fire sword high to reveal any hidden terrors as they entered the gloomy shadows. Thaddeus walked at his side, shoulder to shoulder. They breathed in unison. A step from the entrance, Sam stopped. He swung the blazing steel in an arc to illuminate the shadows. Nothing hindered the entrance.

"Courage, lad." Thaddeus nudged Sam. With right feet first, they inched into the cavern. As they crossed into the shadows, all light was snuffed out, even the sunlight just behind them, as if a door had slammed shut.

Sam stepped lightly, sword out in front to shed light on their surroundings. Eyes shut, he whispered to the sword as if to will it to blaze as brightly as the lights that illuminated the football games back home on Friday nights. "Sword, burn our way ahead." He wasn't sure where those words came from, but the sword responded. Its flame rose higher, but even its orange glow could only provide a limited view of the realm they had entered. The cavern walls were so high that the sword's light failed to reach the ceiling. The smooth walls reflected the glow from the sword, and even sparkled, as if the walls were made of quartz or maybe some kind of gem stone. *If that's the case, Thaddeus may never want to leave this place.*

Sam wondered what Thaddeus thought. Would he really help face Slayer, or at the first discovery of treasure, would he bolt with his newly discovered riches? Sam put that question aside for now. Thaddeus had earned his trust.

"This is no natural cave," Thaddeus whispered.

"I think you're right." Sam pointed his sword forward. Its orange glow reached through the darkness until it hit something. "Is that a—"

"A door," Thaddeus finished Sam's thought. "I suppose we are meant to go through it?"

Each step toward the door took them deeper into the cavern, and the stale air became colder and dank. "This feels like a place where people come to die," Sam whirled around; his sword's flames crackled louder as he spun.

"I have no desire to die today, so no such talk," Thaddeus replied.

They moved the rest of the way in silence. Sam listened for any noise that would indicate Slayer—or anyone else—watched them. The cavern was still. Mist rose from his mouth each time he breathed. Sam shivered and brought the sword closer to his body to warm himself.

As they drew closer to the door, it became clear instead of one massive door, there were two halves welded together as if someone had sealed the entrance closed permanently. The twin doors were made of cut stone shaped into massive rectangles. Sam tilted back his head to see how far the doorway extended, but just like the cavern ceiling, the doorway's highest point was hidden in the shadows. He lowered his head again and studied the twin doors closer. How strange! No doorknob. No handle. No latch. No visible way to open the doors. He reached out with a hand to touch one of the doors. The stone was as smooth as the marble countertops in his kitchen and as cold as an ice cube.

"How do we get in, Thaddeus?"

"Your doorway, not mine."

Sam pushed, but the stone doors refused to give way. He pressed his hands along the stone in search of a secret mechanism to open the portal. Nothing happened. Sam studied his fire sword. *When I jammed it into the rock outside, steps appeared. What might happen if I do the same thing here?*

"Give it a try," Thaddeus agreed as if he understood what Sam contemplated.

As a lump of saliva lodged in his throat, Sam stabbed the burning blade into the stone doors at the point where they were fused together. It sliced into the stone clear up to the handle, but still the door did not budge. "What! Why didn't that work?" Sam pounded a fist against the doors.

"Wait. Be still," Thaddeus insisted. "Look!" The sword's flame caused the doors to pulsate with a red energy. Sam stepped back as the doorway sizzled. A red hot outline of a sword appeared on one door. *Just like my vision!* The glow radiated to the other door where unseen hands scrawled letters into the stone over their heads. Sam followed each burning, crackling letter with his eyes as words formed. "What magic is this?" Thaddeus questioned. "This is not the King's English. That I am sure."

The letters were a mix of lines and circles, swirls and dots that flowed up and down, then reversed back on themselves—as if they could not be read from either right to left or left to right but rather in repetition. Each word had to be read once and repeated before the next word could be read. This repetitive sequence had to be followed through to the end of the sentence.

"I... I can read this," Sam revealed.

"What?"

"I can read this. I know it's an ancient language of magic. I think I need to recite it to open the doors." He closed his eyes and cleared all the clutter from his mind as he visualized the doors. Once the magic was clear, he opened his eyes and read—or chanted—the engraved words. "Mish... Mish Ton... Mish Ton Bur... Mish Ton Bur Norasen... Mish Ton Bur Norasen Ami... Mish Ton Bur Norasen Ami Tranora."

"What meaning do such words have?" Thaddeus asked.

"Shhh," Sam snapped as the doorway moaned. The handle of his sword, which remained wedged in the stone, twisted with a click, as though a lock had been undone. Sam reached for the handle, but quickly recoiled.

"Go on, Samuel," Thaddeus implored.

Sam swallowed a bit of saliva and again reached for the door. His fingertips gently touched the handle. With a nod from Thaddeus, Sam gripped the sword and pulled. The doors parted.

# Chapter 28
## The Protector and The Sword

Sam gasped. Statues of heavily armored knights, built into the walls, at twenty-foot intervals, encircled the round chamber. They numbered at least sixty, each armed with a sword pressed against his chest plate. When Sam peered into one statue's eyes, they seemed to stare back at him. Light trickled in from somewhere high above, but just as in the cavern, dark obscured the chamber's ceiling. A large, rectangular, stone slab occupied the center of the room.

Thaddeus cleared his throat. "Tell me, what did those words mean?"

"Only a conjurer true of heart may enter... I think," Sam's hand throbbed. When he uncurled his fingers from around the handle, the blade slipped from the stone and the sword disappeared.

"How do you know such words?" Thaddeus asked.

"I don't know. I just saw the meaning in my mind."

"Lad, you must be the Chosen One."

"If that's true, who chose me and why? I never asked for this." Sam swallowed. He tried to will his feet to take the first steps into the chamber, but he could not move.

"Do you know what this place is?" Thaddeus also didn't move forward.

"I don't."

Thaddeus sniffed the air. "It reeks of a burial chamber."

"Maybe." Sam's body tensed. He closed his eyes and focused on the beating of his heart. Once... twice... on the third beat, he stepped through the doorway. "Whatever this place is, I know the Sword of Zel-Kar is here, somewhere. I can feel it calling to me."

He chose not to share that if he grasped that sword, he might never be able to put it down. *I think I would use the sword just like Slayer. I could be just as evil as Slayer. Is that my destiny? Am I to conquer the world? No, that can't be. I won't let it be.*

Thaddeus nudged Sam. "Do not fear whatever is inside this place. You are stronger, rest assured."

Sam gave a slight smile and nodded. "All right, let's do this."

Thaddeus aimed his pistol into the chamber. "Just step carefully. This could yet be a trap."

"You think?" Sam stepped heel to toe farther into the chamber. He froze once and held his breath. Eyes wide, ears cocked, his gaze swept around the chamber as he waited for a trap to be sprung. All remained quiet, save for the constant drip of water from somewhere. A foul odor, like the school locker room, permeated the air. *Thaddeus is right—it does seem like a place of death.* An icy chill spread through the chamber. His eyes watered, his shoulders shivered.

Sam scanned the room. Each statute returned his gaze with empty eyes. Their stares weighed heavily on his shoulders and pressed against his chest. He forced himself to breathe despite the icy pain each chilled breath caused. *Come on, you know where you have to go.* Every muscle in his body tugged at him to move to the stone slab in the heart of the chamber. He took cautious steps and flinched as each step echoed, but he inched forward until he stood before the stone slab.

Thaddeus stood right behind him. "Would this be a grave?"

"I was thinking the same thing," Sam answered as he studied the table-like stone slab, which stood as high as his chest. The slab revealed no opening on top or around the edges. The stone was one large smooth block that seemed to have grown from the chamber floor.

Sam reached out to touch it, but the sensation of frost rose from his fingertips into his hand and up his arm. It stung, and he recoiled. Yet he had to make contact with the stone. He had to have whatever was hidden inside. *Do it!* He quieted himself as that feeling crept through him again—like somewhere deep inside his mind lurked something evil. *This is not about you—this about saving Sarah and the children and stopping Slayer. Control it,* he silently urged himself.

He reached again for the stone slab with one hand. His arm again froze, but this time he forced his fingers to continue their journey until they bridged the final few inches to the stone slab. Once in contact, he winced as he waited for an explosion of magic, but all remained still. *Okay, now what.* The icy touch burned his fingertips as they slid over the stone. He disregarded the pain and sought to somehow push through the slab to whatever was hidden inside. *Come, on, I've come so far! Show me the way to open you up! Show me the Sword of Zel-Kar! I demand it!* Wait! Were those his words? *That couldn't have come from me, could it?*

"So?" Thaddeus asked.

Sam did not answer. He placed his other hand on the stone slab—and the chamber reacted. As if a massive earthquake struck, the chamber rattled, stones toppled from above, the walls creaked and cracked. Sam stumbled backward into Thaddeus. Together, they fell to the ground.

"What did you do now?" Thaddeus shouted.

"I don't know!"

"Do we run?"

Sam wanted to. "I think—"

One of the statues turned its head and raised its arms. One leg moved. Its torso twisted and the statue broke free of the wall. It stood tall, its stone sword pointed at Sam, its cold, unblinking eyes locked on him.

Sam tried to stand. "What the…?" The rumble along the wall continued and, one by one, all the statues ripped free and came to life. Sam turned in every direction. Their faces portrayed no emotion, but each knight tipped its sword at him. He and Thaddeus were surrounded.

"What madness is this?" Thaddeus unsheathed his sword and pointed his pistol at each of the statues, one by one.

"But my back."

"What?"

"It's not on fire. My sword isn't warning me of danger."

"That may be, but I would say danger is upon—"

The quake in the chamber quieted. The walls grew still. The statues remained silent and motionless as if their feet had welded to the ground. Thaddeus targeted each of the statues with his pistol, but his hand shook. "What happens now?"

The knights responded as they took their first steps forward; their stone feet struck the ground hard. The step boomed through the chamber. They took yet another step forward and began to form a circle.

"They are moving to surround us!" Thaddeus fired his pistol. The round hit a knight. A chunk of stone broke off from the statue's chest, but the knight continued to advance. "Lad, do not just stand there. Draw that sword of yours."

With a shaky hand, Sam reached behind his back to the mark of his fire sword. Would the sword obey? It had not called to him. *Come on sword, I need you.* His fingers found his birthmark, magically penetrated his skin and gripped the handle. *Thank you, sword.* He raised the burning blade over his head and turned on wobbly legs in every direction to display the weapon to the stone knights. The sight of the fiery steel had no effect. They knights started to close their circle around them.

"Stay by my side. We shall fight our way out." Thaddeus launched himself at one of the knights.

A voice rang out. "Halt!"

The knights stopped their forward march and stood straight and tall with their swords against their stone chests. Since the statues were taller than him, Sam could not see above them or through them to whoever had uttered the command. Thaddeus merely shrugged. The voice spoke again. "Clear a path, my warriors." The statues, in unison, broke from their circle and created a crescent formation around Sam and Thaddeus.

Sam searched the room, but still could not spot the person whose words controlled the statues. "Show yourself."

"Oh, I mean to." From a shadowy corner of the chamber, a man appeared. He walked forward with quiet, fluid steps, as if he floated above the floor. He held his hands behind his back and his head tilted slightly to the right. The shadows concealed his eyes.

"Who are you?" Sam asked.

"I should ask you the same."

"Are you Slayer?" Sam held his fire sword ready to lash out with the blade if necessary.

"I am not."

"Then who?"

"One you should fear much more than the one called Captain Slayer."

The man stopped at the opening the statue warriors had created. He brought his hands to the front. One hand rested loosely on the handle of a sword sheathed at his side. Sam recognized the handle. Shaped like a bird, it was just like the sword the old man in his vision—or hallucination—had when Sam dreamed he was back home at the pier after Slayer blew up *The Mutineer II.*

The man's other hand twisted the end of a long graying mustache that covered both his upper and bottom lips.

With the stone slab between them, Sam pointed the tip of his fire sword at the stranger. The flame cast the man in an eerie yellow glow, but shed enough light to see him better. He was dressed all in white—breeches, long coat, boots, and three-cornered hat. *Again, just like the vision.* The man was tall and lean, his face square and weathered with age. A beard, as gray as the mustache, reached to his chest. Sam guessed he might be fifty. *Could this be the same man from that vision? He's dressed the same, but the man I dreamt of was basically a skeleton. But that wasn't real. I was hallucinating, right? Then again, how do I know what is real and what isn't?*

Finally, the man spoke in a stern and wary voice, his English accent a match to Thaddeus'. He spoke with nobility, like he was from the British Royal Navy. "I see you carry a very particular, very rare weapon. How is it you come to own it?"

The blazing sword's flame generated shadows that danced along the chamber floor and walls. "It, uh, is just there when I need it."

The man strolled around the stone slab and stood just inches from Sam. His eyes were brown, just like Sam's, but much wiser. "I see. And what would your name be, young one?"

"Sam Every, sir." Sam wasn't sure why he said sir. It just seemed like the right thing to say—like somehow the man who stood before him should be shown respect.

"Interesting." The man turned to Thaddeus. "And you—who are you who has accompanied this boy on such a perilous journey?"

Thaddeus bowed. "I am Thaddeus Milan, former British Royal Navy and captain of *The Mutineer*. The boy sought my help."

"Very good. It is a pleasure to make your acquaintances, Samuel and Captain Milan. It has been a long time since I have had guests, but—"

"I believe I am familiar with you," Thaddeus interrupted.

"You dare say." The man frowned. "I suggest you hold your tongue while I speak as I have not decided yet whether you are to live."

Sam spoke. "Sir, we have come for something I think is in this chamber—a sword, a really special sword. It is called the Sword of Zel-Kar."

The man twisted the end of his mustache again. "Tell me what you know of such a weapon."

Thaddeus interrupted again. "I do know you, sir."

The man drew his sword and pointed it at Thaddeus' throat. "Do not try my patience. If I deem it so, I shall reveal my identity."

"My apologies, sir. No disrespect is meant, I assure you." Thaddeus bowed a second time, but kept his eyes on the man's blade.

The man sheathed his sword and motioned to Sam. "Please, share your knowledge."

Sam held the handle of his fire sword tighter. "I know it is a weapon of unlimited power. The one who uses the weapon can, uh, live forever, and cannot be stopped by anyone... ever."

"That is quite remarkable." The man leaned back against the stone slab in the center of the chamber. "If such a weapon exists, why would you seek it? Do you wish to use it to conquer? Do you wish to rule?"

From somewhere deep inside, the urge to say yes wormed its way into Sam's thoughts. "No, sir. I don't want the sword at all. I just need to stop Slayer from getting his hands on it, and I need to stop him from killing children he has kidnapped and to help a friend."

The man nodded. "They say only a magic conjurer can use the weapon."

"Slayer has magic abilities."

"And what of you?"

"He has been called the Chosen One." Thaddeus answered as he fingered the handle of his own sword.

"Then I think I stand in the grace of greatness." The man's words clearly mocked rather than praised.

Sam grew frustrated. "Look, I don't know who you are, but if you have the Sword of Zel-Kar, can you help us? There is no time. Slayer may already be here, and if he gets the sword, we're all in danger."

"More than that," the man suggested. "The future is in jeopardy."

"Yes!" Sam fought the urge to grab the old man by the collar and shake him until he gave up the Sword of Zel-Kar.

The man motioned for Sam to lower his sword. "Young one, if you are a Chosen One, you must have a mark emblazoned on your body. If so, please reveal it to me." At a nod from Thaddeus, Sam removed his vest, now little more than twisted, ripped strands of cloth and turned his back to the man. "Fascinating. You do indeed wear the mark of the sword." The man laughed gently but loud enough to resonate through the chamber.

*Wait a second!* Sam thought. He turned to face the old man. "You used the words *a* Chosen One. Not *the* Chosen One. Why?"

"Oh, did I? My mistake." The man unbuttoned his long coat and his vest to bear his chest. Though covered in gray hair, a dark outline of a sword—a birthmark of a sword—was clearly there. "Then again, perhaps my words ring true."

"What?" This time Sam leaned forward.

"Please allow me to introduce myself. I am Henry Every and we are blood relatives. I have sworn to protect the Sword of Zel-Kar until this day. Now—if fate have it—I would bequeath that duty to you."

# Chapter 29
## Blood Lines

"I knew it to be true!" Excitement tinged Thaddeus' voice. "Sir, it is an honor to stand before the great pirate Henry Every."

Every glowered at Thaddeus. "Perhaps in a former life I lived by the pirate code, but that no longer has any meaning to me."

Sam stood in silence, though a jumble of thoughts spun in his head. *Who is this man? How is it he has my same last name? What's going on? Can he really be like some distant grandfather of mine?* He remembered the words from the skeletal man in his vision—a man who said he was an Every. *It falls upon you to finish what I began. Our family bloodline demands it.* "You came to me in a vision. You knew I was coming, but you spoke in riddles. You could have helped."

"I had a premonition that someday a member of my bloodline would come, but I assure you your vision was entirely of your own doing. If it was me you saw, it was your mind reaching out," the old man responded.

"Lad," Thaddeus reproached, "mind your tone. We are in the presence of a legend. He served in the Royal Navy, fought in the Nine Years' War, sailed the great ship—*Fancy* it was called—and raided the Mughal Empire's grand treasure ship, the *Ganj-i-Sawai*. You became a very rich man from that bounty."

The old man who stood before Sam stared quietly, his face rigid. If he had ever been a pirate, he sure didn't seem like one now. Regret showed in his eyes.

Thaddeus continued. "But you must be a ghost. You disappeared in 1696 when you already were well into your years. No one saw the likes of you again. Why, you should be an old, decrepit man or more likely dead, but here you stand still strong."

The man sighed. "Your words are true. Allow me to continue the story you have begun."

Sam, his fire sword at his side, mouthed, "Go on." If Henry Every disappeared in 1696 and was already old then, wrinkles and age spots should adorn his face since the year was now 1718. Could this be a trick? Another thought crossed Sam's mind. This could still be some crazy dream. But he didn't really believe that anymore. Too much had happened.

With a long sigh and lowered gaze, the old man who claimed to be Sam's distant relative pondered the ground for several moments before he looked Sam square in the eyes. "It is truth to say I served in the Royal Navy. I was loyal to the Crown. I served well. I fought well. It was a terrible time, indeed, the Nine Years' War. So much death. So many friends lost, but how do you think I survived when so many did not?"

Sam shrugged.

"It was my magic." The man paused and moved closer to Sam. "Yes, boy, like you, I have magic. I discovered it when I was a young one, like yourself. My very own sword of fire would come to life at my beckoning."

"And you used it to become a wealthy pirate." Thaddeus, a wide grin on his face, slid the pistol he held into his belt, but kept his hand on the weapon.

"No. I fought and bled like any other man, mostly without my magic." The old man narrowed his eyes on Thaddeus. "However, that is not to say that, from time to time, a little magic did not help in my conquests."

"But why did you become a pirate?" Sam asked.

"Wealth, my boy, the desire for wealth."

"And did magic help in your greatest victory against the *Ganj-i-Sawai*?" Thaddeus asked.

The man showed the smallest glimmer of a smile. "Perhaps. Magic also kept me alive as the Crown began a campaign of death against my fellow pirates."

"But you disappeared." Thaddeus finally eased his hand away from the pistol.

The man walked toward the stone slab. "Yes, from the time I was a boy and discovered my abilities, I felt there was something out there waiting for me, even calling to me."

"The Sword of Zel-Kar," Sam blurted.

The man nodded. "As time pressed on, I encountered other conjurers who spoke of the sword's existence. I came to believe those legends and that only those with the sword marking on their bodies—the Chosen Ones—could reach it. I never disclosed that I had such a birthmark, but I had to possess the sword. I wanted its power, and I was going to use it to conquer empires. I wanted to best the pirate Henry Morgan. He took Panama. I would take the world."

"Just like Slayer." Sam gripped his fire sword and raised it toward Henry Every.

"True. In the year of Our Lord 1696 I headed out to sea on my own and ended up in the middle of nowhere only to find a barrier." Sam glanced at Thaddeus. *Just like us.* "The closer I came to this place," the man continued, "the more my blood boiled to have the sword. I found this chamber. And someone else."

"Who?" Sam asked.

"I discovered an ancient one who was among the Fathers of Magic and a disciple of the great Wizard Zel-Kar. He had sworn to watch over the sword, to protect it."

Sam shook his head. "I don't understand."

"Young one, the Sword of Zel-Kar was created by fusing all the magic in the world together into one piece of steel. It has unlimited power. It was meant to be used for good, but Zel-Kar and his followers knew they had made a mistake. Such a weapon should never have been delivered to the world. They knew it should be destroyed, but none could do it."

"So!" Thaddeus stepped closer to the old man.

"So, they found a bridge to this world—really some strange plain of existence—and hid the sword. And the ancient I discovered had watched over the sword since the beginning. The sword's power kept him alive."

Sam swallowed. "What about the Chosen Ones?"

"I don't fully claim to understand, but some within my family bloodline, like myself, carry the mark that grants us a way to reach the sword. I do not know if there are others outside our family. Very few of us have carried the mark, and I cannot say what became of them. The ancient told me if any with the birthmark are found unworthy, even if they have the mark, this place shall not appear to them."

"And you were worthy?" Thaddeus asked.

"The ancient presented me with a challenge. Choose the right sword or walk away never to return. Choose wrong and he would strike me down as I would be unworthy to possess the sword. I accepted the challenge."

"And?" Sam asked.

"I chose well."

"What happened to the ancient one?" Sam wasn't sure he wanted to hear the answer. The man grew quiet, his gaze dropped. "What happened to him?" Sam trembled as he repeated the question.

"I used the Sword of Zel-Kar to kill him."

"No!" Sam lifted the fire sword higher; the flame blazed brighter as if it reacted to the fury he felt.

Thaddeus grabbed Sam's shoulder. "There is more we need to learn. Besides, I think you would not fare well against this one."

A tear fell from the man's right eye. "I understand your anger, young one. When I killed the protector, power lust warped my thinking. I understood what I would become. I knew the terrible things I would do, and something inside me changed. I dropped the sword and vowed never to hold it again. Although I would not pick up the sword again, I needed to be near its power, and I chose to stay. I became the sword's protector. That is why I appear younger than my years. One touch of the sword can grant longer life, though without constant contact, my time is nearing the end."

Sam broke away from Thaddeus' grip. "What am I supposed to do now?"

The man stood tall. "Young one, you bear the birthmark and carry my family name. We are tied together in blood. That is how you come to be here. Since you have reached this place, you may be worthy. I offer you the same challenge that was offered to me. Choose the right sword, or walk away now. But if you choose wrong, I shall be forced to kill you and your friend. Do not think these old bones lack the will to kill. But remember this—choosing right could be a worse fate."

Sam released the handle of his fire sword, and it vanished. He placed his hands over his eyes. *How could any of this be real? Can I trust this man? Is he who he says he is? Can I really be related to him... a pirate? How can I choose the right sword? How can I make this decision?* "Thaddeus?"

"Only you can decide." Thaddeus responded.

Sam walked around the stone slab in the center of the chamber. He thought of Sarah—her eyes, her words, her belief in him. He thought about Slayer and the kidnapped children. He thought about his life back home. His thoughts returned to Slayer. *If he is able to come after the sword, that must mean he carries the birthmark, too. Are we related, too? Sarah didn't say anything about that. Why?* Sam faced Henry Every. Despite himself, he wanted to believe Henry was something like a grandfather. *I feel it in my gut. Slayer on the other hand—I can't be related to him. There has to be another explanation if he has crossed the barrier. Right now, I can't worry about whether Slayer is a relative. I just have to stop him.* "I accept the challenge."

"As you wish." Henry closed his eyes and extended his hands over the stone slab. He whispered an incantation. The slab exploded in a brilliant blue light. Sam covered his eyes. "You may look now, young one." Sam peeked through his fingers at the stone slab. It glowed softly. The illumination pulsated as if the stone had come to life. With one hand, the old pirate motioned Sam forward. He waved his other hand over the glowing slab and three sword handles rose from inside the stone. The blades remained hidden in the stone.

The handles differed from each other. A jewel-encrusted band, that protected the hand, surrounded a thin, gold handle. A diamond encased the bottom of a silver, T-shaped handle. The bar upon which the blade rested curved upward with smaller diamonds atop both ends. The final handle was much simpler—longer, tarnished and made from some rusted metal. Where the other handles seemed untouched, this one showed signs it had been used in battle. "You must choose," Henry instructed.

Sam took a deep breath and circled the glowing slab. He studied each sword. He stopped once and glanced at Thaddeus, who nodded his support. His hands clutched to his chest, Sam took one step closer to the slab and eyed the old pirate one more time. Henry kept his eyes downcast. *Something isn't right,* Sam thought. *I sense...*

He spun away from the swords and glanced up toward the shadowy layer above. With his next breath, he drew his fire sword from his back and brought it before his face.

"None of these is the Sword of Zel-Kar!" Sam twisted back toward the stone slab and sliced through it with his blazing steel. As the slab split in two, Sam swung his sword like a baseball bat at each half and knocked the halves to opposite ends of the chamber. The three swords embedded in the stone fell to the ground as the sound of steel against the stone floor echoed through the chamber.

"What?" Thaddeus stepped forward.

Sam held out his hand to quiet Thaddeus and peered upward, his fire sword pointed toward the unseen chamber ceiling. "I know you're up there. I can feel you. Show yourself and bring me the real Sword of Zel-Kar."

Silence followed until a growl echoed from the darkness above. The eyes of a familiar dragon burned through the shadows. Its massive wings spread out and, with one mighty thrust, the creature floated down until it landed on the chamber floor behind Henry Every. With its long fluid neck, the dragon lowered its head toward Sam. He was sure it was the same dragon that had spoken to him, the same one that had saved him from the three-headed snake.

Henry smiled and nodded. "Well done. Perhaps you are worthy. Now take hold of the Sword of Zel-Kar, but do so humbly and with great respect, for it shall consume you if you let it."

Sam peered into the dragon's mouth. There, nestled between his fangs, was the true Sword of Zel-Kar. He found the handle and slid the weapon from the dragon's jaw. The clash of steel against fang rang through the chamber.

Finally, Sam held the great Sword of Zel-Kar. The thick blade curved and reflected his image in the crystal-clear steel. There were markings—similar to the writing on the doorway to the chamber—on the steel. Sam read them. "Only the righteous." The handle was of the same steel as the blade, as if the entire weapon had been forged from a single piece of steel.

Sam noticed one more thing. He didn't feel anything. No energy coursed through him to indicate he held a magic weapon of untold power. If the sword had suddenly given him immortality, he didn't feel that either. Then again, maybe he wasn't supposed to feel anything. Maybe the sword didn't work that way. Maybe he just didn't know how to use it. *Maybe I'm not really a Chosen One. Maybe I'm not worthy.*

Thaddeus placed a hand on Sam's shoulder. His eyes focused on the sword. "You have done it, Samuel!"

Sam smiled but did not speak. He glanced at Henry, whose eyes remained locked on the spot the stone slab had occupied before Sam sliced it in two. Sam leaned forward to examine what Henry saw. A face! Faint, as if the waves of time swept it away until only an outline remained. Still he recognized the face. It was—

"I believe that blade is mine." The voice forced Sam to shift his gaze to the doorway where a dozen men stood with swords, pistols and muskets. The man in front held Sarah with a knife to her throat. "I am Captain Slayer."

# Chapter 30
## Slayer Strikes

The dragon roared in anger. Thaddeus drew his sword. Henry pulled his own fire blade from the birthmark across his chest. Fear, but also strength, showed in Sarah's eyes. Sam still clutched the Sword of Zel-Kar. He moved forward with the curved blade aimed at Slayer's heart.

Slayer stood close behind Sarah with his knife still tight against her throat. He perfectly fit the image of someone with an overly inflated sense of power. He was tall—more legs than torso. He dressed in fine clothing, from a long purple coat to a black three-cornered hat with a purple feather bending in a wave-like way from the hat. He wore a heavy, black belt with two pistols tucked inside and a sword with a golden handle sheathed at his side. His boots reached up his knees. A golden pendant hung from his neck, and white gloves hid his hands. His eyes were yellow, streaked with lines of red, and dark shadows formed just below them. A reddish beard and mustache, similar to a lion's mane, accentuated lips curled up in a twisted smile.

"You're too late, Slayer." Sam tried to mask his fear as he spoke. "I have the sword." The searing pain returned to his back, but he did not call forth the fire sword. Instead, he pointed the blade of the Sword of Zel-Kar at Slayer.

"Perhaps, but if you value this little girl's life, you shall make the sword mine in short order." Slayer slid the knife tip along Sarah's cheek. A drop of blood fell from where the knife nicked her skin. Sarah did not flinch.

"Release her at once, infidel!" Henry produced his own fiery blade from his chest and aimed the blade at Slayer. "You do not know the great harm you shall cause."

Henry's chest heaved as he stepped beside Sam. The old pirate's eyes never wavered from Sarah. *Why?* Sam turned his full attention back to Slayer. "If you kill her, you'll never get the sword."

Slayer laughed. "Then I guess we are at an impasse. Hmmm, I wonder how we might reach some kind of accord?"

"Never!" Sam raised the Sword of Zel Kar in both hands as if he stood poised to strike a grand slam with a baseball bat.

Slayer snorted. "Perhaps you are right. Well, then… Captain… what do you have to say about this?"

Sam lowered the sword. "Huh?" From behind him came the sound of a blade as it sliced through flesh. Sam swung around to see the unthinkable. A long blade protruded from Henry's stomach. His mouth agape, but silent, he gazed at the blood that dripped from the sword.

Behind him… *Thaddeus*! He still grasped the handle of the sword he had thrust through Henry's back. "No!" Sam cried. The dragon roared and lowered its head to tear into Thaddeus.

"I would not do that beast, or the girl dies," Thaddeus threatened. The dragon pulled back with a soft, but ferocious, growl.

"What have you done?" Sam aimed the Sword of Zel-Kar at Thaddeus while the fire sword still in his back caused his skin to glow. The burning blade called to him as if it demanded the right to unleash its fury at Thaddeus' treachery.

"I am doing as I have always intended." Thaddeus ripped his sword from Henry's back. The old pirate stood for a moment, then toppled to the ground. "I am claiming what is rightfully mine."

Sam's mind swam at this betrayal. Then the truth struck with the force of lighting. "Why did Slayer call you Captain?"

"There is fine reason for that—I must introduce myself anew." Thaddeus bowed.

"I thought you already did that long ago." Sam's stomach churned. "You're Thaddeus, formerly of the British Royal Navy. You sailed *The Mutineer*. You were my friend."

Thaddeus laughed. "I may have misled you, ever so slightly."

"What do you mean?" Sam took a step back.

"You see, foolish boy, I am the true Captain Slayer. That man holding your girlie is my quartermaster."

"You're lying—"

"Wait, there is more." Thaddeus, who now claimed to be the true Captain Jem Slayer, motioned to Sarah. "Show him, girl." The pretend Slayer no longer held Sarah. Her eyes glowed green as she wiped a line of blood from her cheek. *Sarah, what's going...?* Sam began to ask silently. A shot of green energy flashed from her eyes before he finished that thought. The energy slammed into the unseen chamber ceiling. An explosion echoed high above, then stone and rock rained down on the chamber floor. A large chunk of stone struck the dragon as its size prevented its escape from the debris' path. A second stone, then a third smacked the beast and knocked it to the ground. It lay silently as the rocks buried the beast. "No! Dragon!" Sam cried. *This can't be happening. It just can't.*

Sarah unleashed another stream of green energy that sliced the stone warriors in half in seconds. "Sarah!" Sam slumped to his knees. He let the Sword of Zel-Kar dangle loosely from his hand; the blade clanked as the steel struck the ground. His back glowed bright orange as his fire sword continued to beckon him. It was ready for a fight, but he wasn't. *How could she side with Slayer? All this time, she had been playing me? But why? Why, Sarah?*

In response, she flung her green energy at him. The energy slammed into him. He fell back against the cold, hard chamber floor as The Sword of Zel-Kar slipped from his hand. Flat on his back, he choked and coughed—his chest unable to move air in or out of his lungs. He stared straight into the void that hid the chamber ceiling toward strands of light that poked through where Sarah's energy blasted away stone.

Sarah and Thaddeus—or rather Slayer—walked into view. Slayer picked up the Sword of Zel-Kar. "Magnificent is it not?" he uttered. Sarah nodded.

Sam blinked once, then twice. His vision closed in on itself until sweet darkness came.

# Chapter 31
## The Truth Be Told

Sam coughed. Tears stung as ripples of pain radiated though his body. His chest, charred and blistered, ached and his head was cloudy. Darkness and silence enveloped like a tomb. Sounds slowly filtered in and broke through the fog. A rush of water seemed distant at first, but soon became louder. Waves crashed against a shore. Chains rattled mixed with the sound of children's cries. Laughter—familiar laughter—drifted toward him. *Thaddeus is Slayer!*

Cold water splashed against his face. The darkness broke a little. More water struck his face, and a voice commanded, "Wake up." Sam shook his head. *It can't be true, but it is!* "You are not much of a Chosen One," the voice mocked.

*Thaddeus tricked me. No, Slayer tricked me!* Sam forced open his eyes and blinked against the unexpected burst of sunlight that beamed down on him. At first, his eyes couldn't focus, but then the world cleared. He stood on the island shore, and he was not alone. Two men held his arms from behind. He couldn't see their faces, but their hot breath baked his neck.

About fifty feet away, twenty childen, their wrists chained, knelt in a line on the shore. Several of Slayer's men, armed with muskets, towered over the children. Some of the children cried. Others simply bowed their heads toward the ground. A few gazed at him; their eyes pleaded for help. *If only I could help!*

A few paces in front of him stood the man who had played him like a fool. Slayer had pretended to be Thaddeus, but why? Slayer changed from his ripped and torn clothing to black attire, from the feather in his three-cornered hat to the leather of his high boots. His face was the same. His eyes were the same. They were the eyes Sam had grown to trust. They were the eyes of a trickster, of the man who now held the Sword of Zel-Kar, which made him an even more powerful and dangerous conjurer.

But Sam did not dwell on Slayer. His gaze strayed to Sarah, who stood behind and to the right of Slayer. She no longer wore the scruffy clothing Thaddeus had given her or the dress from her mother—if the story of the dress and her mother had even been true. She now dressed in clean tan breeches, a white shirt, and a tan vest… like a pirate. A ribbon tied her long hair in a ponytail. She avoided his stare, her eyes dark and sad. "Why?" Sam mouthed. She failed to respond. *I should have known. She called him captain for no good reason. He called her by her name. She knew so much about Slayer. She cursed and spoke like she was raised in the streets, but she so quickly shifted to the King's English. I should have known something wasn't right. How could I be so stupid?*

Sam turned his attention back to Slayer. The man he had trusted was the enemy, a con-artist. *I should have seen him for what he was, too. Vane and Hornigold both said they had never heard of him. Because there never was a Thaddeus Milan.* "Why, Thadd… Slayer, why—"

"Why all this deception?" Slayer circled Sam. "It is really quite simple, and quite hilarious, if you ask me."

Sam struggled to break free from the men who held him, but they each clamped a hand on his shoulders and forced him to his knees.

Slayer slid the fingers of his hand along the blade of the Sword of Zel-Kar. "As that old fool pirate said, only those of his bloodline could find and penetrate the barrier to this world. I am not of your blood. The only other member of the Every clan I found with the mark, a distant relative of Henry Every's, though not quite as distant as you, took his own life, rather than guide me here. I imagine that showed some courage."

Slayer grabbed Sam's hair and twisted his head so they were face to face. "That created certain problems as you might imagine. Thus, I had to use the magic abilities of a very special girl to find another member of the Every clan—you, my boy. Her powers led her to you." Sarah returned Sam's stare, blinked, and turned away.

"But why this game?" Sam asked. "Why pretend to be Thaddeus? When Sarah brought me to this time, you could have made me your prisoner and forced me to bring you here. You didn't have to kidnap children. You don't have to kill them. You even killed your own man, Maximilian Black."

Slayer released Sam's hair. "Oh, yes, poor Mr. Black. His death was a necessary loss for the cause. As for the children, I suppose you are right. Then again, I could not take a chance on you killing yourself, too. So I kidnapped the children then schemed to convince you to save them from danger. Thaddeus was born. I must say I enjoyed playing the part. And you are right. I did not need to kidnap children. I have no need to kill them. But I think I shall do it anyway—for fun."

"No!" Sam again tried to break free from Slayer's henchmen, but he couldn't move. *If only I could reach my fire sword.*

Slayer caressed the Sword of Zel-Kar's blade. "And I must thank you for delivering the sword into my hands and for making this moment possible. Such thoughtfulness provided me and my ships safe passage to this land."

Sam gazed beyond Slayer toward the sea where two ships anchored off shore. Pirate flags, with skulls and crossbones, flew over each vessel. "How? Where?"

"They were always there, hidden by my magic. And what I saw, I allowed my men to see. When you held my arm, I saw the barrier and used magic to bring my ships across as well." Slayer laughed. "Not even your pet dragon perceived what my magic hid. Not even your sword could warn you of my ruse. And now I shall use my ships and the Sword of Zel-Kar to return to the Caribbean and conquer all who stand against me."

Sarah gingerly touched the handle of a sword sheathed at her side. "Father, you told me once you had the sword, the children would not be harmed."

He laughed and touched her cheek. "So naïve, child. I still have so much to teach you."

*Father!* A shiver coursed down Sam's spine. "Did she say father?"

Slayer removed his hand from Sarah's cheek. "Yes, this girl you care for so much is my child, my lovely daughter."

"Sarah, tell me it's not true. Tell me none of this is true!"

She finally spoke to him. "I am sorry, Samuel Every, but it is all true. Did you really believe you were some Chosen One who would stop my father? Look at you! You are a weak boy. The only thing you were chosen to be is the fool who would lead my father to that which he longed to possess." Sarah did an about face and dismissed him as if he were no better than a flea. "But Father, the children—"

"Quiet, Daughter. Mind your place." Slayer strolled over to the children. When he patted one head, the boy cowered. A girl flinched as Slayer stroked her long, blond curls. For a moment, he seemed lost in thought then he smiled. "You know, I feel generous this day. I propose a duel."

Sam cringed at the searing sensation in his back, as if the fire sword reacted to the challenge. He lowered his eyes and shook his head. It was a trick. It had to be. Whatever Slayer proposed was nothing more than a new scheme.

"Slayer—"

"Hush, lad! Yes a duel." A grin spread across Slayer's face. "I propose you and I engage in battle. I shall wield the Sword of Zel-Kar. You can wield your burning blade. If you knock the sword from my hand, you shall win the freedom of each and every child. If you strike me down, well then, the sword shall be yours, my men shall be yours, and the world shall be yours to rule." Slayer swung around as if he danced. "What say you?"

Sam raised his eyes. *How can I defeat him? But I have to try. I have to kill him or die trying.* "I'll do it, but if I lose, the children still go free."

Slayer slapped his knee. "Does it really matter? If you are dead, you shall not know what becomes of the children."

Sam turned his gaze toward Sarah. Unless he was mistaken, her eyes showed concern. Since it couldn't be for him since she betrayed him, it had to be for the children. Maybe she would protect them. What choice did he have but to ask her help? Slayer was right. *If I'm dead, I can't help them?* "Sarah, promise me you won't let the children…"

She nodded slightly and Slayer frowned. "Do you truly think you can trust this girl who so easily misled you for so long?"

"Yes." Sam kept his eyes on Sarah.

Slayer snorted. "Then you are still a fool."

"Just tell your goons to let me go, and let's do this."

Slayer motioned to both men, who quickly released Sam. *Finally, free! Don't waste this chance.* Sam rose to his feet, rubbed his arms and stood silently. Slayer pointed the Sword of Zel-Kar at his heart. "Stand ready, Samuel Every."

Sam pulled his fire sword and pointed the tip of the blade at Slayer. The memory of Thaddeus' lecture on how he had to control the blade surfaced. Then he hadn't known enough about the burning blade or his own magic to stop Thad—Slayer. Did he now? The answer lay hidden, but maybe luck would be on his side.

Rather than show fear, Sam delved deep to find the courage to answer without hesitation. "Bring it on, dude."

Slayer snickered. "Then attack."

Sam hefted his sword over his head and ran at Slayer. Their blades connected with a loud ching that echoed across the shore. Sam twisted his body and swung his burning blade to slice Slayer across the chest.

Slayer easily deflected the blow. "You have some fight in you."

"I have a lot of fight in me." Sam swung his fire sword as if he swung wildly at baseballs continually flung by a pitching machine. Flames ripped along his blade, like a roaring fire. Slayer parried. Sam overcommitted and fell as Slayer stuck a leg out to trip him. Sam dropped to his knees, rolled then came up ready to attack again. He gasped. His arms ached already. *I'm losing. I'm losing. I'm losing. No, control yourself. Don't quit. Don't give in to your fear.* He took a deep breath.

Slayer yawned. "Is that all the Chosen One has to offer me?"

Sam fingered the handle of his fire sword. He stared deeply into the blazing steel. *Tell me what to do, sword.* He wasn't sure if his sword answered, but his mind suddenly focused. He pointed the weapon at Slayer's chest and uttered a magical word that flashed in his mind. "Grash-Lan-Tis." A flame shot from the blade and struck Slayer in the chest. He flew backward and landed on his back in the sand. Smoke rose from his chest.

He groggily rose to his knees and onto his feet. His eyes were wild. "You shall pay for that, boy!" Slayer raised The Sword of Zel-Kar over his head and screamed as he charged.

Sam directed another blazing fire stream to surge at Slayer. This time ready, Slayer blocked the fire with the Sword of Zel-Kar's blade and deflected the flame back at Sam.

As the stream of fire rushed back at him, Sam dove then quickly got back to his feet. By then Slayer was already upon him. The pirate conjurer slashed the Sword of Zel-Kar at Sam's head. Sam raised his fire blade to counter, and when the two weapons clashed, they generated a shockwave that threw Sam five feet into the air. He landed on his back, but managed to hold onto the blazing sword. *Get up!* he told himself as Slayer rushed at him one more time. His body responded, and he stood to face Slayer's attack. In a fast and furious assault, Slayer drove his sword at Sam's heart, then his head, then his abdomen.

Sam deflected blow after blow until Slayer stretched out one hand and red energy shot out. It struck Sam's chest at close range. The force lifted him off his feet and slammed him into the sand.

He lost his grip on his fire sword, and the weapon disappeared. He struggled to get to his feet, but the blast of red energy robbed him of his breath. He coughed as he tried to force air in and out, but the movement of air burned. He coughed some more, and drops of blood spewed from his mouth.

Slayer stood over him and placed a black-booted foot on his chest. "You lose, boy, and I am weary of this. But you fight well. I think I might let you live. Perhaps there is a bit of Thaddeus in me. Maybe I feel a certain endearment toward you. But, I cannot have you come after me. I cannot allow you to use that fire sword of yours, so I have a thought. I shall let you live, but I shall take your hands as a memento of our time together. How does that sound?"

"No!" Sam coughed up more blood. "No!"

"Do not worry, Samuel. It shall not hurt… much."

Sam tried to reach his back again, but Slayer's pirates roughly forced him to his feet and dragged him to a boulder.

"Slayer, no!" Sam searched for Sarah. "Sarah, don't let him!"

She turned away.

*Magic, if you're in me, save me. Please!* The pirates pushed Sam to his knees in front of the boulder. They extended his arms across the top. Sam fought to free himself, but it did no good. The more he twisted and squirmed to free his hands, the tighter the pirates held him in place. They were too strong.

Another pirate, the one who had pretended to be Slayer, the one Slayer called his quartermaster, walked around one side of the boulder and grabbed Sam's fingers. The quartermaster smiled from ear to ear. His yellow rotten teeth were exposed. "Do it, Captain," he squealed.

Slayer strutted to the boulder. "I take no joy in this. It simply must be done. But be hardy, for I grant you a chance to live in my new world. Perhaps you can continue to be my fool." Slayer raised his sword over his head.

*Oh God!* Sam's heart pounded, stomach tightened, breathing stopped. He glared at Sarah, who stood behind her father. Her eyes urged him to be calm.

The Sword of Zel-Kar crashed down.

# Chapter 32
## It's All In The Wrists

Sam screamed. He was sure of it, but he didn't hear his own voice. All around him Slayer's pirates laughed. Slayer's quartermaster even fell onto his back he laughed so hard. Some pirates pointed to Sam. Others pointed at his hands. Where were they? Sam scanned the sand around the boulder. They lay together, palms down, a slight piece of bone visible through the blood and flesh.

Were they really his hands? They couldn't be. His hands still felt attached to his wrists. He focused on his wrists, which rested on the boulder. *No!* Where his hands should have been were bloody stumps. His hands had been cleanly sliced and his blood poured from the wounds and traveled across the crevices of the boulder to reach the sand.

Funny, he didn't feel any pain. He was just numb and silent as his arms turned blue. The scenery around him started to spin and his vision clouded. The two pirates behind him released their grips, and Sam toppled onto the sand. *I'm so cold.* Above him, the emerald sky darkened. A few gray clouds rolled in from the sea.

Slayer moved beside him. He spoke, but Sam couldn't hear his words. Slayer held the Sword of Zel-Kar in front of him; blood lined the blade. One of his goons handed him a white rag, and Slayer slowly, carefully wiped the blood from the steel. He dropped the bloodied rag at Sam's side.

Sam shivered. *Why am I so cold?* His eyelids grew heavy as his vision tunneled in on itself. *I'm so tired. I just want to sleep.*

A voice broke through the silence. "Stay awake." It was a familiar voice—Sarah's voice. She knelt beside him and placed her hands against his wrists. "This shall hurt more than my father's blade."

*What did you say? Are you here to finish the job—to kill me? Traitor! How could you betray me?* Sam stared into her dark eyes as she uttered words—magic words. Light erupted from her hands. Though he couldn't hear much, he did hear sizzling. The skin around his wrists burned worse than when the fire sword blazed to life in his back. His wrists were on fire. *What is she doing? Sarah, what are you doing?*

Sam cried out. His body trembled, as if an electric current ran through him, like when he accidentally touched an exposed live wire from his family's Christmas lights. This was ten times worse. He cried out one more time. When the pain subsided, she knelt down until her face was inches from his. She did not speak, but stared into his eyes. A tear may have even formed. She leaned in and kissed his cheek.

As she rose and moved away, Sam eyed his wrists. His hands were still gone... but so were the blood and the exposed bones, as if the wound had healed over time. His chest also had healed; the skin was no longer blackened from the energy blasts. *Her healing powers.* He felt no pain and warmth enveloped him, like his blood started to flow again throughout his body. His vision sharpened, strength returned, but handless, he could not reach his fire sword.

Slowly, Sam climbed to his feet. His legs wobbled until he willed his muscles to obey his commands. He glared at the man who had tricked him. The man he had thought was a friend.

Slayer sheathed the Sword of Zel-Kar and smiled. "You are stronger than I thought. That is good. I have allowed my daughter to heal you because I do not wish you to die... yet. I want you to live and to know that you had a chance to save these children, but failed. Their deaths shall be on your hands." Slayer placed a hand to his mouth and eyed Sam's hands, still in the sand. "Oh, my pardon, their deaths shall not be on... your hands."

"Don't hurt them!" Sam clutched his wrists to his chest. "Sarah, don't let this happen!"

"Father, you promised me!" Sarah fired a bolt of green energy at Slayer. He simply caught the energy in his hands and absorbed it.

"Child, with the Sword of Zel-Kar by my side, you cannot stand against me. Must I teach you a lesson again?" He slapped her with the back of his hand against her cheek. The strike knocked her to the ground. She lay there unconscious. Blood trickled from her cheek.

Slayer turned to his quartermaster. "Pick her up and let us return to our ship." He motioned to his men who stood over the children. "When I am gone, dispose of these little creatures. Then have the boy bury them as best he can. I shall begin the search for the barrier and light the way for you to follow. Oh, and someone please collect the lad's hands. I wish to keep them close."

Sam, his wrists still at his chest, approached Slayer. "Why run away if you have so much power."

"And watch such ugliness? I am above such things now. But you should know our time together has meant a great deal to me. I shall remember all you have done for me. Your name shall be praised in my new world. Your hands shall be worshipped, I assure you."

"Slayer!"

"Good-bye, Samuel. I wish you a very long and sad life."

"Slayer, I still have magic. I will come for you."

"That may be, my boy, but without your hands, without that silly sword of yours, and with my possession of the Sword of Zel-Kar, you shall never be a threat again. And if you do come for me, then I shall deprive you of your life. For now, I strand you on this island, so that you may think on your failure. And as you do, remember this. As I live on long after your death, one day I shall pay a visit to your parents—if they even exist in the world I create—and I shall have their heads."

"Slayer!" Sam yelled for a second time.

Slayer simply waved his hand and vanished as did his quartermaster who held an unconscious Sarah over his shoulder. Several pirates also disappeared. About a dozen men remained to carry out Slayer's orders. Out at sea, the larger of the two ships set sail and it, too, vanished.

Sam lowered his eyes. *I failed everyone. But the children... I can't give up yet. But what can I do? Where is my magic? What powers do I have without my fire sword?*

One of the pirates drew a long, curved sword. "You heard Captain Slayer. These critters are to die." The children cried out as the pirate raised his sword above the head of a boy. He struggled to get away, but the chains around him held him in place. "Stop your squirming," the pirate huffed.

"No!" Sam pointed his wrists at the pirate. He wasn't sure how it happened. He wasn't sure where the power came from, but he felt it deep in his gut. Like a volcano exploded deep inside him and lava poured through his veins. An orange bolt of energy shot from each wrist and struck the pirate in the chest. The blast tore a hole through the pirate's chest and he crumbled to the sand. The sudden surge of power dropped Sam to his knees. Those pirates armed with muskets turned their weapons on him.

"Kill, him!" one shouted.

Shots rang out.

# Chapter 33
## An Unexpected Ally

Sam flinched. Any second a barrage of musket fire would strike him down. He waited and waited... and waited. Nothing! He opened his eyes. Five pirates lay dead or wounded on the shore near the children. Sam scanned the beach. Smoke clouds, those musket fire produced, rose from a line of tropical brush just beyond the shore. *What the...?*

The pirates still standing fired back toward the brush, but another volley erupted from behind the trees and more pirates fell. Sam stood motionless. *Who is firing?* The rest of Slayer's pirates threw their muskets and ran to their longboats to escape the beach.

"Do not let them escape, men!" a voice, large and booming, commanded from the tree line. Sam recognized the voice. A man with a large gut, massive legs, and a bushy beard emerged from the jungle. The golden handle of his sword protruded from a scabbard and a pistol was wrapped in a ribbon that hung around his neck.

"Captain Hornigold," Sam whispered.

Five of his men rushed from the jungle brush toward Slayer's pirates as they attempted to cast off. They didn't get very far. Another volley killed the pirates instantly.

"Captain Hornigold!" This time Sam shouted the name.

The Captain nodded. "Get these children off the beach. It is still quite dangerous out in the open."

Sam blinked and shook his head. Was the Captain real? How could it be? Hornigold walked toward him. As he approached, cannon fire exploded from the one Slayer ship still off shore. "Cover!" Hornigold yelled. His men shielded the children with their own bodies, but the cannonballs struck the trees beyond the beach. Hornigold laughed. "Now it is my turn."

From the sea more cannon fire erupted, but not from Slayer's ship. A second vessel sailed into view. Her cannons boomed like thunder as she attacked. Her volleys ripped into Slayer's ship. *Ranger*, Hornigold's ship, hugged the shoreline. Her first round of cannon fire cut through the masts of Slayer's ship. Before the pirates could turn their cannons around to fire on Hornigold's ship, *Ranger* unleashed another barrage that splintered planks all over Slayer's ship. A third round nearly split the ship in two. The screams of men echoed from Slayer's ship as it exploded and tipped over.

Sam lowered his head to the sand. *Thank God.* He eyed his wrists and sighed. *At least the kids are safe.* When he looked up, Captain Hornigold stood over him. "By God, son! What did that beast do to you?"

"I'll live."

Hornigold gripped Sam's shoulder. "Let us get you to my ship. We have a doc aboard."

Sam shook his head. "Don't worry about me."

Hornigold frowned at Sam. "Where are your friends—that slippery fellow, Thaddeus, and the nice young lass? Did Slayer kill them?"

Sam laughed. "I was tricked. As it turns out, Thaddeus was Slayer in disguise."

"Treacherous beast!" Hornigold spit into the sand. "He deceived both of us then. And what of the girl?"

"The girl… well… she stood with Slayer. They both played me, like I was some fool. I guess I was a fool." Sam didn't tell Hornigold the complete truth. For some reason, he decided it best not to let anyone know Sarah was Slayer's daughter, if it was even true. He didn't know what to believe anymore.

"Many a man has been a fool when it comes to women, boy." Hornigold lamented. "And where are they now?"

Sam raised his wrists. "After Slayer did this to me, they sailed off."

Honigold placed his arm around Sam's waist. "All right then, let us help you to your feet and at least fill your belly with some rum."

Sam broke free. "You don't understand. I let Slayer get away with a very dangerous weapon called the Sword of Zel-Kar. Right now, he's out there somewhere crossing some magical barrier back to our world to conquer it, and I let it happen. I brought him to this place, and I handed him the sword. It's all because of me." Sam took a deep breath. "Wait a minute! How is it you're here in this world, wherever this world is?" Hornigold scratched his beard and smiled, but did not immediately answer. "Captain, do you have magic abilities, too? Do you carry the mark of the sword?"

"My goodness, no boy." Hornigold shook his head. "I have no use for magic. I believe in steel, a fair wind and a strong ship."

"So how then?"

"I believe they might have your answer." Hornigold pointed toward the tropical jungle. "Boys, step lively and show yourselves."

Sam's eyes widened with surprise. "What?"

"I would like you to meet the newest members of my crew." Hornigold winked. From the jungle brush appeared four teens. Sam recognized them all—his friends, Greg, Dean and John and his cousin, Zack.

Hornigold laughed. "I found them in the sea and scooped them up like fish. I would have left them on some island somewhere if they did not have quite the tale—a tale I found myself believing, though I cannot say why. It involved you, my boy, so I heeded their words."

His cousin and friends reached him by the end of Hornigold's explanation.

"Cuz, your hands," Zack sniffed and blinked. He wiped his eyes with his fists. Before Sam could respond, his cousin threw his arms around Sam. "I'm so sorry."

Sam glanced at his friends. They shrugged. *Is this the same Zack who has always bullied me? Why the change of heart?* Sam pushed those thoughts away. He had no great love for his cousin, but right now that didn't matter. It was good to see somebody— anybody—from home. He returned Zack's embrace. "This isn't your fault, Zack. Well, maybe a little."

Sam's friends also joined in the embrace. It lasted until Hornigold spoke. "What is this now? We have business to attend to."

Sam broke away. He placed his arms behind his back. "I don't understand. How did you get here?"

Zack sighed. "I've never shown anyone this before."

"Shown what?"

"You're not the only one with a strange birthmark." Zack turned and lowered his pants. On his right butt cheek was a birthmark—in the shape of a sword. It was just like Sam's.

"I don't believe it!" Sam stared too long at his cousin's butt and looked away.

"Sometime after you disappeared, that same girl haunting you visited me. She told me you were in danger and that I had to return to the water. I didn't know what to think, but something compelled me to listen. I didn't know what else to do. So many people were looking for you, cuz. I thought maybe you drowned. I told them all what had happened. They searched for you... for your body, but found nothing. They're still searching. Your parents are a mess. So I had to listen to that girl. Maybe she knew something."

Sam missed his parents and his little brothers. He had to let them know he was all right. He wanted to go home to them, but if he didn't stop Slayer there would be no home to return to. But maybe that had all been part of Sarah's lie. Maybe he could go home and everything would be all right. Of course, this could all still be a wild dream. He couldn't rule that out. If this was a dream, for some reason he couldn't wake up from it. If it was real, he had to face Slayer again before he could go home. Sarah may have told a bunch of lies, but Slayer was a clear danger and had to be stopped. Sam stared at his wrists. *Like this, what can I do against him?* He refocused on his cousin's story. "So what happened?"

"I went to the pier and found them." Zack pointed to Sam's three friends.

"We went to the water every day since you went missing," Greg explained. "It just seemed like the right thing to do."

"Well, I told them about my dream," Zack continued. "I told them I was supposed to jump from the pier into the water, just like before when I saved you."

"We weren't going to let him go without us," John interrupted.

"We jumped off the pier and that's when I saw her," Zack described. "She told me I was the blood of the Chosen One and that you needed my help. Oh God, man, I never meant for anything like this to happen to you. All those times I hassled you I never really meant you harm. I just didn't think, you know. It's kind of like what I'm expected to do. I'm so sorry man."

Sam sighed. After all he'd been through, Zack's bullying no longer mattered, but he scoffed when his cousins said it was what he was expected to do. Still, now was not the time to work out their differences. "Zack, whatever—just tell me what happened next."

Zack wiped his eyes. "But your hands—"

"Zack!" Sam glared at his cousin.

"We all followed her through some doorway in time." Zack gazed toward the crimson sea.

"We ended up in the middle of the ocean," Dean cut in. "But the girl was gone."

"And that's when I found them." Hornigold lifted his three-cornered hat farther up on his head. "They told me about you, and I remembered our meeting. I decided perhaps these boys could help lead me to Slayer. Somehow the one with the mark on his backside found some cloudbank that led us here. We arrived on the opposite side of this island."

"Jeez, cuz, I'm sorry I didn't believe you." Zack kicked the sand. "I've been such a jerk."

"Yeah you have been," Sam agreed, "but none of it matters now. I'm glad to see you guys, all you guys, but I blew it. That girl who brought you here was using me. She let Slayer do this to me." He stretched out his arms. "I guess she's… evil."

Zack placed a hand on Sam's shoulder. "She can't be all bad. I mean she brought me to help you."

"I don't know what to say to that." Sam bowed his head. "Maybe she wanted to hurt—or kill—you, too, because you have the same sword mark. Then again…"

"What, boy?" Hornigold asked.

"I saw something in the—"

A roar vibrated throughout the island. Something big flew from the skull peak and soared into a sky that darkened with the onset of dusk. Hornigold drew his pistol. His men pointed their muskets.

"Don't shoot!" Sam urged. The dragon swooped down onto the beach. Blood speckled its head where the stones had struck the beast.

A man rode atop the dragon. As it landed, he slowly slid from its back and stood hunched over in the sand. Blood soaked his shirt.

It was the pirate Henry Every.

# Chapter 34
## The Scroll's Truth

The old pirate fell to his knees and onto his back.

"Henry!" Sam ran to him and knelt by his side. He stared at the old pirate, as if he stared into the face of his grandfather. "Henry, you're alive."

"Not for long, young one." The old pirate coughed up blood. It ran down the side of his chin and into the sand.

"Henry, no, you can't die. I need you. I didn't stop Slayer. He has the sword, Henry. You have to stop him."

Henry coughed and wheezed between words. "No, young one, my time has passed. You are stronger than you know. The blood in our family is strong. You can defeat Slayer."

"How? He has the Sword of Zel-Kar because of me."

Henry smiled as he coughed again. "All is not as it seems."

"What do you mean?"

"Inside the chamber on the ground you saw something did you not?" Henry's eyes drooped, closed and opened again.

Sam nodded. "Y—yes. I saw the face of a girl."

"Not just any girl." Henry clarified.

Sam quieted for a moment. His gaze shifted to the skull peak. "I saw Sarah's face."

"Yes. I have brought this for you." Henry wheezed as he struggled to catch his breath. He spit blood from his mouth before he spoke again. "It was hidden in the floor underneath the image of the girl." Henry lifted his arms. On his chest was a scroll covered in his blood.

Sam took it. "What is this?"

"The truth."

Sam held the scroll close to his chest. "I don't—"

"Slayer has the Sword of Zel-Kar? That is true to a point," Henry whispered, his voice faint. "The Sword of Zel-Kar is a lie."

"I don't understand." Sam leaned closer to Henry.

"Oh, it is a magic sword and it is indeed powerful." The old pirate's chest convulsed and he gritted his teeth before he spoke again. "It can even grant longer life. But it is not all powerful. It cannot give immortality."

Sam glanced once at Zack then turned back to the old pirate. "What are you saying?"

Henry coughed for several moments. His words were broken and came slower. "In the ancient scroll… the truth. The words are clear but forgotten. The words fade, perhaps to protect her. The words read Sworsha Zel-Kara."

Sam understood the words. "Yes, Sword of Zel-Kar."

Henry shook his head. "Must read the full passage. Appeared to me, for I bare the mark. The full passage reads… Sworsha Zel-Kara, Sworsha Zel-Kara Anira, Sworsha Zel-Kara Anira Illusa, Sworsha Zel-Kara Anira Illusa Manuta."

Sam held his breath. The words doubled back on each other, just like the writing on the doorway to the skull chamber, and he understood them. "The Sword of Zel-Kar Shall Be The Bringer Of The Light."

Henry's breathing grew shallow. "Yes."

Sam licked his lips. His heart beat fast. "The Sword of Zel-Kar is a person."

"Yes."

"It's—it's Sarah!"

"Yes."

Sam gazed out to sea then back at the old pirate. *Yes, it's true. I think I felt it all along. But she's Slayer's daughter, and she sided with him. What can this all mean? What am I supposed to do now? She's the enemy, isn't she?* "Does she know? Does Slayer?"

"No." Henry's eyes opened wide. "I learned the truth when I came for the sword. The one before me... passed on the responsibility... to me. He shared the scroll... showed me the image."

Henry coughed again. "Scroll tells that a girl shall be born. Guarded her identity. Recognized her with you. Now you must. She shall bring light to the world. Must save her."

"That's why you focused on her in the chamber," Sam reasoned.

"Yes."

"But she's Slayer's daughter, Henry. She's chosen him. She's evil."

"You do not believe that."

"I don't know what to believe."

"Save her. Slayer shall abuse her power or kill her. Save her, Chosen..." Henry Every slowly closed his eyes and was silent.

"Henry, no! Henry, please!"

"He's gone, boy." Hornigold removed his three-cornered hat.

Sam lowered his head to the old pirate's chest. Why did his death hurt so much? He barely knew Henry Every. But it did hurt. Tears fell, and Sam unleashed a yell as loud as the dragon's roar.

# Chapter 35
## The Fight Must Continue

Lighted by a full moon now in the western sky, they buried Henry Every on the beach. They marked his grave with his sword. Sam, unable to help, sat in the sand and watched. Mostly, he stared at his wrists. "What do I do now?" He didn't expect an answer, but got one anyway.

"You heard what the old man said," Zack casted a shadow in the moonlight. "He said it's up to you to save her. Let's do it. We'll help."

"How am I supposed to do that?" Sam spread his arms wide. "Look at me. Look what Slayer did to me. Just leave me here and go off on your own. Save her without me. You have the mark. You're a Chosen One, too."

"Not like you, cuz."

"Then don't save her. If Slayer doesn't know who she is and she doesn't know, then who cares what happens. Leave me here and find your way home. I just want to sleep."

Hornigold walked up behind them. "Chances are, Slayer shall learn the truth soon enough. He shall know that blade is useless. When he learns the girl has the real power, he shall exploit her. Now, I have a ship, a crew, and I am ready to join this little expedition. But we need a leader."

"Sam, we're with you, too," Greg offered.

"For sure," John nodded.

"You know I'm in." Dean linked his arms around John and Greg. "What do you say, Sam? Let's go save your girlfriend."

The dragon, resting nearby, growled as if to offer its support.

Sam laughed. "Do you know what we're up against? Slayer has an entire fleet and an army of pirates. What do we have?"

"You," Hornigold retorted. "And this winged beast."

Sam shuffled his feet in the sand and gazed at the dragon. "Even with a dragon for help, I'm not enough."

"Try." Hornigold's eyes grew large and serious. "We shall not let this pirate have the victory. I swear I shall do all I can to help you defeat him."

Sam focused on his wrists. Where had the energy come from that he fired at the pirate with a gun? Could he do it again? It had felt good.

"Boy, the doc aboard my ship is really more of a carpenter," Hornigold pointed toward his ship. "I am sure he can fix you up some hands."

*A carpenter? I'm glad Sarah healed my wounds first.* Sam glanced from his friends to Henry's grave to the sea where the crimson water met the emerald sky. Somewhere out there the two worlds touched. Had Slayer already found the way back home? Was he still in this strange world? Had he fled into space to one of the planets now in the western sky?

"And what about Sarah?" Was she friend or foe? She had saved him. That was for sure. But why had she chosen him in the first place? Why not Zack if he had the same birthmark? One answer eclipsed all others. *He's the strong one, not me. She chose me because I'm weak—because she could play me for a fool more than Zack.* And so what if she had saved him. She still sided with Slayer, her father.

Sam Inhaled deeply and studied his friends' faces. His course was clear. *I have to save her if only to save everyone else.*

Before anyone could respond, Sam stood. "All right, I'm in. But this is not about saving my *girlfriend*. This is about saving the world and making sure when we do go home—to our time—it's still there."

"Good show, boy," Hornigold wrapped an arm around him. "But, one more point you must gnaw on. If the girl cannot be saved, you must be ready to kill her—for the good of all."

Sam stared at the pirate hunter for several moments then nodded. "I'll do what I have to do."

# Chapter 36
## A Vision of the Future

*Sam stood in a factory where flames and smoke choked off the flow of air. Hammers pounded steel all round him. Coughs from workers echoed through a dimly lighted building as large as a football field. Just how many workers toiled in this inhospitable environment was impossible to tell. It could have been hundreds, maybe a thousand. Sam also couldn't tell what they built until he bumped into a mound of weapons—guns of all sizes—piled onto car-length containers. As he scanned the building, he counted maybe a hundred containers all piled with guns.*

*What was this place? How did he get here? Hadn't he just been on an island where his cousin, friends and a pirate hunter rescued him after the pirate Jem Slayer had severed his hands? He looked at his hands. They were attached.*

*A monitor—something like a large television screen—dropped from the ceiling and blazed to life. On the screen was an image of an ornately decorated office. It reminded Sam of the Oval Office at the White House. He obviously had never been there, but he had seen the President on the news give speeches from the Oval Office. As he kept his eyes on the screen, a man dressed in a black suit walked into view and sat down at a chair behind a large desk.*

*Sam recognized the face immediately. Slayer! It was the same face, the same black hair with slightly graying sides, and the same gray beard, only now it was nicely trimmed. He no longer looked like a pirate from 1718. He dressed in modern clothing—a suit and tie. In fact, Sam thought in terror, he looks like a president. Slayer spoke like a president, too, as if he addressed the nation—maybe the world.*

*"My good people, your blood and sweat and sacrifice—under my rule, of course—have made this world a safer place, and now there is a universe out there that we must conquer. I assure you your labor shall make my vision of a united universe possible. Many of you shall probably die as a result of my vision, but it shall be well worth it, and I shall honor your deaths, I promise you. So continue to work, parent to parent, child to child, brother to brother—all of you, my good people—to honor those who have come before and those who shall build on the foundations of your bones."*

*Slayer held the smile of a concerned world leader, but his eyes shined in the same way they did when he sliced off Sam's hands. As the screen went dark, and the monitor slid back into the ceiling, Sam felt a tap on his shoulder.*

*He turned to face his cousin Zack and his friends, Greg, John and Dean. All wore dirty, greasy overalls and their faces were covered in grime. "You failed us, Chosen One," Zack declared, his voice hoarse and tired. "You failed us all."*

*Sam closed his eyes. "I'm sorry," he shouted. When he opened his eyes, he no longer stood in the factory. He stood on a hillside over the city where he was raised, but the city he knew was gone. His school, his street, the mall—everything he cared about had vanished. In their place stood factories, like the one he had been inside; all belched out smoke and ash into a sky where the sunlight was blocked by dark clouds of vile pollution. He was back in his time, but it wasn't the world he had left behind. He had failed. "No, it can't be!" he cried.*

"Wake up, lad… wake up. You are having a nightmare." Sam blinked his eyes as he recognized the voice of Doc O'Malley, *Ranger's* doctor. *That's right. I'm aboard Captain Hornigold's ship, Ranger, and Doc is fitting me with new hands. That means I was having a dream or a vision of the future. It wasn't real—at least I hope it wasn't real. The truth is I don't know what's real or dream anymore. At least, if this time and this place are real, I still have a chance to stop Slayer.* Sam tried to rise from Doc's operating table, but *Ranger's* doctor held his shoulders.

"Don't get up too fast. You have been out for a few hours. That actually proved helpful, giving me time to finish your new hands. Take a look. I have attached them." Doc stood back and studied his work. His green eyes gleamed. His Scottish accent resonated throughout his cabin inside *Ranger's* belly. His smile, which showed through his long red beard, and the kind tone to his voice, would be infectious enough to lift anyone's dark spirit—anyone but Sam.

The hands were better than he had expected—since he hadn't expected anything more than steel hooks, like in most pirate stories he had read. Doc had to be an expert craftsman. His creations looked like hands. Both artificial limbs were wooden. The one on the left had four fingers and a thumb outstretched as if to shake hands. The hand was covered in a long brown glove that stretched up his arm to his elbow. Strings from the glove wrapped several times around his forearm and were tied into a knot near his elbow to hold the hand in place. The one on the right was shaped into a grip large enough to hold the handle of a sword. Wooden posts were built into the glove and rose up the sides of the forearm to reinforce the hand's strength so that it might support a sword.

Yes, the hands were fine. They were not the reason Sam's brow was furrowed. He had gotten over the loss of his hands from Slayer's cruel strike. The vision of the future troubled him, for one. But he also questioned why Slayer let him live. It would have made more sense for Slayer to kill him and be done with the *Chosen One.*

"You're quiet, young man." Doc patted Sam on the back. "Do you not like your new hands?"

"No, sir… I mean, yes, thank you. I was just thinking. Sorry. These hands are perfect."

"Perfect might be an overstatement, my boy, but you are fortunate in a way. Carving hands, feet, even legs and arms from timber has become something of an art I have been dabbling with, since in battle too many good men end up maimed. It is an ugly reality of life aboard a ship. I figured why not try to help. As it so happens, I had just finished the pair of hands you now wear."

"Again, thank you." Sam moved toward the door to Doc's cabin. "I will try to hold on to these hands—keep them safe."

Doc laughed. "I think not. I see wildness in you. I am quite sure you shall lose these hands in battle just as you lost your own. Never fear. I have already started another pair. Just hold on to your head. I cannot replace that."

Sam gulped and walked from Doc's cabin up to *Ranger's* deck. The ship had cast off hours ago from the island and they had sailed across the crimson sea in search of a barrier that would lead them back home—at least back to the Caribbean. The day-and-night halves of the sky had completed their shift. A large orange moon was high in the western half of the sky over this magical world, and an array of planets—so close you could see mountains and deep canyons—marked the night. A massive sun brightened the eastern half of the sky where white clouds were painted against an emerald canvas, the color of this world's daylight.

Sam stood against *Ranger's* port railing and stared out to sea. A strong wind blew across the ship and pushed against the sails. He closed his eyes and lifted his head into the wind, felt it toss his hair in every direction. Whispers from behind caused him to open his eyes. They were the whispers of *Ranger's* crew. He was aware of their stares. *They don't know what to make of me—what to make of any of this*, he thought. *They might even be scared of me. I wonder if they have any idea of what they've become mixed up in— I wonder how long until they mutiny against Hornigold for dragging them into this magic mess.*

His thoughts returned to the question of why he still lived when Slayer should have killed him. His mind lingered on one reason. *When I was in the cave and still believed the Sword of Zel-Kar was some all powerful weapon, I wanted it for myself. I wanted it bad— thought I could rule with it. But that's no different than what Slayer wants to do. Could he see evil in me? Did he let me live because he thinks I might join him? And now that I know Sarah is the true Sword of Zel-Kar, the bringer of the light, do I want to save her or control her like Slayer would if he knew the truth?* Sam wrestled with those questions until his head hurt. A friendly voice interrupted his thoughts.

"Hey, dude, shouldn't you be resting," Zack asked.

"Can't," Sam answered. "Have to find the barrier."

"What, you don't think I can find it? I have the blood in me, too." Zack placed an arm around Sam.

"I know—I thought together we might have a better chance of finding it faster." Sam wasn't so sure he liked his cousin placing an arm around him. They had been enemies until just a few hours earlier. Sam still wasn't sure how he felt about Zack. None of this would have happened if Zack hadn't chased him into the water. Then again, maybe it would have happened with or without Zack. *That is, of course, if any of this is real.* He still prayed he might wake up at some point from this nightmare and still have hands.

"Oh, so cute, you guys are hugging it out," Greg joked as he, Dean and John joined them by the railing.

Zack snapped his arm away from Sam. "Shut up, Greg."

"Touchy," John said.

"Not sure I like sweet Zack as much as Zack the surfer jerk," Dean added.

"I like your new hands." Greg reached out as if to shake Sam's left hand. "I think they're actually an improvement over the originals."

Sam laughed slightly. "Nice joke, doofus. You want to try having someone chop off your hands. It's a lot of fun."

"I know, dude—sorry," Greg pulled his hand back.

"Did you guys just come from below deck," Sam asked.

"Yeah." John rubbed his belly. "Captain Hornigold had the ship's cook prepare a meal of some stew or soup or something. It was supposed to be beef, but I swear there were living things crawling inside my bowl."

"Didn't stop you from eating," Dean blurted.

"How are the kids?" Sam hadn't seen them since they were brought aboard.

"Captain Hornigold is with them now below deck." Greg's tone was serious, which was unusual for him. "I think he's telling them a story, trying to get them to go to sleep."

Sleep sounded good. Sam lowered his head. Troubling thoughts returned. "I'm really glad you guys are here, but you know you never should have come. You're all in danger now. And what about your families? They won't know what happened to you, just like mine. They'll go crazy searching for you."

Zack answered for the group. "Cuz, think about it. If we stop Slayer and are able to return home, they won't even know we were gone, right? Isn't that how this time travel stuff works?"

Sam shrugged. "I guess."

"By the way," Greg jumped in. "Is there any way to make time traveling not suck so much. I haven't felt so sick to my stomach in my life. When we crossed over, I couldn't stop spewing. Half the ocean must be filled with my vomit." Dean and John nodded their agreement.

"Yeah, and I had crazy hallucinations," John added. "It was really freaky. We were back home, but it was different. Our school was gone. The mall was gone. We were working in some factory. I don't know what we were making, but the whole city was filled with factories."

Sam shivered. *My God, the same vision!*

"Dude," I saw the same thing." Dean's eyes grew wide.

Sam's stomach cramped. He didn't tell them he had the same vision. "Wow—that is freaky," was his only response.

Zack stood silently as if he contemplated the visions John and Dean spoke of. *Did he have a similar vision?* Sam wondered. Zack blinked his eyes several times before he spoke. "So how do we stop Slayer and save the world?"

"And not die while trying," Greg chimed in.

Sam paced the deck. "I don't know. I just don't know, but we have a ship, a dragon and we have each other. Maybe that will be enough."

# Chapter 37
## A Storm is Coming

*Ranger* sliced silently through the water. Sam stood alone on deck, except for a few crew members who performed their duties. Zack and his friends had gone to sleep as had the children they had rescued from Slayer. Even Hornigold was fast asleep in his cabin. His snores could be heard from every corner of his ship.

The darkened western sky showed the first signs of morning light as golden rays splintered the night and the eastern sky drifted toward a purple dusk. The only sounds came from the wind as it danced with the sails and the water that splashed against the hull.

Sam leaned against the railing. He thought about the question Zack had asked. *So how do we stop Slayer and save the world?* He wished he knew how to answer the question and how to protect his friends as they risked everything to help him face Slayer. At that moment, loneliness crept into his thoughts. He wasn't alone, but he missed the one person he had come to rely on—Thaddeus. But there never was a Thaddeus. It was always Slayer. Sam held his head with his wooden hands and fought back tears.

"Does the Chosen One cry?" The words came from the ocean as if the sea had whispered in his ears.

Sam backed away from the railing and whirled in every direction. "Slayer!"

"Yes, boy," said the disembodied voice.

"Where are you?" Sam backed into one of *Ranger's* masts.

"I'm everywhere, and I can see you."

Sam tried to sound brave. "Then show yourself."

"In time. We shall face each other again, when I deem the time right. For now, continue your chase."

'You should have killed me, Slayer."

"I can easily rectify that."

"Then…"

"Oh, and lad, I know your little secret."

"What secret?" Sam dropped to his knees. The air spilled from his lungs and he struggled to take another breath. Slayer never answered. His voice faded away as though it slunk back over the sea from wherever it had originated. "Slayer!" Sam shouted. Still no answer. *What does he mean by that? Does he know about Sarah? Is that the secret? Or is it something else? Do I tell the others? No, not now. They'll lose hope, and without hope, we're lost.*

Sam stood and returned to the railing, his eyes toward the sea. *I need to find some reason to hope.* He lifted his shirt over his head and threw it on the deck. With soft breaths, he concentrated on the sword-shaped birthmark across his back. Words flashed through his mind in a strange language but the words were clear to him. *I summon you, sword. Do my bidding.*

With his right-gloved hand—the one shaped into a grip—he reached around to his back and repeated the phrase, *I summon you.* The wooden hand touched skin. Another deep breath and the hand slipped through the skin and found the handle of the burning sword. *Please! I need you!* The sword heeded his plea. As he removed his right hand from his back, the sword followed. Despite a shaky arm, he lifted the fiery blade and brought it before his eyes.

The blade burned bright; its flame rose into the early morning sky. "Thank you," Sam proclaimed. He had done what Thaddeus said he must. He had controlled the sword. Thaddeus had said that was the only way to stop Slayer. Sam smiled. "You were right, Thaddeus."

His eyes followed the flame toward the sky until his gaze found the dragon. The creature sliced a trail through the last remaining moments of darkness to the west. It roared as it soared past *Ranger* and climbed back into the sky. From its mouth, it spewed its own flame.

Sam waved. *Maybe there is reason to hope.* He held that thought until his eyes caught a glimpse of dark clouds gathered in the east. A gusty wind blew across *Ranger's* bow. A voice rose from behind him—this time a friendly voice, but it brought a warning. "Quite the squall is kicking up," Captain Hornigold announced. "Looks like a storm is coming."

Sam didn't bother to look back at *Ranger's* captain. He lifted the flaming blade toward the sky. "It's already here."

# About the Author

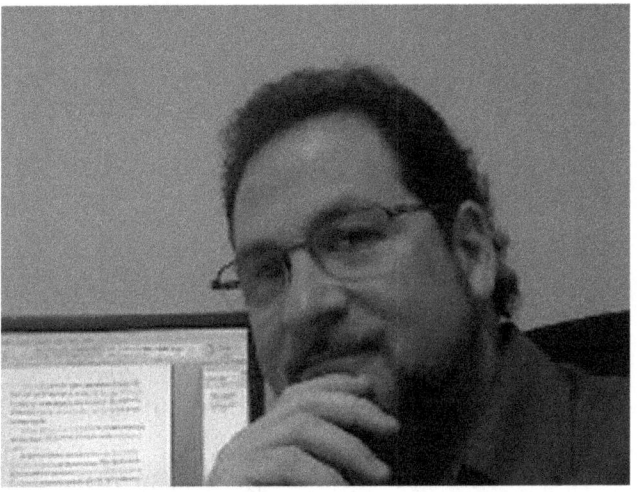

Darren Simon has been a writer for much of his life. His career has included working as a journalist in Los Angeles, Israel and Southern California along the Mexican and Arizona borders. He presently works in government affairs on California water issues, teaches college English for the California Community College system, and does free-lance writing for regional magazines. His work as an author focuses on middle grade and young adult readers to inspire them to read the way he was inspired, first by comic books and then the science fiction and fantasy novels that were so important to his youth. He resides in California's Desert Southwest with his wife and sons.

For more information, and to contact Darren, visit his website at:

www.darren-simon.com